LIPPINCOTT'S REVIEW SERIES

Pediatric Nursing

LIPPINCOTT'S REVIEW SERIES

Pediatric Nursing

J.B. LIPPINCOTT COMPANY
Philadelphia

New York • *London* • *Hagerstown*

Sponsoring Editor: **Donna L. Hilton, RN, BSN**
Coordinating Editorial Assistant: **Susan Perry**
Project Editor: **Melissa McGrath**
Indexer: **Alexandra Nickerson**
Designer: **Doug Smock**
Production Manager: **Helen Ewan**
Production Coordinator: **Maura Murphy**
Compositor: **Pine Tree Composition, Inc.**
Printer/Binder: **R. R. Donnelley & Sons Company**
Cover Printer: **The Lehigh Press, Inc.**

6 5 4

Library of Congress Cataloging-in-Publication Data

Lippincott's review series : pediatric nursing.
   p.   cm.
  Includes bibliographical references and index.
  ISBN 0-397-54774-9
  1. Pediaric nursing—Examinations, questions, etc. 2. Pediatric
nursing—Outlines, syllabi, etc. I. J.B. Lippincott Company.
  II. Title: Pediatric nursing.
  [DNLM: 1. Pediatric Nursing—examination questions. WY 18 L765]
RJ245.L57 1991
610.73'62—dc20
DNLM/DLC
for Library of Congress   91–25662
                                                CIP

CONTRIBUTING AUTHORS

Nu-Vision, Inc.
Paula S. Cokingtin, RN, EdD, President
Kathy D. Robinson, RN, MSN, Vice President
Carolyn H. Brose, RN, EdD, Vice President
Linda N. Kohlman, RN, MN, Associate

Karen Chung, RN, MSN
Associate Professor
St. Louis University
School of Nursing
St. Louis, Missouri

Roberta K. Olson, RN, PhD
Associate Dean for Undergraduate Nursing
University of Kansas
School of Nursing
Kansas City, Kansas

Judith A. Vinson, RN, MSN
Coordinator, Nursing Education
St. Louis Children's Hospital
St. Louis, Missouri

REVIEWERS

Julie Stier LaMothe, RN, BSN, MSN, CPNP

Professor of Nursing
Indiana University
School of Nursing
Indianapolis, Indiana

Mary Ann Ludwig, RN, PhD

Associate Professor
State University of New York/Buffalo
School of Nursing
Buffalo, New York

M. Thayer Wilson, RN

Associate Professor
Medical College of Georgia
Augusta, Georgia

INTRODUCTION

Lippincott's Review Series is designed to help you in your study of the key subject areas in nursing. The series consists of four books, one in each core nursing subject area:

Medical-Surgical Nursing
Pediatric Nursing
Maternal-Newborn Nursing
Mental Health and Psychiatric Nursing

Each book contains a comprehensive outline content review, chapter study questions and answer keys with rationales for correct and incorrect responses, and a comprehensive examination and answer key with rationales for correct and incorrect responses.

Lippincott's Review Series was planned and developed in response to your requests for outline review books that address each major subject area and also contain a self-test mechanism. These books meet the need for comprehensive subject review books that will also assist you in identifying your strong and weak areas of knowledge. Each book is a complete source for review and self-assessment of a single core subject—all four together provide an excellent comprehensive review of entry-level nursing.

Each book is all-inclusive of the content addressed in major textbooks. The content outline review uses a consistent nursing process format throughout and addresses nursing care for well and ill clients. Also included are such necessary additional topics as developmental and life-cycle issues, health assessment, patient teaching, and other concepts including growth and development, nutrition, pharmacology, and anatomy, physiology, and pathophysiology.

You can use the books in this series in several different ways. Overall, you can use them as subject reviews to augment general study throughout your basic nursing program and as a review to prepare for the National Council Licensure Examination (NCLEX-RN). How you use each book depends on your individual needs and preferences and on whether you review each chapter systematically or concentrate only on those chapters whose subject areas are particularly problematic or challenging. You may instead choose to use the comprehensive examination as a self-assessment opportunity to evaluate your knowledge base before you review the content outline. Likewise, you can use the study questions for pre- or post-testing after study, followed by the comprehensive examination as a means of evaluating your knowledge and competencies of an entire subject area.

Regardless of how you use the books, one of the strengths of the series is the self-assessment opportunity it offers in addition to guidance in studying and reviewing content. The chapter study questions and comprehensive examination questions have been carefully developed to cover all topics in the outline review. Most importantly, each question is categorized according to the components of the National Council of State Boards of Nursing Licensing Examination (NCLEX).

▸ Cognitive Level: Knowledge, Comprehension, Application, or Analysis
▸ Client Need: Safe, Effective Care Environment (Safe Care); Physiological Integrity (Physiologic); Psychosocial Integrity (Psychosocial); and Health Promotion and Maintenance (Health Promotion)
▸ Phase of the Nursing Process: Assessment, Analysis (Dx), Planning, Implementation, Evaluation

For those questions not related to a client need or to a phase of the nursing process, NA (not applicable) will be used, as in questions that test knowledge of a basic science.

Unlike the NCLEX examination that tests the cumulative knowledge needed for safe practice by an entry-level nurse, these practice tests systematically evaluate the knowledge base that serves as the building block for the entire nursing educational process. In this way, you can prepare for the NCLEX examination throughout your course of study. Good study habits throughout your educational program are not only the best way to ensure on-going success, but also will prove the most beneficial way to prepare for the licensing examination.

Keep in mind that these books are not intended to replace formal learning. They cannot substitute for textbook reading, discussion with instructors, or class attendance. Every effort has been made to provide accurate and current information, but class attendance and interaction with an instructor will provide invaluable information not found in books. Used correctly, these books will help you increase understanding, improve comprehension, evaluate strengths and weaknesses in areas of knowledge, increase productive study time, and as a result help you improve your grades.

MONEY BACK GUARANTEE—Lippincott's Review Series will help you study more effectively during coursework throughout your educational program, and help you prepare for quizzes and tests, including the NCLEX exam. If you buy and use any of the four volumes in Lippincott's Review Series and fail the NCLEX exam, simply send us verification of your exam results and your copy of the review book to the address below. We will promptly send you a check for our suggested list price.

Lippincott's Review Series
J. B. Lippincott Company
227 East Washington Square
Philadelphia, PA 19106-3780

CONTENTS

Pediatric Nursing

Overview

I. Evolution of pediatric health care

A. Early milestones

1. 1870: Abraham Jacobi, the "father of pediatrics," was awarded the first pediatric professorship in the United States; he later established pediatric departments in several New York City hospitals.

2. 1889: The first milk distribution center providing pasteurized milk opened in New York City as a result of Dr. Jacobi's recommendations; proliferation of these centers led to a marked decline in infant mortality.

3. 1900: Lillian Wald, considered the founder of community health nursing, began providing preventive health care information aimed at children, at Henry Street Settlement, a facility she founded in 1893 to provide medical and other services to the poor in New York City.

4. 1902: Public school nursing in the United States began with the appointment of Lina Rogers as the first full-time public school nurse in New York; Ms. Wald was instrumental in establishing this position.

5. 1907: The first professional courses in pediatric nursing were instituted at the Teacher's College of Columbia University.

B. Important federal programs

1. 1909: The first White House Conference on Children was convened by President Theodore Roosevelt to address the poor working and living conditions of many children in the United States.

2. 1912: The U. S. Children's Bureau was established to oversee children's health and environmental conditions.

3. 1921: The Sheppard-Towner Act provided grants to states to establish maternal and child health divisions in state health care departments.

4. 1935: The Social Security Act provided for aid to dependent families and children (ADFC), maternal and child health services, and child welfare services.

5. 1965: Title XIX, the Medicaid program, provided block grants to states to improve access to health care for pregnant women and young children.

6. 1966: The federal WIC (Women, Infants, and Children) Program was established to supplement the nutritional needs of low-income families.

7. 1969: The U. S. Children's Bureau was transferred to The Office of Health, Education, and Welfare (HEW), Office of Child Development.

8. 1975: The Education for All Handicapped Children Act (PL94-142) established federally mandated special education in public schools.

9. 1975: Title XX, Social Services, began providing block grants for day care, emergency shelter, counseling, family planning, and other services for children.

10. 1981: Alcohol, Drug Abuse, and Mental Health block grants began funding services for mentally disturbed children and adolescents.

II. Principles of growth and development

A. Growth

1. The term *growth* denotes an increase in body size. In pediatric nursing, focus is on the child's height and weight.

2. Growth occurs as cells divide and synthesize new proteins.

3. Nutrition represents the most important variable influencing a child's growth.

B. Development

1. Development refers to a gradual growth and change from a lower to a more advanced state of complexity.

2. It involves expansion of the child's capacities through growth, maturation, and progressive gains in functional ability.

C. **Stages of growth and development**
1. Child growth and development commonly is categorized into five approximate age stages.
2. The *prenatal* stage extends from conception to birth.
3. *Infancy* runs from birth to about 12 months and encompasses two periods:
   a. Neonatal: birth to age 28 days
   b. Infancy: age 29 days to about 12 months
4. Age 1 to 6 years, the *early childhood* stage, commonly is subdivided into:
   a. Toddler: age 1 to 3 years
   b. Preschool: age 4 to 6 years
5. *Middle childhood*, or the school-age period, extends from about age 6 to 11 or 12 years.
6. *Later childhood* encompasses:
   a. Prepubertal period: about age 11 to 13 years
   b. Adolescence: about age 13 to 18 years

D. **Patterns of growth and development**
1. Growth and development occurs in definite and predictable patterns, or trends: directional trends, sequential trends, and secular trends.
2. *Directional trends* occur in regular directions, or gradients, reflecting the development and maturation of neuromuscular functions; these trends apply to physical, mental, social, and emotional development and include:
   a. *Cephalocaudal* (or head-to-tail) development, occurring along the body's long axis, in which control over head, mouth, and eye movements precedes control over the upper body, torso, and legs
   b. *Proximodistal* (midline-to-peripheral) development, progressing from the center of the body to the extremities, in which the child develops arm movement before fine motor finger ability. Proximodistal development is symmetrical; each side develops in the same direction at the same rate as the other
   c. *Mass-to-specific* development, sometimes referred to as *differentiation*, in which the child masters simple operations before complex functions and moves from broad general patterns of behavior to more refined patterns
3. *Sequential trends* involve a predictable sequence of growth and development stages through which a child normally passes; these trends have been identified for motor skills, such as locomotion (e.g., a child crawls before creeping, creeps before standing, and stands before walking), and behaviors such as language and social

skills (e.g., a child first plays alone, then with others in increasing numbers and in progressively complex activities).

4. *Secular trends* refer to worldwide trends in the rate and age of maturation. In general, children are maturing earlier and growing larger at each age as compared to preceding generations.

E. Implications for nursing

1. The nurse must understand that the pace of normal growth and development varies from child to child.
2. The nurse provides parents with necessary information to promote the birth and normal growth and development of healthy children.
3. The nurse provides health promotion education for families within constraints imposed by illness, disease, or disability.
4. Developmental assessment involves consideration of physiologic, neuromotor, cognitive, and psychosocial parameters; a systematic approach is necessary to ensure coverage of all significant areas.

III. Family and cultural influences

A. Family influences

1. Important functions of the family include:
   a. Childbearing and childrearing
   b. Providing basic maintenance for the child in the form of food, clothing, shelter, and health care
   c. Providing emotional, social, and psychological support for family members
   d. Providing safety and protection from harm to the child
   e. Providing status to the child as a member of a family and a larger community
   f. Providing socialization for the child by facilitating acquisition of beliefs, values, and behaviors considered culturally desirable or appropriate
2. Because the family is the child's primary resource, pediatric nursing must include the family in various aspects of nursing management. The family should be involved directly in decisions and activities related to the child's care, and the nurse should treat the family itself as a client in potential need of nursing care.

B. Cultural influences

1. The child is acculturated by the family to the traditional views and practices of their culture.
2. Culturally derived health beliefs influence how the child and family respond to preventive, maintenance, and restorative practices.

C. Implications for nursing

1. The challenge of providing culturally sensitive nursing care involves adapting ethnic practices to the child's health needs instead of trying to change long-standing values and beliefs.

2. Family participation in positive health care practices is enhanced when nursing interventions accommodate their belief systems.
3. The nurse should assess for these health-related beliefs and collaborate with the family to develop an optimal plan of care.
4. The nurse also must consider the family's religious and spiritual beliefs and values when developing a plan of care.
5. To provide culturally sensitive nursing care, the nurse needs to explore his or her own values and the relation between personal values, beliefs, and actions.
6. The nurse plays an important role in interpreting a family's traditional folkways system and resolving conflicts with the modern western medical system, helping to expand the family's understanding and decrease their fear and mistrust.

IV. Pediatric health assessment
A. General considerations
1. For the child:
   a. Maintain eye contact; bend to the child's level as appropriate.
   b. Use language appropriate for the child's cognitive level; include the child in the assessment interview as appropriate.
   c. Keep in mind that a child is perceptive of caregivers' non-verbal communication and body language.
   d. Allow the child some warm-up time to become acquainted with the caregivers and the environment; introduce yourself, and explain the purpose of your presence (e.g., interview, procedure, play time).
   e. Respect the child's responses and need for privacy as appropriate for age.
   f. Incorporate play into the assessment as appropriate (e.g., let the child pretend to examine you, use puppets to explain procedures).
2. For the family:
   a. Develop a family-oriented approach that encourages parents to participate in the child's assessment.
   b. Choose a quiet setting for assessment and any teaching sessions.
   c. Ask open-ended questions to elicit responses beyond yes or no answers.
   d. Focus on the information needed or problem to be solved.
   e. Listen attentively, respect responses, and provide appropriate feedback. Use silence judiciously.
   f. Communicate the importance of the parents' role in planning and providing care for the child in conjunction with the health care team.
   g. Encourage parents to express concerns and ask questions.

B. **Health history**
  1. Purpose: to collect subjective data about the patient's health status and provide insights into actual or potential health problems
  2. Components include:
     a. Identifying (or biographical) information
     b. Chief complaint
     c. History of present illness
     d. Past health history
     e. Review of systems
     f. Family health history
     g. Sexual history
  3. Identifying information includes:
     a. Name, address, telephone number
     b. Mother's and father's names
     c. Date and place of birth
     d. Sex
     e. Race, nationality, or cultural background
     f. Religion
  4. Chief complaint: the child's reason for seeking health care or the parent's (informant's) reason for seeking health care for the child
  5. Current health status: the sequence of events leading up to the chief complaint and other related information, including:
     a. Symptom analysis of the chief complaint
     b. Other current or recent illnesses or problems
     c. Any other health concerns
     d. Current medication use
  6. Past health status: information concerning past health status, previous problems, and health promotion practices, including:
     a. Birth history (pregnancy, labor and delivery, perinatal history)
     b. Previous illnesses, injuries, or operations
     c. Allergies
     d. Immunization status
     e. Growth and development milestones
     f. Habits (e.g., sleeping and waking, eating, elimination)
  7. Review of systems: focused questions about body system function, covering:
     a. General: overall health status
     b. Integument: lesions, bruising, care habits
     c. Head: trauma, headaches
     d. Eyes: infection, drainage, visual acuity
     e. Ears: infection, drainage, hearing acuity
     f. Nose: bleeding, congestion
     g. Mouth: lesions, soreness, pattern of dental care
     h. Throat: sore throat frequency, hoarseness, difficulty swallowing

      i.   Neck: stiffness, tenderness

      j.   Chest: pain

      k.   Respiratory: cough, wheezing, shortness of breath, history of pneumonia or other infection

      l.   Cardiovascular: history of murmurs, exercise tolerance, dizziness

      m. Gastrointestinal: appetite, changes in bowel habits, food intolerances, nausea, vomiting

      n.   Genitourinary: urgency, frequency, dysuria, enuresis, history of urinary tract infections or sexually transmitted diseases

      o.   Gynecologic: age at menarche, menstrual history, sexual activity

      p.   Musculoskeletal: pain, swelling, fractures

      q.   Neurologic: ataxia, unusual movements, tremors, history of seizures

      r.   Endocrine and metabolic: growth patterns, polyuria, polyphagia, polydipsia

  8. Family medical history: assessment of family genetic traits or diseases with familial tendencies or any communicable diseases in family members

  9. Sexual history: assessment of child's concerns or activities and data pertinent to adult sexual activities that affect the child

C. **Physical assessment**

  1. Purpose: to obtain objective findings on body systems functioning and overall health status

  2. General principles

      a.   In most cases, physical assessment involves a head-to-toe examination that covers each body system.

      b.   Complete less threatening and least uncomfortable procedures first to gain the child's trust.

      c.   Explain what you will be doing and what the child can expect to feel; allow the child to manipulate unfamiliar equipment before its use.

      d.   Allow the parent of an infant or a young child to be present during the examination.

      e.   Provide an adolescent with the option of having a parent present or not.

  3. Head-to-toe sequence should cover:

      a.   Vital signs

      b.   Anthropometric measurements: height, weight, head circumference (in infants)

      c.   Skin: color, pigmentation, turgor, temperature, sensitivity, lesions

      d.   Hair: distribution, characteristics

      e.   Nails: texture, color, shape, condition

      f.   Lymph nodes: swelling, mobility or fixation, temperature

      g. Head: symmetry, condition of fontanels

      h. Eyes: visual acuity, external eye examination, internal eye (ophthalmoscopic) examination

      i.   Ears: hearing acuity, external ear examination, internal ear (otoscopic) examination

      j.   Nose and sinuses: discharge, pain or tenderness on touch

      k. Mouth: condition of lips and gums, teeth, hard and soft palate, tonsils, tongue, and buccal mucosa

      l.   Chest: shape, anatomic landmarks, lungs (breath sounds), breasts (developmental stage, nipple discharge), heart sounds

      m. Abdomen: appearance of umbilicus, bowel sounds, inguinal area (for herniation), size and characteristics of liver, spleen, kidneys, bladder

      n. Genitalia: in girls—vulva, urinary meatus, internal vaginal examination (as appropriate), secondary sex characteristics; in boys—penis, scrotum and testes, urinary meatus, secondary sex characteristics

      o. Extremities and musculoskeletal system: muscle size and strength, posture and body alignment, symmetry, range of motion, balance, gait

      p. Neuromuscular: cranial nerve function, coordination, deep tendon and superficial reflexes, sensory function, cerebral function (language, cortical sensory function, cortical motor integration)

D. **Nutritional assessment**

    1. Purpose: to obtain information confirming good nutrition or altered nutritional status

    2. Determine the quantity and types of foods or formula ingested daily: use 24-hour recall, food diary for 3 days (2 weekdays and 1 weekend day), or food frequency record

    3. Evaluate nutritional status based on:

      a. Height, weight, and head circumference compared with norms for child's curve and norms for agemates

      b. Triceps skin-fold thickness (to assess body fat)

      c. Weight to height or length ratio

      d. Pertinent laboratory test results (e.g., hemoglobin, serum iron, iron-binding capacity, free erythrocyte porphyrin, transferrin saturation, serum ferritin)

    4. Assess for clinical signs of altered nutrition, including:

      a. Hair: dry, dull, easily plucked, thin, sparse, color change

      b. Face: edema, pallor, change in skin pigmentation, scaling skin

      c. Eyes: pale conjunctivae, dull corneas, redness and fissures in corners of eyelids

    d.   Tongue: edema, redness, rawness, fissures, sores

    e.   Teeth: mottling

    f.   Gingivae: swelling, sponginess, easy bleeding, sores

    g.   Neck: thyroid enlargement

    h.   Skin: dryness, hyperpigmentation or hypopigmentation, lesions, easy bruising, poor turgor, decreased subcutaneous fat

    i.   Nails: spoon shaped, brittle, ridged

    j.   Muscles: atrophy, weakness

    k.   Skeleton: epiphyseal swelling, knock-knees, bowlegs

    l.   Neurologic: irritability, tetany, mental confusion, sensory changes

E.   Developmental assessment

    1.   Purpose: to confirm normal achievement of growth and developmental milestones and identify any problems or areas of possible concern

    2.   Assess and record developmental milestones in:

        a.   Gross motor skills

        b.   Fine motor skills

        c.   Language development

        d.   Cognitive development

        e.   Social and affective development

        f.   Independence

    3.   Observe the child's behavior before structured interaction for spontaneous activity; observe the child's responses to the environment

    4.   Administer developmental tests as appropriate for age (e.g., Denver Developmental Screening Test, Brazelton Neonatal Behavioral Assessment Scale, Goodenough-Harris Draw-a-Person Test, temperament questionnaires)

F.   Family assessment

    1.   Purpose: to assess family structure and function for factors that could affect the child's health status

    2.   Structural assessment includes:

        a.   Composition of family, home, and community environment

        b.   Occupation and education of family members

        c.   Cultural and religious background

    3.   Assessment of family function involves:

        a.   Communication patterns, including expression of feelings and individuality

        b.   Personal interactions

        c.   Roles, including sources of power, decision making, and problem solving in the family

        d.   Health care function (health care practices, values, and beliefs)

        e.   Economic function (financial status)

4.   Available family assessment tools include the Home Observation for Measurement of the Environment, Family APGAR, and Neonatal Perception Inventory

Bibliography

Brunner, L. S., and Suddarth, D. S. (1991). *Lippincott manual of nursing practice* (5th ed.). Philadelphia: J. B. Lippincott.

Foster, R. L., Hunsberger, M. M., and Anderson, J. J. (1989). *Family-centered nursing care of children*. Philadelphia: W. B. Saunders.

Mott, S. R., James, S. R., and Sperhac, A. M. (1990). *Nursing care of children and families* (2nd ed.). Menlo Park, CA: Addison-Wesley.

Whaley, L. F., and Wong, D. L. (1991). *Nursing care of infants and children* (4th ed.). St. Louis: C. V. Mosby.

STUDY QUESTIONS

1. One result of the first White House Conference on Children was the establishment of the Children's Bureau in 1909. Although the Bureau evolved to address health, welfare, education, social, economic, and psychologic needs of the nation's children, its initial function was to
   a. mandate a childhood immunization schedule
   b. establish guidelines for the position of school nurse
   c. establish standards for milk pasteurization
   d. regulate child labor

2. The WIC program, enacted in 1966, provides
   a. food and nutrition education to low income, pregnant, postpartum, and lactating women and their infants and children up to age 5
   b. funds to states for projects to support prevention, treatment, and rehabilitation related to substance abuse
   c. funds to states for public education for all handicapped children
   d. block grants for various health services for low-income women, infants, and children

3. The Denver Developmental Screening Test (DDST) assesses a child's
   a. intelligence quotient
   b. psychological development
   c. eye muscle coordination and vision
   d. social, motor, and physical development

4. The fact that infants achieve structural control of the head before the trunk and extremities is an example of which universal principle of development?
   a. Development proceeds in a cephalocaudal direction.
   b. Development proceeds in a proximodistal direction.

   c. Development proceeds from the simple to the complex.
   d. Development proceeds from the general to the specific.

5. In developing a culturally sensitive plan of care for Joseph, age 5 months, whose mother speaks Spanish and little English, the nurse should be sure to
   a. provide written information in Spanish
   b. speak slowly and enunciate clearly so that Joseph's mother can understand
   c. determine when an English-speaking family member could be present to interpret for her
   d. request that a bilingual staff member act as an interpreter

6. Which of the following statements about a child's cultural background is correct?
   a. A child's physical characteristics mark him or her as part of a particular culture.
   b. Patterns of behavior are learned from ancestors and passed along to future generations.
   c. Heritage dictates a group's shared cultural values.
   d. Cultural background usually has no bearing on a family's health practices.

7. Assessment of family structure includes all the following *except*
   a. composition of family, home, and community environment
   b. occupation and education of family members
   c. cultural and religious background
   d. communication patterns among family members

8. Which of the following is *not* a component of a pediatric health history?
   a. identifying information
   b. review of systems
   c. vital signs
   d. current health status

ANSWER KEY

1. *Correct response: d*
   In 1909, President Theodore Roosevelt convened the first White House Conference on Children to address the poor working and living conditions of many children in the United States.
   a. Immunization was not part of the Bureau's original mandate.
   b. Lillian Wald was instrumental in establishing the role of school nurse.
   c. Milk pasteurization was not part of the Bureau's original responsibilities.
   Comprehension/NA/NA

2. *Correct response: a*
   In 1966, the federal WIC (Women, Infants, and Children) Program was established to supplement the nutritional needs of low-income families.
   b. This is the purpose of the 1981 Alcohol, Drug Abuse, and Mental Health Act.
   c. This describes PL94-142, Education for All Handicapped Children Act.
   d. This describes Title XX.
   Comprehension/Physiologic/NA

3. *Correct response: d*
   The DDST evaluates the developmental level of motor, social, and language skills in children age 1 month to 6 years.
   a, b, and c. The DDST does not evaluate these components. Various other tests are available to evaluate these parameters.
   Knowledge/Psychosocial/Assessment

4. *Correct response: a*
   Gaining control of the head before control of the trunk and extremities is an example of cephalocaudal development.
   b, c, and d. These principles of development are not applicable.

Knowledge/Physiologic/Assessment

5. *Correct response: c*
   This is the most appropriate measure to ensure good nurse–parent communication and proper teaching.
   a. Written instructions alone do not ensure good communication.
   b. These measures will not ensure Joseph's mother's understanding.
   d. A family member would be a better interpreter than a staff member.
   Application/Psychosocial/Implementation

6. *Correct response: b*
   Behavioral patterns and values of the family are passed from one generation to the next.
   a. Physical characteristics do not determine cultural values.
   c. Heritage plays a part in culture, but the behavior patterns are stronger.
   d. Cultural background often has a great bearing on a family's health practices.
   Comprehension/Health promotion/Analysis (Dx)

7. *Correct response: d*
   Evaluating communication patterns among family members is a part of assessing family function.
   a, b, and c. These are all aspects of family structure.
   Application/Psychosocial/Assessment

8. *Correct response: c*
   Measuring vital signs is part of the physical assessment not the health history.
   a, b, and d. These are all components of the pediatric health history.
   Application/Psychosocial/Assessment

Infant Growth and Development
(Age 1 Month to 1 Year)

I. Physical growth and development
A. General characteristics
1. The best indication of good overall health in an infant is steadily increasing height, weight, and head and chest circumference.

2. Growth and development is monitored by plotting measurements on a standardized growth chart from birth to age 2 years.

B. Height and weight changes

1. The nurse measures an infant's height and weight and plots the values on a standardized growth chart.
2. Sequential measurements should demonstrate a pattern conforming to normal growth curves.
3. Normal height changes include:
   a. Growth of ½ to ¾ inch (1.3 to 1.9 cm)
   b. Increase of 50% over birth length by age 12 months
4. Normal weight changes include:
   a. Gain of 5 to 7 oz (125 to 175 g) per week
   b. Doubling of birth weight by age 6 months
   c. Tripling of birth weight by age 12 months

C. Head and chest circumference changes

1. At birth, normal head circumference is about 13.7 inches (35.1 cm), normal chest circumference about 12.9 inches (33 cm).
2. Head and chest circumferences equalize during the first year after birth.
3. After age 2 years, chest circumference increases substantially more than head circumference.
4. Normal head circumference changes include:
   a. Increase of ½ inch (1.3 cm) per month between ages 1 to 6 months
   b. Increase of ¼ inch (0.64 cm) per month between ages 7 to 12 months
5. Normal chest circumference changes include:
   a. Smaller than head circumference at birth
   b. Equal to head circumference at age 12 months, then becoming significantly larger in subsequent years

D. Cranial suture changes

1. The posterior fontanel measures 1 × 1 cm at birth and normally closes by age 2 months.
2. The anterior fontanel measures 3.5 × 3.5 cm at birth and normally closes by age 18 months.

II. Developmental theories

A. Psychosocial development (Erikson)

1. Erikson terms the psychosocial crisis faced by an infant (from birth to age 1 year) *trust vs. mistrust.*
2. In this stage, the infant's significant other is the "maternal" person.
3. The psychosocial theme is "To get; to give in return."
4. Developing a sense of trust in caregivers and the environment is a central focus for an infant.
5. This sense of trust forms the foundation for all future psychosocial tasks.

6. The quality of the caregiver–child relationship is a crucial factor in the infant's development of trust.

7. The development of mutual reciprocity between a caregiver and an infant is the desired outcome to enhance the infant's sense of trust.

8. An infant who receives attentive care learns that life is predictable and that his or her needs will be met promptly; this fosters trust.

9. In contrast, an infant experiencing consistently delayed needs gratification will develop a sense of uncertainty, leading to mistrust of caregivers and the environment.

10. An infant commonly seeks comfort from a security object (e.g., a blanket or favorite toy) during times of stress.

B. Psychosexual development (Freud)

1. In the *oral stage* of development, extending from birth to age 18 months, the erogenous zone is the mouth, lips, tongue, and teeth, and sexual activity takes the form of sucking, swallowing, chewing, and biting.

2. In this stage, the infant meets the world by:
    a. Crying, tasting, sucking, eating, and early vocalization
    b. Biting, to gain a sense of having a hold on and having greater control of the environment
    c. Grasping and touching, to explore tactile variations in the environment

C. Cognitive development (Piaget)

1. The *sensorimotor stage*, from birth to around 18 months, involves the development of intellect and knowledge of the environment gained through the senses.

2. During this stage, development progresses from reflexive activity to purposeful acts.

3. The sensorimotor stage consists of five substages:
    a. Substage 1 (birth to age 1 month), characterized by innate and predictable survival reflexes
    b. Substage 2 (age 1 to 4 months), marked by stereotyped repetition and the infant's focus on his or her own body as the center of interest
    c. Substage 3 (age 4 to 8 months), characterized by acquired adaptation and a shifting of attention to objects and the environment
    d. Substage 4 (age 8 to 12 months), marked by intentionality and consolidation and coordination of schemes
    e. Substage 5 (age 12 to 18 months), characterized by an interest in novelty and creativity and discovery of new means through active experimentation

4. At the completion of this stage, the infant achieves a sense of object permanence:

> a. Retains a mental image of an absent object
> b. Sees self as separate from others

5. An emerging sense of body image parallels sensorimotor development.

III. Social development

A. Language

1. During infancy, language development begins.
2. Crying represents the infant's first means of verbal communication.
3. As early as age 5 to 6 weeks, an infant vocalizes with short throaty sounds.
4. By age 2 months, the infant typically makes single vowel sounds; by age 3 to 4 months, consonant sounds; by age 8 months, more consonants and combined syllables, such as "mama" and "dada" (although without comprehension of meaning); and by age 1 year, several short words with meaning.

B. Play

1. Play is the infant's "work"; it facilitates learning.
2. The infant learns about the environment through the senses of touch, taste, hearing, smell, and sight.
3. The infant develops motor skills through manipulating toys and other objects.
4. An infant's play is basically solitary (noninteractive with peers).

C. Socialization

1. Attachment to the significant other begins at birth and becomes increasingly evident after age 6 months.
2. Between ages 4 and 8 months, the infant progresses through the first stage of separation–individuation, gaining a sense of self and his or her significant other as separate persons, and begins to acquire a sense of object permanence, recognizing that the significant other can be absent.
3. The infant makes major strides in personal–social behavior during the first year, learning to shape his or her environment and elicit specific responses from others (e.g., by smiling in response to pleasurable stimuli).

IV. Health promotion

A. Fears

1. Infants exhibit a reflexive startle response to loud noises, falling, and sudden movements in the environment.
2. Stranger anxiety typically begins around age 6 months.
3. A caregiver's cuddling and warmth can help ease fears.

B. Temperament

1. Temperament theory attempts to account for individual differences among infants in behavior, reactions, and manner of thinking.

2.   The better the fit between parental expectations and infant responses, the more mutual reciprocity the parent–infant relationship has.

C.   Communication
1.   Talking in a soothing tone can be comforting to an infant.
2.   Regularly talking to an infant also stimulates the infant to imitate sounds and words.

D.   Discipline
1.   Spoiling an infant with too much attention is difficult; meeting the infant's needs promptly always takes precedence over promoting discipline.
2.   An infant has no ability to accept delayed gratification; learning to wait develops progressively after infancy. For this reason, disciplinary actions for an infant often seem fruitless.
3.   Nevertheless, discipline and setting limits should begin in infancy; the earlier effective disciplinary methods are instituted, the easier they are to continue as the child ages.
4.   Effective disciplinary methods may include negative voice, stern eye contact, timeout, and at times, *one* slap on the hand or buttocks.

E.   Nutrition and feeding
1.   Consistent oral intake of sufficient calories provided by a caring parent sets a positive pattern for an infant's future eating behaviors.
2.   Feeding schedule suggestions for an infant from birth to age 6 months receiving breast milk or formula on demand include:
   a.   Age 1 month: 4 oz six times a day
   b.   Age 2 months: 4 oz five times a day (one night feeding is eliminated)
   c.   Age 5 months: 5.8 oz five times a day
   d.   Age 6 months: 4.2 oz five times a day (as solid food feedings begin, milk feedings decrease)
3.   At age 6 to 12 months, solid food becomes appropriate because of the infant's developmental readiness (e.g., the infant can assume an upright position, the extrusion reflex lessens, and the digestive tract matures).
4.   Solid food should be introduced progressively: first, cereal with iron, followed by pureed fruits, then vegetables, then meats. Each new food should be added to the infant's diet separately at intervals of 4 to 7 days each to determine allergies.
5.   Ideally, weaning an infant from breast or bottle begins at age 6 months.
6.   Suggestions for weaning include:
   a.   Eliminate one breast or bottle feeding at a time for one cup feeding.

      b. Begin practicing with sips from a cup at age 4 to 5 months, when motor ability has developed.

      c. Introduce juice in a cup rather than a bottle to help prevent dental caries.

F. Sleeping patterns

1. During the first month after birth, an infant sleeps most of the time not spent eating. With age, daily sleep time decreases as awake and alert times increase.

2. In the first year of life, an infant typically takes morning and afternoon naps.

3. Bedtime rituals begun in infancy help prepare the infant for sleep and prevent future bedtime and sleeping problems.

4. Parents should establish that the infant's crib is for sleeping, not for playing, and prevent reinforcing wakefulness during the night by picking up the infant whenever he or she wakes and cries.

G. Dental health

1. An infant's primary (deciduous) teeth erupt at about age 6 months. Assessment guide: age of child in months minus 6 months equals number of primary teeth.

2. Clean an infant's teeth with a damp cloth; brushing is too harsh for the infant's tender gums.

3. Assess the need for a fluoride supplement; consult with the physician.

4. Despite a widespread belief to the contrary, fever, vomiting, and diarrhea usually are not associated with teething but rather indicate illness.

H. Immunization

1. Infant immunization helps prevent the spread of communicable disease and decreases morbidity and mortality of infants and children.

2. Generally, immunizations should follow an age-based schedule (Table 2–1).

TABLE 2–1.
Immunization Schedule for Infants and Children*

AGE	RECOMMENDED VACCINATIONS
2 months	DTP-1, OPV-1
4 months	DTP-2, OPV-2
6 months	DTP-3, OPV-3 in endemic areas
15 months	MMR
18 months	DPT-4, OPV-3 (if not given earlier), PRP-D
4 to 6 years	DPT-5, OPV-4
14 to 16 years	Td (repeat every 10 years thereafter)

Recommended by the American Academy of Pediatrics, 1988.

3. Contraindications for infant immunization include:
   a. Severe febrile illness (other than the common cold)
   b. Immunodeficiency stemming from a malignant condition or from chemotherapy
   c. Known allergy to the vaccine, to egg white, or to poultry
4. Pregnant women should not receive live vaccines (e.g., measles, mumps, and rubella [MMR]) because a live attenuated virus may cross the placenta.
5. Administering a live vaccine to a child whose mother is pregnant seems to carry no risk to the developing fetus.
6. Parents should understand that the benefits of immunization usually far outweigh any potential risks.

I. Injury prevention

1. Accidental injuries are a major cause of death during infancy; common causes include:
   a. Falls off of beds and down stairs
   b. Aspiration of small objects
   c. Poisoning from overdose of medications or ingestion of toxic household substances
   d. Suffocation due to inadvertent covering of the nose and mouth, pressure on the throat or chest, or prolonged lack of air such as in a closed, parked car
   e. Burns from hot liquids or foods, scalding bath water, excessive sun exposure, or electrical injury
   f. Motor vehicle accidents, most commonly linked to improper use or nonuse of an infant car seat
2. Nursing considerations associated with accident prevention include:
   a. Instruct parents to maintain a safe environment for the infant by keeping breakables, sharp objects, and harmful substances out of reach.
   b. Alert parents to age-specific potential injury sources and accident-prevention strategies.
   c. Encourage parents to avoid repetitive negative expressions for the sake of safety and to stress positive aspects of the infant's behavior, such as playing with suitable toys.

J. Toy selection

1. Infant toys serve several purposes, including:
   a. Stimulation for psychosocial development
   b. Diversion for relieving boredom, pain, and discomfort
   c. A means of communicating and expressing feelings
   d. Aid in the development of sensorimotor skills
2. Infant toys should be safe and age appropriate.
3. Toy safety considerations include:
   a. No sharp part edges
   b. No detachable parts (e.g., wheels, tops)

4. Age-appropriate toys take into account an infant's short attention span with such features as bright colors to provide visual stimulation.

5. Examples of safe, age-appropriate infant toys include:
   a. Age 1 to 3 months: mobile, mirror, music box, stuffed animal with no detachable parts, and rattle
   b. Age 4 to 6 months: squeeze toys, busy box, and play gym
   c. Age 7 to 9 months: various cloth textures, splashing bath toys, blocks, and balls
   d. Age 10 to 12 months: durable books with large pictures, building blocks, nesting cups, large puzzles, and push–pull toys

V. Selected health problems of infants

A. Fever

1. Description: abnormal body temperature elevation
2. Etiology
   a. Common causes of fever in infants include upper and lower respiratory tract infection, pharyngitis, otitis media, and generalized and enteric viral infections.
   b. More serious causes of fever include urinary tract infection, pneumonia, bacteremia, meningitis, osteomyelitis, septic arthritis, cancer, poisoning or drug overdose, immunization reaction, and dehydration.
3. Pathophysiology
   a. Fever most commonly results from disruption of the hypothalamic set point due to infection, allergy, endotoxins, or tumor.
   b. This disrupted thermoregulation leads to increased heat production and decreased heat loss.
   c. Associated clinical findings provide important indications of the seriousness of fever (e.g., an active, alert child with a fever of 104°F [38.8°C] generally is of less concern than a listless, lethargic infant with a temperature of 102°F [40.5°C]).
4. Assessment findings
   a. Temperature 102° to 105°F (38.9° to 40.6°C) measured by the axillary route
   b. Skin flushing, diaphoresis, chills
   c. Restlessness or lethargy
5. Nursing diagnoses
   a. Altered Body Temperature
   b. High Risk for Injury
6. Planning and implementation: Teach parents measures to control fever, such as:
   a. Antipyretics: acetaminophen, 1 grain (60 mg) administered five times in 24 hours

        b.   Sponge baths: light friction rub with lukewarm water for 20 to 30 minutes

    7.   Evaluation

        a.   Temperature decreases by no more than 1°F each hour.

        b.   The infant appears to feel more comfortable.

B. **Iron-deficiency anemia**

    1.   Description: a microcytic, hypochromic anemia resulting from inadequate supplies of iron to synthesize hemoglobin adequately

    2.   Etiology: causes include inadequate dietary intake of iron and insufficient iron stores

    3.   Pathophysiology

        a.   In a full-term infant, iron stores are adequate for the first 5 to 6 months after birth.

        b.   In a premature infant or an infant from a multiple birth, iron stores are adequate for only 2 to 3 months.

        c.   The signs and symptoms of *normal physiologic anemia* commonly develop after 2 to 3 months. This physiologic anemia should not be confused with iron-deficiency anemia.

    4.   Assessment findings

        a.   Pallor, weakness, lethargy

        b.   Hemoglobin level less than 9 g/dL

        c.   Increased susceptibility to infection

        d.   Impaired cognitive ability (long-term consequence)

    5.   Nursing diagnoses

        a.   Altered Nutrition: Less than Body Requirements

        b.   Activity Intolerance

        c.   High Risk for Infection

    6.   Planning and implementation

        a.   Promote an adequate intake of iron-rich formula or foods; limit milk after 6 months when solid foods are begun.

        b.   Provide an iron supplement if necessary; when giving oral iron supplement, avoid contact with the infant's teeth to prevent discoloration.

        c.   Minimize the physical demands of activity and emotional stress; encourage quiet play rather than active play.

        d.   Institute infection-prevention measures (e.g., keep the infant isolated from others with infections, carefully monitor temperature and laboratory test results).

    7.   Evaluation

        a.   Diet modifications are implemented.

        b.   The infant's energy level increases.

        c.   The infant remains free of infection.

        d.   The infant's hemoglobin level rises.

C. **Candidiasis**

    1.   Description: a usually mild, superficial fungal infection affecting the skin and mucous membranes

2. Etiology: the causative organism is the yeastlike fungus *Candida albicans*
3. Pathophysiology
    a. The infant may contract infection during the birth process through contact with an infected person, most commonly the mother.
    b. Infection also may result after birth; the most common predisposing factor is an alteration in the normal GI tract flora due to ingestion of prescribed broad-spectrum antibiotics.
4. Assessment findings
    a. Oral involvement: white patches on the tongue, palate, and inner aspects of cheeks
    b. Perianal involvement: dermatitis in inguinal folds and on the buttocks and lower abdomen
5. Nursing diagnoses
    a. Impaired Skin Integrity
    b. High Risk for Infection
6. Planning and implementation
    a. Institute infection prevention measures (e.g., wash hands thoroughly, ensure that all caretakers are free of infection, boil reusable nipples for bottles).
    b. Rinse the infant's mouth with water after feedings.
    c. Cleanse the perianal area with soap and water with each diaper change and dry thoroughly before applying topical medication.
    d. Apply topical nystatin to oral surfaces four to six times daily, and to the affected perianal area with each diaper change.
7. Evaluation
    a. Oral thrush and perianal dermatitis resolve.
    b. No further spread of infection occurs.

D. Impetigo
1. Description: a progressive, superficial, highly contagious skin infection marked by vesicopustular eruptions
2. Etiology: causative organisms include streptococci and staphylococci
3. Pathophysiology: the mode of transmission is exudate from lesions
4. Assessment findings
    a. Ubiquitous staphylococcus or streptococcus infection
    b. Lesions progressing from macules to vesicles to crusts
    c. Itching
5. Nursing diagnoses
    a. High Risk for Injury
    b. High Risk for Infection

   c. Impaired Skin Integrity

  6. Planning and implementation: Teach parents to:

   a. Wash hands well to prevent spread of infection

   b. Isolate the infant and his or her belongings from other family members

   c. Apply compresses with Burow's solution (aluminum acetate) 1:20

   d. Administer prescribed antibiotics (parenteral or oral) and topical bactericidal ointment

   e. Cut the infant's fingernails short and cover his or her hands with socks during sleep to prevent scratching and spread of infection

  7. Evaluation

   a. Infection does not spread.

   b. No scarring or secondary infection occurs.

VI. Hospitalization of infants

A. Infant's response to hospitalization

  1. Fears associated with hospitalization commonly include:

   a. Separation from parents and significant others

   b. Pain

  2. Typical behaviors differ according to age and may include:

   a. Age 1 to 6 months: global reactions, primarily to changes in routine and handling

   b. Age 7 to 12 months: protest, despair, and detachment; total body rigidity to protect from pain; crying

B. Parents' response to their infant's hospitalization

  1. For many parents of a firstborn infant, hospitalization is a new, frightening experience carrying an uncertain outcome.

  2. Variables that influence parents' responses to their infant's hospitalization include:

   a. The seriousness of the threat to their child

   b. Experience with illness or hospitalization

   c. The nature of the procedures involved in diagnosis and treatment

   d. Availability of support systems

   e. Previous coping abilities

   f. Personal ego strengths

   g. Additional stresses on the family system

   h. Cultural and religious beliefs and influences

   i. Communication patterns among family members

C. Nursing considerations

  1. Primary nursing care helps provide consistent care, which may help reduce the infant's and parents' anxiety and fear.

  2. The nurse should encourage parents' presence and involvement in their infant's care and arrange for rooming-in when possible.

3. The nurse can help minimize separation reaction by spending time with the infant when parents or significant others are not present.
4. Smooth, unhurried movements, gentle touching, and soothing talk help increase the infant's trust in the caregiver.

Bibliography

American Academy of Pediatrics (1988). *Report of the committee on infectious diseases* (21st ed). Elk Grove Village, IL: American Academy of Pediatrics.

Houdlin, A. D. (1987). Infant temperament and the quality of the childrearing environment. *Maternal-Child Nursing Journal, 16,* 131–143.

Jarrett, G. (1982). Childrearing patterns of young mothers: Expectations, knowledge, and practices. *American Journal of Maternal/Child Nursing, 1,* 24–32.

Mott, S. R., James, S. R., and Sperhac, A. M. (1990). *Nursing care of children and families* (2nd ed.). Menlo Park, CA: Addison-Wesley.

Whaley, L. F., and Wong, D. L. (1991). *Nursing care of infants and children* (4th ed.). St. Louis: C. V. Mosby.

Wink, D. (1985). Getting through the maze of infant formulas. *American Journal of Nursing, 85,* 388–392.

STUDY QUESTIONS

1. During the first year after birth, an infant's birth weight normally
   a. remains stable
   b. doubles
   c. triples
   d. quadruples

2. Which of the following represents the most age-appropriate toy for an infant aged 5 months?
   a. balloon
   b. teddy bear with button eyes
   c. push–pull toy
   d. busy box

3. Which of the following statements about infant feeding (breast or formula) between ages 1 and 3 months is correct?
   a. Feedings should be scheduled every 4 hours.
   b. About 6 oz of breast milk or formula should be given at each feeding.
   c. Burping should be encouraged after each 4 oz.
   d. The infant should be placed on the abdomen or the right side after feeding.

4. In an infant aged 6 to 12 months, bottle-mouth caries syndrome commonly results from
   a. prolonged sucking on a too-hard nipple
   b. habitual sucking on a bottle of milk or juice while lying down
   c. addition of sugar to infant formula
   d. too-frequent breast-feeding

5. Because weight gain is a reliable indicator of infant health, the nurse needs to know that an infant normally doubles his or her birth weight by age
   a. 2 months
   b. 6 months
   c. 7 months
   d. 9 months

6. Mrs. Jones expresses concern that she might spoil her 2 month-old daughter, Amy, by picking her up when she cries. Which of the following would be the nurse's best response to Mrs. Jones's concerns?
   a. "Babies need cuddling and holding. Meeting these needs will not spoil Amy."
   b. "If she isn't wet or soiled, leave her alone, and she will fall asleep."
   c. "At 2 months when babies cry, they are usually hungry. Try feeding her."
   d. "Leave her alone for 15 minutes; if she hasn't stopped crying, then pick her up."

7. When exploring Mrs. Jones's knowledge of injury prevention in an infant, the nurse should recommend all the following measures *except*
   a. placing safety gates across stairways once Amy begins to crawl
   b. keeping all toxic substances out of Amy's reach
   c. safe diapering practices (i.e., keeping a hand on Amy at all times)
   d. avoiding using a car seat until Amy is at least 6 months old

8. Mrs. Jones wants more specific information about introducing solid foods in Amy's diet. Which of the following instructions is appropriate?
   a. "Introduce solid foods when Amy is age 8 and 10 months, when her extrusion reflex disappears."
   b. "Introduce solid foods one at a time for a period of 4 to 7 days each."
   c. "When you think Amy is ready for solids, mix the food in her bottle to ease the transition."
   d. "Introduce fruits and vegetables first, when Amy is age 3 to 4 months."

9. During a well-baby check, Mrs. Smith mentions that since her daughter Cindy, age 10 months, sits so well by herself, they have "loosened up" on some of the child safety measures they had instituted earlier. Which of the following statements by Mrs. Smith should the nurse *not* be concerned about?

a. "We still have all the medicines locked in the cabinet in the bathroom."

b. "She plays by herself in the bathtub for no more than 5-minute intervals so I can make some quick telephone calls."

c. "She sleeps so soundly during her naps, I have left her alone to run next door to the neighbors, just to get a break."

d. "We stopped using the car seat because she sits so well in the seat belt."

10. Communication with an infant before any procedure should include all the following *except*

a. explaining the procedure even if you do not believe the infant can understand

b. allowing a parent or significant other to be present

c. providing pictures of the procedure for an older infant

d. arranging for a primary nurse to perform all procedures

11. Which method provides the most accurate assessment of an infant's pulse rate?

a. palpating the radial pulse for 1 full minute

b. palpating the apical pulse for 10 seconds, then multiplying the result by 6

c. palpating the apical pulse for 1 full minute

d. palpating the radial pulse for 10 seconds, then multiplying the result by 6

12. Which is the optimal technique for measuring infant height?

a. measuring standing height with the infant held upright

b. measuring recumbent height with the infant prone

c. measuring recumbent height with the infant supine

d. measuring recumbent height with the infant lying on his or her side

13. Which of the following statements concerning blood pressure assessment in an infant is *not* correct?

a. Blood pressure measurement is not done until age 9 months because it provides inaccurate data in younger infants.

b. A Doppler instrument provides the most accurate blood pressure measurements in an infant.

c. The blood pressure cuff should measure one half to two thirds of the infant's upper arm or thigh circumference.

d. In a young infant, it is acceptable practice to record the systolic value and record *P* (for palpated) for the diastolic reading if it is undetectable by auscultation.

14. Which of the following statements about an infant's and family's cultural background is correct?

a. An individual's physical characteristics indicate his or her membership in a particular culture.

b. Certain behavioral patterns are learned from ancestors and passed along to present and future generations.

c. Heritage dictates the particular cultural values that groups of persons share.

d. A culture is defined as "a division of mankind possessing traits that are transmissible by descent and sufficient to characterize a distinct human type" (*Webster's New Collegiate Dictionary*).

ANSWER KEY

1. *Correct response: c*
An infant's birth weight normally should triple by age 12 months.
  a. An infant normally experiences rapid weight gain (5 to 7 oz/wk).
  b. Birth weight normally doubles by age 6 months.
  d. Birth weight normally quadruples by age 24 months.
Knowledge/Physiologic/Assessment

2. *Correct response: d*
A busy box facilitates the hand and finger development that occurs between ages 4 and 6 months.
  a. Broken balloons carry a risk of aspiration.
  b. Button eyes on a teddy bear can detach and be aspirated.
  c. An infant of this age cannot walk, so he or she will not use a push–pull toy.
Application/Health promotion/
Implementation

3. *Correct response: d*
The stomach empties to the right; this position facilitates emptying and helps prevent aspiration of any vomitus.
  a. An infant should be fed on demand, about every 2 to 5 hours.
  b. The infant will eat only as much as he or she needs, usually 4 to 5 oz per feeding.
  c. Burping should be encouraged after every 1 to 2 oz to help reduce spitting up.
Analysis/Safe care/Implementation

4. *Correct response: b*
Lying down while drinking milk or juice results in fluid pooling on the teeth, predisposing to dental caries.
  a. Sucking on a hard nipple improves mouth and jaw muscles and does not result in dental caries.
  c. Although adding sugar to formula could increase the risk of dental caries, this is not a common practice and thus not a common cause.

  d. Because an infant breast-feeds in a sitting position, milk does not pool on teeth.
Application/Physiologic/Analysis (Dx)

5. *Correct response: b*
An infant weighing 7 lb at birth should weigh about 14 lb by age 6 months.
  a. An infant normally gains 5 to 7 oz/wk, so by age 2 months he or she would have gained only about 1½ lb.
  c and d. An infant who does not double his or her birth weight until age 7 or 9 months requires a comprehensive nutritional assessment.
Application/Physiologic/Assessment

6. *Correct response: a*
A young infant needs to be comforted when he or she cries. Until a child can make appropriate cognitive connections—which usually does not occur until late infancy or early toddlerhood—it is difficult to spoil the child with too much attention.
  b. A gentle touch may be necessary until he or she falls asleep.
  c. Infants cry for many reasons other than hunger.
  d. Crying for 15 minutes wears out an infant; ignoring the infant promotes mistrust in caregivers and the environment.
Analysis/Psychosocial/Implementation

7. *Correct response: d*
A child weighing under 40 lb should always be secured properly in a safe car seat.
  a. Safety gates can help prevent falling down stairs, a major cause of injury in infants.
  b. An infant cannot recognize unsafe substances and can easily ingest them if allowed access.
  c. Keeping a hand on the infant while changing helps prevent him or her from rolling off the changing table.
Analysis/Safe care/Implementation

8. *Correct response: b*
   Introducing new foods in this manner allows caregivers to detect any food allergies.
   a. Solid foods generally are begun at age 6 months; the infant learns to eat despite the extrusion reflex.
   c. Solid foods should be fed separately with a spoon so the infant learns to eat from a spoon.
   d. Cereal is the first solid food given, beginning at age 6 months.

   Knowledge/Physiologic/Implementation

9. *Correct response: a*
   The nurse should compliment Mrs. Brown on keeping the medicines locked and out of reach.
   b. The nurse should remind Mrs. Brown that even though Cindy sits well and enjoys playing in the bath water, this practice carries a real risk of drowning.
   c. The nurse should point out that leaving Cindy alone during a nap or a bath can easily stretch into more than a "moment" and that an infant is too young to be left unsupervised.
   d. The nurse should stress that a car seat provides more protection than a seat belt alone and should be used until Cindy is about 4 years old.

   Application/Health promotion/Assessment

10. *Correct response: c*
    Pictures are not useful because they are beyond an infant's comprehension; they are more appropriate for school-age children.
    a. Talking with the infant before and during the procedure is soothing and helps hold his or her attention.
    b. The presence of a parent or significant other can help comfort the infant.
    d. A consistent caregiver promotes the infant's trust.

    Application/Psychosocial/Implementation

11. *Correct response: b*
    Listening to the heart rate apically for 1 full minute is the most accurate.
    a, c, and d. Measurements obtained through these methods are not as reliable.

    Knowledge/Physiologic/Assessment

12. *Correct response: c*
    When measuring an infant's length, placing him or her in a supine position provides the most accurate measurement.
    a. Standing measurements are inaccurate until the child can stand straight on his or her own.
    b. The prone position would yield an inaccurately long measurement by including the length of the foot.
    d. The side-lying position also would yield inaccurate results.

    Knowledge/Physiologic/Assessment

13. *Correct response: a*
    Accurate blood pressure measurements are possible in a young infant.
    b. The Doppler instrument, which amplifies the systolic and diastolic sounds, provides the most accurate readings for young infants.
    c. A too-narrow cuff will result in falsely elevated readings; a too-wide cuff, in falsely low readings.
    d. This is an accepted clinical practice.

    Application/Physiologic/Analysis (Dx)

14. *Correct response: b*
    The behavior patterns and values of the family are passed from one generation to the next.
    a. Physical characteristics do not determine cultural values.
    c. Heritage plays a part of the culture, but the behavior patterns are stronger.
    d. This is *Webster's* definition of race.

    Comprehension/Health promotion/Analysis (Dx)

Toddler Growth and Development (Age 1 to 3 Years)

I. Physical growth and development

A. General characteristics

1. Height and weight increase in a steplike rather than a linear fashion, reflecting the growth spurts and lags characteristic of toddlerhood.
2. A toddler's characteristic protruding abdomen results from underdeveloped abdominal muscles.
3. Bow-leggedness typically persists through toddlerhood since the legs must bear the weight of the relatively large trunk.

B. Height and weight changes

1. Normal height changes include:
   a. Growth of about 3 inches (7.7 cm) per year
   b. Average height of 34 inches (87.1 cm) at age 2 years
   c. Reaching about half of expected adult height at age 2 years
2. Normal weight changes include:
   a. Considerably slower rate of gain than in infancy, about 4 to 6 lb (1.8 to 2.7 kg) per year
   b. Average weight of 27 lb (12.3 kg) at age 2 years

C. Head circumference and fontanel changes

1. Head circumference normally increases about 1 inch (2.6 cm) between ages 1 and 2 years.
2. Thereafter, head circumference increases about ½ inch (1.3 cm) per year until age 5.
3. The anterior fontanel closes between ages 12 and 18 months.

D. Psychomotor milestones

1. By age 3, a toddler usually achieves fairly good bowel and bladder control.
2. Sensory changes increase as proximodistal sensations heighten; the toddler enjoys holding and cuddling with soothing motions from caregivers.
3. The toddler typically begins to walk by age 12 to 15 months, to run by age 2 years, and to walk backward and hop on one foot by age 3 years.
4. The toddler usually cannot alternate feet when climbing stairs; instead, he or she puts one foot on a step, then brings the other foot to the same level.
5. Mastery of fine motor skills increases for building, undressing, and drawing simple lines.

II. Developmental theories

A. Psychosocial development (Erikson)

1. Erikson terms the psychosocial crises facing a child between ages 1 and 3 years *autonomy vs. doubt and shame*.
2. At this stage, the child's significant other is the "paternal" person.
3. The psychosocial theme is "To hold on; to let go."

4. The toddler has a developed a sense of trust and is ready to give up dependence to assert his or her budding sense of control, independence, and autonomy.
5. The toddler begins to master:
    a. Individuation (differentiation of self from others)
    b. Separation from parent(s)
    c. Control of bodily functions
    d. Communication with words
    e. Acquisition of socially acceptable behavior
    f. Egocentric interactions with others
    (*Note:* Some of the interaction skills that the toddler is starting to develop may not be mastered until adolescence when the child revisits uncompleted tasks associated with early periods of development. Erikson refers to this as the "psychosocial moratorium.")
6. The toddler has learned that his or her parents are predictable and reliable; now the toddler begins to learn that his or her own behavior has a predictable, reliable effect on others.
7. The toddler learns to wait longer for needs gratification.
8. The toddler often uses "no," even when he or she means yes, to assert independence (negativistic behavior).
9. A sense of doubt and shame can develop if the toddler is kept dependent in areas where he or she is capable of using newly acquired skills or if made to feel inadequate when attempting new skills.
10. A toddler often continues to seek a familiar security object, such as a blanket, during times of stress.

B. Psychosexual development (Freud)
1. In the *anal stage*, typically extending from age 8 months to 4 years, the erogenous zone is the anus and buttocks, and sexual activity centers on expulsion and retention of body waste.
2. In this stage, the child's focus shifts from the mouth to the anal area, with emphasis on bowel control as he or she gains neuromuscular control over the anal sphincter.
3. The toddler experiences both satisfaction and frustration as he or she gains control over withholding and expelling, containing and releasing.
4. The conflict between "holding on" and "letting go" gradually resolves as bowel training progresses; resolution occurs once control is firmly established.

C. Cognitive development (Piaget)
1. The *sensorimotor phase* (between ages 12 and 24 months) involves two stages:
    a. Tertiary circular reactions (age 12 to 18 months), involving trial-and-error experimentation and relentless exploration

b. Beginning of thought (age 18 to 24 months), during which the toddler begins to devise new means for accomplishing tasks through mental calculations

2. In the *preconceptual phase*, extending from about age 2 to 4 years, the child uses representational thought to recall the past, represent the present, and anticipate the future (see Chapter 4, section II.C, for more information).

D. Moral development (Kohlberg)

1. Moral judgment is a cognitive process that develops gradually at three levels:
   a. Preconventional
   b. Conventional
   c. Postconventional

2. Each level of moral development can be further divided into two substages.

3. A toddler typically is at the first substage of the preconventional stage, involving punishment and obedience orientation, in which he or she makes judgments on the basis of avoiding punishment or obtaining a reward.

4. Discipline patterns affect a toddler's moral development:
   a. Physical punishment and withholding privileges tend to give the toddler a negative view of morals; withdrawing love and affection as punishment leads to feelings of guilt in the toddler.
   b. Appropriate disciplinary actions include providing simple explanations why certain behaviors are unacceptable, praising appropriate behavior, and using distraction when the toddler is headed for danger.

III. Social development

A. Play

1. For a toddler, play is the major socializing medium.
2. Play typically is parallel—beside rather than with another child.
3. Push–pull toys help enhance walking skills.
4. A toddler's short attention span causes him or her to change toys often.
5. Safe toys provide opportunities for exploring the environment; good examples include:
   a. Play dough
   b. Blocks
   c. Housekeeping toys
   d. Containers
   e. Toy telephone
   f. Wooden puzzles
   g. Cloth books
   h. Simple musical instruments

B. Language

1. A toddler typically begins to use short sentences and has a vocabulary of about 300 words by age 2.
2. A toddler tends to ask many "what" questions.

C. Socialization

1. A toddler's social interaction is dominated by ritualism, negativism, and independence.
2. Confidence in separating from parents continues to grow.

IV. Health promotion

A. Fears

1. Common fears of toddlers include:
   a. Loss of parents—separation anxiety
   b. Stranger anxiety
   c. Large animals
   d. Loud noises (e.g., vacuum cleaner)
   e. Going to sleep
2. Emotional support, comfort, and simple explanations may help allay a toddler's fears.

B. Temperament

1. An infant with an "easy" temperament usually becomes more challenging as a toddler but still may be easier to discipline than a toddler with a more intense temperament.
2. A toddler with an intense temperament may have more temper tantrums with greater activity but also may experience more intense "happy" times.
3. Temper tantrums are typical for toddlers until they learn how to deal with frustration by engaging in different actions and verbalizing their feelings.
4. Parents need to take behavioral cues from their child to help limit activity that is frustrating and necessitates quicker intervention such as "friendly warnings" or an activity change.

C. Communication

1. Frequent, repetitive naming helps the toddler learn appropriate words for objects.
2. When preparing a toddler for a stressful event, such as a surgical procedure, caregivers should provide simple explanations immediately before the event.
3. The presence of a parent during a stressful event will help the toddler cope.

D. Discipline

1. Because a toddler can move swiftly and skillfully, a caregiver must watch the toddler at all times and provide a child-proof environment for safe exploration.
2. General guidelines for implementing discipline for a toddler in-

clude consistency, timing, commitment, and an age-appropriate approach.

E. Nutrition and feeding

1. A toddler typically masters these psychomotor skills associated with feeding:

   a. Skillful at handling finger foods but messy with soft foods as he or she learns to use a spoon

   b. Drinks well from a cup held with both hands

   c. Chews with mouth closed

2. Most toddlers prefer to feed themselves.

3. A toddler is at risk for aspiration of small foods that are not easily chewed (e.g., popcorn, peanuts, and corn on the cob).

4. Many toddlers experience ''food jags'' and episodes of physiologic anorexia as the result of alternating periods of fast and slow growth.

5. A toddler generally does better eating several small, nutritious meals each day rather than three large meals.

6. Eating habits continue to build throughout toddlerhood. Mealtime struggles now may set negative patterns that prove difficult to change later.

7. Feeding suggestions for toddlers include:

   a. Provide the basic four food groups in small portions four times per day; caloric needs are 100 kcal/kg/day.

   b. Offer only a limited number of foods at any one time.

   c. Prepare nutritious food in an attractive manner.

   d. Understand that breakfast is commonly a toddler's favorite meal, at which he or she ''tanks up,'' then eats little the rest of the day.

   e. Limit concentrated sweets and empty calories.

   f. Sit the child in a high chair at the family table.

   g. Allow sufficient time to eat, but take food away when the toddler begins playing with it; this likely indicates fullness.

   h. Avoid using food as a reward or punishment.

F. Sleeping patterns

1. Toddlers' sleep needs average 12 hours per day.

2. A toddler typically sleeps through the night and has one daytime nap.

3. A child typically discontinues daytime naps around age 3.

4. A consistent bedtime ritual helps prepare a toddler for sleep (e.g., same bedtime, a light snack, reading, and tucking into bed). A security object, such as a blanket or stuffed toy, may aid the transition to sleep.

G. Dental health

1. A child should begin brushing with a small soft-bristled toothbrush, with parental assistance, around age 2.

    2. Dentist visits should begin at age 2½.

H. **Bowel and bladder control**

    1. Signals indicating that a toddler is ready for toilet training include:

        a. Walks well (Muscle coordination indicates that sphincter control can be gained.)

        b. Communicates with parents

        c. Has awareness of a wet or soiled diaper

        d. Can hold urine for 2 hours

        e. Is interested in pleasing parents

    2. Bowel control develops before bladder control; the toddler may stay dry during the day but need a diaper at night until age 4.

I. **Immunization**

    1. A toddler should receive appropriate immunizations, including:

        a. Age 15 months: MMR (measles, mumps, and rubella)

        b. Age 18 months: DTP, OPV

        c. Age 24 months: HBPV (*Hemophilus influenzae* type b polysaccharide vaccine) (see Chapter 2, Table 2-1)

    2. Parents should receive information about the need for, and side effects of, immunizations.

J. **Sibling rivalry**

    1. A toddler commonly develops feelings of sibling rivalry after a new baby is born, stemming from a sense of "dethronement" since he or she no longer is the sole focus of his parents' attention.

    2. Caregivers may help reduce a toddler's sense of sibling rivalry by beginning preparation 1 month before the new baby's scheduled birth; discussing the baby's feeding, diapering, and sleeping needs; and reassuring the toddler that his or her routine will stay much the same (e.g., meals, bedtime rituals).

    3. After the baby's birth, parents should allow and encourage the toddler to help care for the new baby whenever possible so that the toddler feels included and important.

K. **Injury prevention**

    1. Toddlers are prone to the same injuries as infants, including:

        a. Falls

        b. Aspiration

        c. Poisoning

        d. Suffocation

        e. Burns

        f. Motor vehicle accidents

        g. Other accidental injuries

    2. Nursing considerations associated with accident prevention include:

        a. Falls: Instruct parents to keep crib rails up, place gates across stairways, keep screens secure on all windows, and supervise the toddler at play.

b. Aspiration and poisoning: Teach parents to place all toxic substances up high and locked (child can now climb and open); secure safety caps on medications; and remove all small, easily aspirated objects from the child's environment. Urge them to keep the phone number of a poison control center by the telephone at all times.

c. Suffocation: Encourage parents to teach the toddler water safety to help prevent accidental drowning in bathtubs and pools; instruct them to avoid storing plastic bags and balloons within the toddler's access.

d. Burns: Instruct parents to avoid using table cloths (a curious toddler may pull the cloth to see what is on the table, possibly spilling hot foods or liquids on himself or herself); to teach the toddler what "hot" means; to store matches and cigarette lighters in a locked cabinet out of reach; and to secure safety plugs in all unused electrical outlets.

e. Motor vehicle accidents: Instruct parents to continue using an appropriate-sized car seat at all times.

f. Other accidental injuries: Teach parents to lock cabinets and drawers that contain hazardous items, such as knives, firearms, and ammunition; encourage parents to teach the toddler to avoid playing in the street and how to cross the street safely; and urge parents to supervise tricycle riding and outdoor play.

L. Anticipatory guidance

1. Anticipatory guidance involves intervening, through providing guidance to parents, to addressing common problems of toddlers before health problems develop.

2. An understanding of potential hazards and conflicts associated with each developmental period enables the nurse to provide guidance to parents regarding childrearing practices aimed at preventing potential problems.

3. Important anticipatory guidance issues for parents of toddlers commonly include:

   a. Preparing parents for expected behavioral changes (i.e., negativism and ritualism)

   b. Assessing feeding patterns and caloric intake; as necessary, counseling parents to decrease the toddler's milk intake and increase solid food intake; and explaining that although they should not expect the toddler to have table manners, they can set limits on playing with food

   c. Assessing bedtime rituals and sleep patterns and suggesting changes as appropriate

   d. Discussing ways to child-proof the home

  e. Discussing cues that indicate the toddler's readiness for toilet training: ability to walk and communicate verbally, desire to please, and awareness of wet or soiled diaper

  f. Explaining disciplinary guidelines, including providing structured firmness for meeting reasonable expectations, ignoring temper tantrums, praising accomplishments, and providing brief explanations of why certain behavior is unacceptable

  g. Pointing out that play and activity selection should be guided by the child's psychomotor needs, short attention span, and safety considerations

  h. Emphasizing the need for safety teaching (e.g., crossing the street, water play, and climbing and riding activities)

  i. Assessing the parents' need for information regarding emergency telephone numbers and care for poisoning and burns

  j. Encouraging short periods of separation with the toddler left with a trusted caregiver

  k. Explaining that the toddler may experience emotional regression during periods of stress, such as separation and hospitalization

  l. Assessing the child's readiness for a nursery school experience as he or she reaches age 3

  m. Discussing sibling rivalry and suggesting strategies for minimizing it

V. Selected health problems of toddlers

A. Lead poisoning

  1. Description: a toxic condition caused by the ingestion or inhalation of lead or lead-containing compounds

  2. Etiology

   a. Lead poisoning can result from chronic ingestion of lead-based paint or caulking chips, inhalation of fumes from leaded gasoline, use of unglazed pottery, or drinking water traveling through old lead-containing plumbing.

   b. Deficient parental interaction and supervision (i.e., insufficient feedings, poor hygiene practices) is a major contributing factor.

   c. Lead poisoning affects 4% of children aged 6 months to 5 years, with peak incidence at age 2 to 3 years; it is six times more prevalent in blacks than in whites.

  3. Assessment findings

   a. Serum lead levels above 19 μg/dL

   b. Behavioral changes (e.g., pica [ingestion of nonedible substances] lethargy, slowness, decreased curiosity)

   c. Failure to gain weight or develop

  4. Nursing diagnosis: High Risk for Injury

5. Planning and implementation
   a. Administer chelating medications: dimercaprol (BAL) and calcium disodium edetate (CaEDTA) on planned rotation sites or IV, as ordered.
   b. Teach the parents how to eliminate sources of lead from the child's environment.
   c. As appropriate, instruct the parents in medication administration (e.g., dosage schedule, injection site rotation).
   d. Discuss with the parents the child's age-appropriate growth and development needs, and suggest strategies for meeting those needs.

6. Evaluation
   a. Serum lead level is reduced to less than 1 μg/dL.
   b. The child's environment is free from potential sources of lead poisoning.
   c. The child does not ingest lead-containing substances.
   d. Safety teaching is integrated by parents.

B. Salicylate poisoning

1. Description: a toxic condition caused by the ingestion of salicylate, most often in the form of aspirin

2. Etiology
   a. Until recently, salicylate poisoning most commonly resulted from accidental ingestion of aspirin by a young child.
   b. In recent years, with the advent of child-proof containers and the increased use of acetaminophen and other nonaspirin antipyretics, the incidence of accidental aspirin overdose by children has declined.
   c. Today, about half the cases of salicylate poisoning result from a dosage error made by a parent or other caregiver.

3. Pathophysiology
   a. The principle toxic effects of salicylate poisoning include stimulation of the respiratory center and alteration of carbohydrate and lipid metabolism, leading to altered acid–base balance and both respiratory and metabolic acidosis; inhibition of oxidative phosphorylation, resulting in fever, increased oxygen consumption and CO_2 production, and possibly altered glucose metabolism; and, in chronic overdose, inhibition of platelet aggregation and prothrombin production, resulting in bleeding tendencies.
   b. Toxicity is dose related (Table 3–1).
   c. Salicylate effects peak in 2 to 4 hours (although symptoms may not occur for up to 6 hours) and persist for 12 to 18 hours or longer in chronic poisoning.

4. Assessment findings
   a. Hyperpnea

b. Vomiting

c. Hyperpyrexia

d. Lethargy

e. Altered level of consciousness ranging from confusion to coma

5. Nursing diagnoses

a. High Risk for Injury

b. Altered Comfort

c. Altered Health Maintenance

d. Knowledge Deficit

6. Planning and implementation

a. Administer syrup of Ipecac within one half hour of ingestion if the victim is awake; perform gastric lavage otherwise.

b. Administer fluid and electrolyte replacement therapy—including sodium bicarbonate, calories, and vitamin K—as ordered.

c. Observe for latent effects of chronic intoxication: bleeding tendencies, subtle onset of dehydration, coma, or seizures.

d. Monitor vital signs frequently.

e. Provide parent teaching as indicated (e.g., safe storage of medications, appropriate aspirin dosages, cumulative effects of aspirin in a child who is dehydrated due to persistent vomiting and diarrhea).

7. Evaluation

a. The child's serum salicylate level drops to normal.

b. The child's fluid and electrolytes levels are balanced.

c. The child is free of complications.

d. The child's environment is altered as necessary to decrease the risk of recurrence.

C. Child abuse and neglect

1. Description: acts of commission or omission by caregivers that prevent a child from actualizing his or her potential for growth and development

2. Etiology

a. An estimated 25% of fractures in children under 3 years stem old from child abuse.

b. Parental characteristics linked to child abuse include a history of being abused themselves, low self-esteem, and difficulty controlling aggressive impulses. .

c. Factors that may predispose a child to abuse include the child's temperament, birth order, and sex; in addition, an illegitimate or ''imperfect'' (i.e., mentally or physically impaired) child is often at risk for abuse.

d. Family characteristics that may contribute to child abuse include chronic stress, financial or emotional crises, and major life changes.

3. Assessment findings
   a. Physical evidence of abuse or neglect (e.g., bruises, fractures, burns, underweight, poor hygiene)
   b. Conflicting reports from caregivers and child on how injuries occurred
   c. Inappropriate delay in seeking treatment
   d. History inconsistent with the child's developmental level
   e. Absent or exaggerated parental response to injury
   f. Inappropriate response of the child to injury

4. Nursing diagnoses
   a. High Risk for Injury
   b. Powerlessness
   c. Altered Parenting
   d. Altered Family Processes

5. Planning and implementation
   a. Demonstrate acceptance of the child during physical assessment.
   b. Carefully assess the child's emotional status and behavior.
   c. Provide the child with positive attention and age-appropriate play activities.
   d. Document your assessment findings carefully and objectively.
   e. Collaborate with the multidisciplinary health care team concerning immediate and long-term therapies to help prevent further abuse.
   f. Work with caregivers on changing the situation that led to abuse.
   g. Report abuse to local authorities, following protocols.

6. Evaluation
   a. The child's physical injuries heal.
   b. The child's emotional injuries are healing in progress with therapy with an appropriate health care worker.
   c. The suspected child abuse victim is removed from the abusive environment.
   d. Appropriate interventions aimed at effecting behavioral changes in caregivers are in progress.

VI. Hospitalization of toddlers

A. Toddler's response to hospitalization

1. Common fears of hospitalized toddlers include:
   a. Separation from parents
   b. Loss of control
   c. Pain
2. Typical behaviors include:

      a.   Protest, despair, and detachment associated with separation from parents

      b.   Regression, negativism, temper tantrums, resistance to new caretakers and procedures, and physical and verbal aggressiveness

B.   **Parents' response to their toddler's hospitalization**

    1.   Parents typically experience anxiety and dread at leaving their child in the care of strangers.

    2.   They also may feel intense emotional stress as their child protests their leaving or expresses pain and fear associated with a procedure.

C.   **Nursing considerations**

    1.   Primary nurse: Become familiar with the child's rituals and routines, and encourage their continuance during hospitalization.

    2.   Encourage the parents' presence and participation, as appropriate.

    3.   Provide rooming-in accommodations for parents, as possible.

    4.   Provide parents with information about plans, and include in collaboration with implementation, as appropriate.

    5.   Teach parents not to sneak away from the child's bedside but to confront issues surrounding separation openly so as to convey respect for the child.

Bibliography

Lutz, W. J. (1986). Helping hospitalized children and their parents cope with painful procedures. *Journal of Pediatric Nursing, 1,* 24–32.

Mott, S. R., Fazekas, N. F., and James, S. R. (1985). *Nursing care of children and families: A holistic approach.* Menlo Park, CA: Addison-Wesley.

Triplett, J., and Arneson, S. (1979). The use of verbal and tactile comfort to alleviate distress in young hospitalized children. *Research in Nursing and Health, 2,* 17–23.

Weeks, H. (1980). Administering medications to children. *American Journal of Maternal/Child Nursing, 5,* 63–66.

Whaley, L. F., and Wong, D. L. (1991). *Nursing care of infants and children* (4th ed.). St. Louis: C. V. Mosby.

STUDY QUESTIONS

1. Why does a toddler typically experience temper tantrums?
   a. It is the only way the toddler can gain attention from his or her mother.
   b. More than likely, the toddler is spoiled and needs a spanking.
   c. The toddler cannot express his or her frustration verbally.
   d. The toddler is expressing his or her need for identity.

2. Appetite lags occur in toddlers for all the following reasons *except*
   a. a form of rebellion against parents
   b. physiologic anorexia
   c. preference for one type of food
   d. high activity level

3. Popcorn and nuts should not be given to a toddler primarily because they
   a. will spoil the child's appetite
   b. are easily aspirated
   c. have very little food value
   d. can cause tooth decay

4. In a toddler, regression occurs during periods of stress primarily because
   a. the child forgets the skills he or she has learned
   b. the child's parents may prefer less mature behaviors
   c. the child returns to a level of behavior that increases his or her sense of security during stressful events
   d. the child experiences growth promotion as he or she regresses, regroups, and then forges ahead

5. The primary purpose of a toddler's ritualistic behavior patterns is to
   a. manipulate and control adults in his or her environment
   b. establish learning behaviors
   c. provide a sense of security in an inconsistent world
   d. reestablish a sense of identity

6. Kevin and Patrick, both age 2½ years, are fighting over a toy truck. Which of the following interventions would be the most appropriate in this situation?
   a. Find another truck and tell them that they can each have one.
   b. Admonish them for fighting and tell them to share or you will put the truck away.
   c. Take the truck and place the boys in separate parts of the room, saying nothing.
   d. Explain that they must not fight and that there are enough toys to go around, and give Kevin a ball.

7. Which of the following characteristics are *not* typical of a toddler's language development between ages 1 and 2 years?
   a. comprehends more than he or she is able to express in words
   b. increases vocabulary from 4 to 300 words
   c. answers questions with multiword sentences
   d. progresses from holophrases (expressive words) like "up" to multiword sentences like "mama go byebye"

8. Toy selection for a toddler should take all the following principles into consideration *except*
   a. durability
   b. safety
   c. weight
   d. expense

9. Appropriate principles for disciplining a toddler include all the following *except*
   a. explanation
   b. admonishment
   c. distraction
   d. praise

10. Reasonable limits set by parents for toddlers are important because limits provide
    a. toddlers with a sense of security
    b. parents with a feeling that they are "right"
    c. clearly defined rules that toddlers understand and consistently follow
    d. parents with control over the toddler

11. A toddler's temperament affects discipline strategies. Which of the following disciplinary approaches likely would be the most effective for a "difficult" child?
    a. time for gradual introduction to new situations
    b. a stern voice and sustained eye contact
    c. a quick spanking with explanation for misbehavior
    d. a friendly warning to curtail activities with structured time out if necessary

12. Which of the following characteristics most closely describes a toddler's typical eating patterns?
    a. "food jags"
    b. preference for eating alone
    c. consistent table manners
    d. increased appetite

13. Analyzing a toddler's daily nutritional needs from the basic four food groups should include all the following information *except*
    a. 3 cups of milk or milk products
    b. two servings from the meat group— 2 tablespoons each serving
    c. four servings from the fruit and vegetable group—2 tablespoons each serving
    d. eight or more servings of breads and cereals—1 slice of bread or ¾ to 1 cup of cereal each serving

ANSWER KEY

1. **Correct response: c**
   When a child learns to express himself or herself in words, temper tantrums usually decrease in frequency.
   a. Toddlers use many methods to gain their parents' attention (e.g., touching, acting out).
   b. Spanking is not an appropriate intervention for temper tantrums; it only calls attention (negative) to the behavior. Generally, a better strategy is to ignore the tantrum.
   d. Identity is not yet important to the toddler; he or she needs to learn separation–individuation first.
   Comprehension/Psychosocial/Analysis (Dx)

2. **Correct response: a**
   Appetite lag is not a conscious rebellion; a toddler does not have cognitive desire.
   b. Growth rate slows, so the toddler is not hungry.
   c. Narrow food preferences do interfere with trying new foods.
   d. The toddler is too busy exploring the limits of his or her new autonomy to sit down to eat.
   Analysis/Physiologic/Assessment

3. **Correct response: b**
   These foods pose a risk of aspiration because the toddler cannot easily chew them.
   a. The safety issue is the overriding concern.
   c. Peanuts and popcorn both have good food value.
   d. These foods have a low sugar content and would not contribute to tooth decay.
   Application/Safe care/Implementation

4. **Correct response: c**
   Stress can trigger a return to a level of successful behaviors from earlier stages of development.
   a. Although the toddler's skills remain intact, a high stress level prevents their use.

   b. Parents rarely desire less-mature behavior.
   d. Growth promotion occurs when the child does *not* regress backward.
   Application/Psychosocial/Evaluation

5. **Correct response: c**
   Autonomy is possible when the toddler has familiar rituals (family, sleep, eating) to return to for security.
   a. A toddler's immature cognitive level does not allow him or her to manipulate others to this degree.
   b. No theory supports this statement.
   d. The child masters a sense of identity during adolescence.
   Application/Psychosocial/Evaluation

6. **Correct response: a**
   Children at age 2½ are too egocentric to share. Providing a truck for each would be the optimal intervention.
   b. The children are not yet capable of sharing; this ability begins during the preschool years.
   c. If the children receive no explanation, they will not have any idea what was wrong.
   d. Kevin is not interested in a ball, he is interested in a truck.
   Analysis/Safe care/Implementation

7. **Correct response: c**
   In response to a parent's questions, a 2-year-old frequently exhibits a blank stare or points.
   a. Comprehension may be evidenced by bringing a requested item to mother, but no words are spoken.
   b. A toddler's vocabulary is constantly expanding.
   d. "Up" can mean "pick me up" or "see the plane."
   Application/Psychosocial/Evaluation

8. **Correct response: d**
   Although expense may be an economic consideration for the family, it is not a criteria for safe, appropriate toy selection.

a. Toys must be durable to allow rough play.

b. Age appropriateness is an important safety factor.

c. Toys must be lightweight to help prevent injury but durable enough not to fall apart.

Analysis/Safe care/Planning

9. *Correct response: b*

Admonishment leads to a sense of doubt and shame because of the toddler's cognitive limits.

a. A brief explanation of the misbehavior benefits a toddler's learning.

c. Distraction often is effective in changing a toddler's direction.

d. Praise provides positive reinforcement for good behavior.

Comprehension/Safe care/Planning

10. *Correct response: a*

Unrestricted freedom is an overwhelming threat to a toddler's safety and security.

b. It is more important for the toddler to be safe than for the parents to be "right."

c. Although the rules may be few, the toddler still will test the limits of control.

d. The goal is to move the toddler toward rudimentary inner control in learning limits.

Comprehension/Safe care/Evaluation

11. *Correct response: d*

A "difficult" child is persistent, frequently has a high activity level, and needs structured time out.

a. A "slow-to-warm-up" child needs time to become comfortable in new situations.

b. An "easy" child who responds quickly to the authority figure will benefit from this approach.

c. Spanking conveys the message that violence is acceptable because an authority figure uses it.

Comprehension/Safe care/Planning

12. *Correct response: a*

A toddler's food jags express a preference for the ritualism of eating one type of food for several days and excluding others.

b. A toddler typically enjoys the socialization provided by the family meal and enjoys imitating others.

c. A toddler cannot be expected to have proper table manners.

d. A toddler's appetite generally is decreased because of a slow growth rate.

Application/Physiologic/Analysis (Dx)

13. *Correct response: d*

Four servings of breads and cereals daily is recommended; eight servings would provide excessive carbohydrates.

a. This is the correct amount to provide sufficient calcium and phosphorus but not too much to exclude solids.

b. 2 tablespoons is a reasonable amount of cut-up chicken, hot dog, tuna, egg, etc.

c. Fruits and vegetables offer a variety of finger foods; 1 tablespoon per year of age for a child.

Analysis/Physiologic/Analysis (Dx)

Preschool Growth and Development (Age 3 to 6 Years)

I.   Physical growth and development
A.   General characteristics
1.   A healthy preschooler is slender, graceful, and agile, with good posture.
2.   Major development occurs in fine motor coordination, as demonstrated by improved ability to draw.

3. Gross motor skills also improve; the child can hop, skip, and run more smoothly. Athletic abilities such as skating and swimming can be developed.

B. Height and weight changes
1. Normal height changes include:
   a. Growth of 2½ to 3 inches (6.5 to 7.8 cm) per year
   b. Average height of 37 inches (96.2 cm) at age 3, 40½ inches (103.7 cm) at age 4, and 43 inches (111.8 cm) at age 5
2. Normal weight changes include:
   a. Gain of 5 lb (2.3 kg) per year
   b. Average weight of 32 lb (14.5 kg) at age 3, 37 lb (16.8 kg) at age 4, and 41 lb (18.6 kg) at age 5

C. Psychomotor milestones
1. A preschooler demonstrates increased skill in balancing; by age 4 or 5, he or she can balance on alternate feet with eyes closed.
2. A preschooler alternates feet when climbing stairs, indicating increased balance and coordination.
3. A preschooler also can use scissors successfully and tie shoelaces.

II. Developmental theories
A. Psychosocial development (Erikson)
1. Between ages 3 and 6, a child faces a psychosocial crisis that Erikson terms *initiative vs. guilt*.
2. The child's significant other is the family.
3. The psychosocial theme is "To make, to make like, to play."
4. At this age, the child normally has mastered a sense of autonomy and moves on to master the task of initiative.
5. A preschooler is an energetic, enthusiastic, and intrusive learner with an active imagination.
6. Conscience (an inner voice that warns and threatens) begins to develop.
7. The child explores the physical world with all of his or her senses and powers.
8. Development of a sense of guilt occurs when the child is made to feel that his or her imagination and activities are unacceptable. Guilt, anxiety, and fear result when the child's thoughts and actions clash with parents' expectations.
9. A preschooler begins to use simple reasoning and can tolerate longer periods of delayed gratification.

B. Psychosexual development (Freud)
1. In the *phallic stage*, extending from about age 3 to 7, the child's pleasure centers on the genitalia and masturbation.
2. The *Oedipal stage* occurs, marked by jealousy and rivalry toward the same-sex parent and love of the opposite-sex parent.
3. The Oedipal stage typically resolves in the late preschool period with a strong identification with the same-sex parent.

      4. At this stage, the child's superego begins to develop, and conscience emerges.

C. **Cognitive development (Piaget)**
    1. This stage of *preconceptual thought* consists of two phases.
    2. In the *preconceptual phase*, extending from age 2 to 4, the child:
      a. Forms concepts that are not as complete or logical as an adult's
      b. Makes simple classifications
      c. Reasons from specific to specific
      d. Exhibits egocentric thinking
    3. In the *intuitive phase*, extending from age 4 to 7, the child:
      a. Becomes capable of classifying, quantifying, and relating objects but remains unaware of the principles behind these operations
      b. Exhibits intuitive thought processes (is aware that something is right but cannot state why); unable to see viewpoints of others
      c. Uses many words appropriately but without a real knowledge of their meaning

D. **Moral development (Kohlberg)**
    1. A preschooler is in the *preconventional phase* of moral development, which extends from age 4 to 10 years.
    2. In this phase, conscience emerges, and the emphasis is on external control.
    3. The child's moral standards are those of others, and he or she observes them to either avoid punishment or reap rewards.

III. **Social development**
  A. **Language**
    1. A preschooler's vocabulary typically increases to about 900 words by age 3 and 2100 words by age 5.
    2. A child this age may talk incessantly and ask many "why" questions.
    3. By age 3, a child usually talks in three- or four-word sentences.
  B. **Play**
    1. By preschool age, a child's play becomes more cooperative.
    2. The child understands the concept of sharing and is able to interact with peers.
    3. A preschooler needs regular socialization with agemates.
    4. This is the typical age of imaginary playmates.
    5. Play and activity suggestions include:
      a. A large space for running and jumping
      b. Dress-up clothes, paints, paper, and crayons for creative expression
      c. Field trips to museums and parks to expand the child's horizons

       d.   Swimming and other individual sports to aid gross motor development

       e.   A variety of puzzles and toys to aid fine motor development and stimulate imagination

C. **Socialization**

    1.   In the preschool years, a child's radius of significant others expands beyond parents to include grandparents, siblings, and preschool teachers.

    2.   The child needs regular interaction with agemates to help develop social skills.

IV. **Health promotion**

A. **Fears**

    1.   A child commonly experiences more fears during the preschool period than at any other time.

    2.   Common fears of preschoolers include:

       a.   The dark

       b.   Being left alone, especially at bedtime

       c.   Animals, particularly large dogs

       d.   Ghosts

       e.   Body mutilation

       f.   Pain; objects and people associated with painful experiences

    3.   The preschooler is prone to parent-induced fears stemming from his or her parents' remarks and actions; parents often are unaware that their behavior is instilling fear in their child.

    4.   Allowing the preschooler to have a night-light and encouraging him or her to play out fears with dolls or other toys may help give the child a sense of control over the fear.

    5.   Exposing the child to a feared object in a controlled setting can provide an opportunity for desensitization and reduction of fear.

B. **Temperament**

    1.   Characteristics observed in infancy and toddlerhood persist in the preschool period.

    2.   The child's temperament now must begin to adapt to group situations; observation provides an idea of how the child will adapt to a more structured school setting.

C. **Communication**

    1.   By age 3, a child typically can speak in short phrases; by age 4, in five- or six-word sentences; and by age 5, in longer sentences that contain all parts of speech.

    2.   By preschool age, a child's speech should be readily understood by others, including nurses and other health care providers. The child also can clearly understand what others are saying to him or her.

D. **Discipline**
1. Authority figures must apply discipline fairly, firmly, and consistently.
2. The child needs simple explanations of why certain behavior is not appropriate.
3. In a conflict situation, a short time out (e.g., 1 minute per year of age) can help the child relieve intensity, regain control, and think about his or her behavior.

E. **Dental health**
1. The preschooler's fine motor development enables him or her to use a toothbrush properly; the child should brush twice a day.
2. Parents should supervise the child's brushing and perform flossing.
3. The child should avoid cariogenic foods to help prevent dental caries.

F. **Nutrition and feeding**
1. A preschooler's daily caloric requirement is 85 kcal/kg, or about 1,700 kcal/day.
2. Daily fluid intake should average 100 mL/kg, depending on activity level.
3. Most 3- and 4-year-olds exhibit food "fads" and strong taste preferences. Emphasis should be placed on the quality rather than the quantity of foods eaten.
4. A 5-year-old tends to focus on the "social" aspects of eating: table conversation, manners, willingness to try new foods, and help with meal preparation and cleanup.

G. **Preschool program**
1. Preschool's primary purpose is to foster the child's social skills.
2. Criteria to consider when selecting a preschool program include:
    a. Accreditation; standards followed
    b. Daily schedule of activities
    c. Teachers' qualifications
    d. Environment: safety, noise level, teacher:child ratio, and sanitary practices
    e. Recommendations of other parents
    f. Observations of the children at play and work and their interactions with teachers

H. **Sex education**
1. Because preschoolers are keen observers but poor interpreters, the child may recognize but not understand sexual activity.
2. Before answering a child's questions about sex, clarify:
    a. What the child is really asking
    b. What the child already thinks about the specific subject
3. Answer questions simply and honestly, providing only the information the child requests; additional details can come later.

I. **Sleeping patterns**
1. On average, a preschooler needs about 12 hours of sleep each day.
2. In many children, sleeping problems that apparently were solved during toddlerhood now reappear, manifested as:
   a. Nightmares stemming from a vivid imagination
   b. Difficulty settling in after an active day
   c. Stretching bedtime rituals to delay going to sleep
3. Continuing reassuring bedtime rituals with relaxation time before bedtime should help a child settle in.
4. The daytime nap may be eliminated if it seems to interfere with nighttime sleep.
5. For many preschoolers, a security object and night-light continue to provide help with sleep.

J. **Bowel and bladder control**
1. By age 4, the child usually has daytime control but may experience bedwetting accidents at night and occasionally during the day resulting from a delay in getting to the bathroom.
2. By age 5, the child normally achieves both bowel and bladder control although accidents may occur in stressful situations.

K. **Immunization: The child should receive DTP and OPV boosters between ages 4 and 6 years, before starting school (see Table 2–1 in Chapter 2).**

L. **Injury prevention**
1. Although preschoolers are somewhat less accident prone than toddlers, they still are at risk for the same types of injuries and require many of the same safety precautions (see Chapter 3, section IV.K).
2. Parents and other caretakers should emphasize safety measures; preschoolers listen to adults and can understand and heed precautions.
3. Because preschoolers are keen observers and imitate adults, parents and other caretakers need to ''practice what they preach'' regarding safety.
4. When a child reaches 40 lb and 40 inches tall, a seat belt can safely replace a child car seat.

V. **Selected health problems of preschoolers**
A. **Tonsillitis**
1. Description: inflamed, infected tonsils
2. Etiology and pathophysiology
   a. Tonsils and adenoids consist of lymphoid tissue.
   b. In young children, tonsils commonly are enlarged; they diminish in size with aging.
   c. Enlarged tonsils are vulnerable to viral or bacterial infection.
   d. Nonbacterial exudative tonsillitis is a mild disorder charac-

      terized by gradual onset, low-grade fever, mild headache, sore throat, hoarseness, and productive cough.

  e. Bacterial tonsillitis, most often caused by beta-hemolytic streptococcal infection, is a more dramatic disorder marked by rapid onset of high fever, headache, generalized muscle aches, and vomiting.

  f. Sequelae of bacterial tonsillitis may include skin rash and extension of infection to include peritonsillar abscess, middle ear infection, and involvement of the mastoids or meninges. Late sequelae may include rheumatic fever and acute glomerulonephritis.

  g. Marked tonsil and adenoid enlargement may occlude the airway, requiring surgical removal.

  h. Removal of the tonsils, adenoids, or both is indicated in chronic enlargement that interferes with swallowing or breathing, or in recurrent group A beta-hemolytic streptococcal infections, otitis media, peritonsillar abscess, or retropharyngeal abscess.

3. Assessment findings

  a. Difficulty eating and breathing because of tonsil enlargement

  b. Frequent sore throats and ear infections

  c. History of allergic disorders

4. Nursing diagnoses (preoperative and postoperative)

  a. High Risk for Fluid Volume Deficit

  b. High Risk for Injury

  c. Knowledge Deficit

  d. Pain

5. Planning and implementation (preoperative)

  a. Prepare the child for hospitalization and surgery (see section VII.C).

  b. Explain to the child and parents that the child will have a sore throat after surgery but will be able to talk and swallow.

  c. Explain postoperative care measures (e.g., proper positioning, ingestion of cool liquids, use of an ice collar).

6. Planning and implementation (postoperative)

  a. Observe for and report unusual bleeding.

  b. Intervene for bleeding as appropriate.

  c. Monitor vital signs.

  d. Assess skin color.

  e. Observe for frequent swallowing and restlessness.

  f. Help prevent bleeding by avoiding gargling and discouraging the child from coughing.

  g. Position the child on the side or abdomen to facilitate drainage from the throat.

  h. Teach the child and parents activity restrictions, including when the child can return to school, the need to avoid persons with infections, the importance of a soft diet with adequate fluid intake, and the need to avoid acidic foods and other foods and liquids that can irritate the throat.

    7.   Evaluation

        a.   Vital signs are within normal limits (based on the child's baseline and age-appropriate values).

        b.   The child does not exhibit restlessness or frequent swallowing.

        c.   No signs of bleeding are evident.

B.   **Chickenpox (varicella)**

    1.   Description: an acute, highly contagious viral infection common in childhood

    2.   Etiology and pathophysiology

        a.   The varicella zoster virus is transmitted though respiratory secretions and lesions in the vesicle stage.

        b.   The communicable period extends from 1 day before lesions erupt to 6 days after the first crop of vesicles appear, when crusts have formed.

    3.   Assessment findings

        a.   Slight fever

        b.   Skin rash mainly on the trunk and face, progressing from macules to pustules to vesicles to crusting with pruritus

    4.   Nursing diagnoses

        a.   High Risk for Infection

        b.   Pain

        c.   High Risk for Impaired Skin Integrity

    5.   Planning and implementation

        a.   Collaborate with parents to keep the child isolated for 7 to 10 days until crusts have formed.

        b.   Provide skin care: Bathe and change clothes daily; remove crusts; apply calamine lotion; keep fingernails short; encourage the child to avoid scratching; place clean socks on the child's hands at night to prevent scratching.

        c.   Avoid administering aspirin for fever because of the risk of Reye's syndrome sequelae.

        d.   Keep the child occupied with activities to distract him or her from scratching.

    6.   Evaluation

        a.   Lesions remain free of infection and subsequent scarring does not occur.

        b.   Isolating the child prevents spread to high-risk persons.

VI.   **Hospitalization of preschoolers**

   A.   **Child's response to hospitalization**

      1.   Typical fears of hospitalized preschoolers include:

        a.   Separation

        b.   Loss of control

        c.   Bodily injury and pain from intrusive procedures, mutilation, and castration

   2.   Common behaviors include:

        a.   Protest, despair, and detachment related to separation (similar to that of a toddler but less intense)

        b.   Aggression (physical and verbal)

        c.   Regression to earlier behaviors, marked by dependency; withdrawal; feelings of fear, anxiety, guilt, shame; physiologic responses; immature behavior

   3.   The preschooler's ability to understand the reason for hospitalization and details of the hospital experience is limited by egocentricity and magical thinking.

B.   **Parents' response to their child's hospitalization**

   1.   The response of parents of preschoolers requiring hospitalization may be affected by various factors, including:

        a.   Seriousness of the child's condition

        b.   Experience with illness or hospitalization

        c.   The diagnostic procedures and treatments their child is undergoing

        d.   Available support systems

        e.   Personal ego strengths

        f.   Previous coping abilities

        g.   Additional stressors on the family system

        h.   Cultural and religious beliefs

        i.   Communication patterns among family members

   2.   Parents of a seriously ill child commonly progress through the following phases:

        a.   Disbelief, usually accompanied by denial

        b.   Anger, guilt, or both

        c.   Fear, anxiety, and frustration

        d.   Some degree of depression after the acute stage passes

C.   **Nursing considerations**

   1.   Provide primary nursing care, if possible.

   2.   Provide time for therapeutic play.

   3.   Keep in mind that a preschooler is unaware of invisible physical or mechanical forces that make things operate and has a vivid imagination that can give rise to many fears; allow time for expressing fears and clarifying misunderstandings.

   4.   Also remember that the child is most interested in how a procedure will feel ("Will it hurt?"); to minimize fears, use words like "fix" rather than "take out" or "remove."

   5.   Provide visual, tactile, auditory, and motor images when preparing a preschooler for a procedure; specific suggestions include:

     a.   Using puppets, dolls, and teddy bears to demonstrate procedures

     b.   Allowing the child to handle equipment before the procedure

     c.   Explaining unusual sights, smells, and sounds

6.   Provide the child with simple explanations just before the procedure; the level of detail depends on the child's coping needs and need to gain mastery over the situation.

7.   Allow the presence of parents and security objects, when possible, to provide comfort.

Bibliography

Hansen, B., and Evans, M. (1981). Preparing a child for procedures. *American Journal of Maternal/Child Nursing, 6,* 392–397.

Mott, S. R., Fazekas, N. F., and James, S. R. (1985). *Nursing care of children and families: A holistic approach.* Menlo Park, CA: Addison-Wesley.

Pidgeon, V. (1981). Function of preschool children's questions in coping with hospitalization. *Research in Nursing and Health, 4,* 229–235.

Pontious, S. (1982). Practical Piaget: Helping children understand. *American Journal of Maternal/Child Nursing, 7,* 114–117.

Whaley, L. F., and Wong, D. L. (1991). *Nursing care of infants and children* (4th ed.). St. Louis: C. V. Mosby.

STUDY QUESTIONS

1. Piaget describes the main characteristic of the 2- to 7-year-old child's intellectual development as egocentric. This means
   a. selfishness
   b. inability to see another's point of view
   c. self-centeredness
   d. preferring to play and assume responsibilities by oneself

2. At age 3½, Susie is ready to begin an experience in a preschool setting. When choosing a preschool program, her mother considered the environmental features of several programs. Which of the following is the *most* important environmental aspect of a preschool setting?
   a. height of the sinks for handwashing
   b. educational and experiential qualifications of the teachers
   c. number of agemates with different cultural backgrounds
   d. daily schedule of work and play activities

3. The major psychomotor advances for the child aged 3 to 6 include all the following *except*
   a. swimming
   b. drawing recognizable figures
   c. hopping on one foot
   d. playing baseball

4. In a preschooler's mind, parents typically are viewed as
   a. a necessary evil
   b. persons that keep order
   c. omnipotent
   d. too rigid

5. Which of the following is the most accurate description of cognitive development in Wendy, aged 5?
   a. thinks abstractly
   b. has magical thinking
   c. comprehends conservation of matter
   d. sees more than one dimension of an object

6. Patrick, aged 4, resists going to bed at night. Which of the following suggestions should the nurse offer Patrick's parents?
   a. Allow him to go to sleep in your room, then move him to his own bed.
   b. Tell him that you will lock him in his room if he gets up one more time.
   c. Provide for active play before bedtime so that he'll be tired and fall asleep easily.
   d. Read him a story and allow him to play quietly in his bed until he falls asleep.

7. Patrick's 5-year-old brother, Eric, believes that there are "bogeymen and monsters" in his bedroom at night. What advice can the nurse give to Eric's parents to help Eric cope with his fears?
   a. Let Eric sleep with his parents.
   b. Tell Eric that bogeymen and monsters do not exist.
   c. Keep a night-light on in Eric's room.
   d. Tell Eric that no one else sees any monsters, so he must not see them either.

8. Richard, aged 3, is resisting eating lunch. Which of the following strategies might the nurse find helpful in encouraging Richard to eat?
   a. Use colorful, child-size plates and cups.
   b. Let Richard feed himself.
   c. Have Richard sit at an appropriate-sized table for his height.
   d. Serve small portions of cut-up food.

9. A preschooler's nutritional needs change from those of toddlerhood. Which of the following statements most accurately reflects preschool age nutritional requirements?
   a. Caloric requirements per kilogram of body weight increase slightly during this period.
   b. Nutritional requirements are very different from those of the toddler.

c. The quality of the food consumed by the preschooler is much more important than the quantity.

d. Protein should account for 25% of the child's total daily caloric intake.

10. The most common initial reaction of parents to an illness in their child is
    a. anger or guilt
    b. fear and anxiety
    c. depression and fear
    d. denial and disbelief

11. Daniel, aged 5, has begun to use "swear words." His mother is concerned about how to stop this behavior. Which of the following suggestions by the nurse likely would be the most helpful?
    a. Ignore the behavior; he will soon outgrow it.
    b. Try to instill a sense of guilt about this unacceptable behavior.
    c. Inform Daniel that swearing is not acceptable and that if he continues to do so he will be disciplined.

d. Point out that good boys and girls do not use swear words.

12. The family's culture, ethnic origin, and value system do *not* directly influence the 4-year-old child's ability to
    a. learn table manners
    b. ride a bicycle or throw a ball
    c. master the tasks of toilet training
    d. participate in household chores

13. A child can be safely restrained in regular seat belts when he or she reaches
    a. 35 lb or age 3 years
    b. 30 lb or 30 inches tall
    c. 40 lb or 40 inches tall
    d. 60 lb or age 6 years

14. By the end of the preschool period, a 6-year-old usually has mastered the developmental task of
    a. identity
    b. industry
    c. initiative
    d. autonomy

ANSWER KEY

1. Correct response: b
The preschool child tends to believe that everything is just the way he or she sees it and that there is no other way.
  a and c. A preschooler usually is willing to share and take turns.
  d. A preschooler usually enjoys socializing in cooperative play with others.
Knowledge/Psychosocial/Assessment

2. Correct response: b
The teaching staff's theoretical and practice background and approach to the children is the most important factor influencing a child's learning experience.
  a. Good sanitation practices for the children and staff facilitate infection prevention.
  c. Early interaction with children of various cultures is enriching.
  d. A schedule of varied activities enhances learning.
Comprehension/Safe care/Analysis (Dx)

3. Correct response: d
Baseball requires coordinated skills and stamina that preschool children have not yet developed.
  a. Swimming is an excellent activity for the preschool child.
  b. As fine motor coordination improves, scribbles become recognizable objects.
  c. Hopping on one foot demonstrates coordination, interest, and gross motor ability.
Application/Physiologic/Implementation

4. Correct response: c
The preschooler typically believes that his or her parents can do no wrong and enjoys their guidance.
  a. This more accurately describes the typical view of an adolescent.
  b. The preschooler usually has not yet developed this view of his or her parents.
  d. A preschooler is not bothered by rigidity and guidelines; rather, such

discipline provides a needed sense of security.
Analysis/Health promotion/Evaluation

5. Correct response: b
Magical thinking is part of the intuitive phase of cognitive development, in which the child believes that he or she can make things happen the way he or she wishes.
  a. Abstract thinking in formal operations typically develops after age 11.
  c and d. Both conservation and centering occur during concrete operations in development between ages 7 and 11.
Application/Psychosocial/Assessment

6. Correct response: d
Quiet play and time with parents is a positive bedtime routine that provides security and readies the child for sleep.
  a. The child should sleep in his or her own bed.
  b. The child will likely test this threat; locking the door is frightening and promotes insecurity.
  c. Active play stirs up the child, increasing the time it takes to settle down to sleep.
Application/Safe care/Implementation

7. Correct response: c
A night-light helps decrease "spooky" shadows in the room.
  a. Sleeping with parents is not an optimal solution; it will impede the child's developing sense of independence.
  b and d. Denying that "bogeymen and monsters" exist does not acknowledge the child's fear of what he or she imagines.
Analysis/Psychosocial/Implementation

8. Correct response: b
Autonomy is important to the 3-year-old and should be encouraged; this is an area over which the child can gain mastery and control at an age when other

tasks are not yet under his or her control.

a, c, and d. These aspects are all important but less so than encouraging autonomy.

Analysis/Health promotion/Analysis (Dx)

9. Correct response: c

The quality rather than quantity of foods consumed is most important; high caloric intake may consist of mainly "empty" calories.

a. A preschooler's daily caloric requirements decrease slightly from a toddler's, to 85 kcal/kg.

b. A preschooler's nutritional requirements are similar to a toddler's.

d. A preschooler's daily protein requirement is 1.5 g/kg, optimally satisfied by two meat servings, three milk servings, and four bread and fruit and vegetable servings.

Analysis/Physiologic/Planning

10. Correct response: d

Initially, parents usually respond with disbelief that this could be happening to their child. Denial often gives parents time to develop coping strategies.

a, b, and c. Parents may experience any or all of these subsequent responses, depending on their coping mechanisms and their child's condition. A common sequence of responses following disbelief and denial is anger, fear, and anxiety, and some degree of depression.

Comprehension/Health promotion/Evaluation

11. Correct response: c

By explaining their objections and expectations, Daniel's parents will teach him why the behavior is unacceptable and help him understand that he must stop it.

a. Ignoring the behavior will not help Daniel learn why it is unacceptable and that it must cease.

b. Harsh warnings will not teach Daniel about the inappropriateness of his behavior.

d. This strategy will only give Daniel the impression that he is "bad" and will adversely affect his self-esteem while doing little to change his behavior.

Application/Health promotion/Implementation

12. Correct response: b

The ability to ride a bicycle is developmentally, not culturally, determined.

a, c, and d. All these are influenced by family value systems, in terms of how frameworks for these areas are patterned in these identity-building years of the child.

Application/Physiologic/Evaluation

13. Correct response: c

A child of this weight and height has sufficiently developed bone structure and muscle mass to use regular restraints.

a. A child of this size is too small to use seat belts safely.

b. A child of this size also is too small to use seat belts safely.

d. Although a child of this size can use seat belts safely, use of a car seat can be discontinued much earlier.

Knowledge/Safe care/Planning

14. Correct response: c

Initiative is a normal developmental milestone for a preschool child.

a. Identity is a developmental task of an adolescent.

b. Industry is a developmental task of a school-age child.

d. Autonomy is a developmental task of a toddler.

Knowledge/Psychosocial/Evaluation

School-Age Growth
and Development
(Age 6 to 12 Years)

I.   Physical growth and development
A.   General characteristics
   1.   During this period, girls often grow faster than boys and commonly surpass them in height and weight.

2. During preadolescence, extending from about age 10 to 13, a child commonly experiences rapid and uneven growth as compared to agemates.
3. The preschool period normally is a time of good health; the child leaves the preschool period of increased susceptibility to communicable disease and has yet to enter the period of susceptibility to adult disease, which begins with adolescence.

B. **Height and weight changes**
1. Normal height changes include:
   a. Growth of about 2 inches (5.2 cm) per year between ages 6 and 12.
   b. Average height of 45 inches (115.2 cm) at age 6 and 59 inches (151 cm) at age 12.
2. Normal weight changes include:
   a. Weight gain of $4\frac{1}{2}$ to $6\frac{1}{2}$ lb (2 to 2.9 kg) per year between ages 6 and 12
   b. Average weight of 46 lb (20.9 kg) at age 6 and 88 lb (40 kg) at age 12

C. **Psychomotor milestones**
1. This period encompasses a wide range of achievements; obviously, a 6-year-old and a 12-year-old have very different capabilities.
2. The child continues to refine his or her fine motor skills, as demonstrated by mastery of printing, then cursive writing.
3. Gross motor skills continue to develop, and strength and endurance increase profoundly, enabling participation in team sports.

II. **Developmental theories**
A. **Psychosocial development (Erikson)**
1. Erikson terms the psychosocial crisis faced by a child aged 6 to 12 *industry vs. inferiority.*
2. During this period, the child's radius of significant others expands to include school and instructive adults.
3. This period's psychosocial theme is "To make think; to make together; to make complete."
4. A school-age child normally has mastered the first three developmental tasks—trust, autonomy, and initiative—and now focuses on mastering industry.
5. A child's sense of industry grows out of a desire for real achievement.
6. The child engages in tasks and activities that he or she can carry through to completion.
7. The child learns rules and how to compete with others and to cooperate to achieve goals.
8. Social relationships with others become increasingly important sources of support.

9. The child can develop a sense of inferiority stemming from unrealistic expectations or a sense of failing to meet standards set for him or her by others. Because the child feels inadequate, his or her self-esteem sags.

B. **Psychosexual development (Freud)**

1. The *latency period*, extending from about age 5 through 12, represents a stage of relative sexual indifference before puberty and adolescence.
2. During this period, development of self-esteem is closely linked with a developing sense of industry in gaining a concept of one's value and worth.

C. **Cognitive development (Piaget)**

1. A child aged 7 to 11 is in the stage of *concrete operations*, marked by inductive reasoning, logical operations, and reversible concrete thought.
2. Specific characteristics of this stage include:
    a. Movement from egocentric to objective thinking—seeing others' points of view, seeking validation, and asking questions
    b. Focus on immediate physical reality with inability to transcend the here-and-now
    c. Difficulty dealing with remote, future, or hypothetical matters
    d. Development of various mental classifying and ordering activities
    e. Development of the *principle of conservation*—of volume, weight, mass, and numbers
3. Typical activities of a child in this stage may include:
    a. Collecting and sorting objects (e.g., baseball cards, dolls, marbles)
    b. Ordering items according to size, shape, weight, and other criteria
    c. Considering options and variables when problem solving

D. **Moral development (Kohlberg)**

1. A child at the conventional level of the *role conformity* stage (generally, from age 10 to 13) has an increased desire to please others.
2. The child observes and to some extent internalizes the standards of others.
3. The child wants to be considered "good" by those persons whose opinions matter to him or her.

III. **Social development**

A. **Play**

1. Play becomes more competitive and complex during the school-age period.
2. Characteristic activities include team sports, secret clubs, "gang"

activities, scouting or other organizations, complex puzzles, collections, quiet board games, reading, and hero worship.

3. Rules and rituals are important aspects of play and games.

B. **Socialization**

1. The school-age years are a period of dynamic change and maturation as the child becomes increasingly involved in more complex activities, decision making, and goal-directed activities.

2. As a school-age child becomes more knowledgeable about his or her body, social development centers on the body and its capabilities.

3. Peer relationships gain new importance.

4. Group activities, including team sports, typically consume much time and energy.

C. **School adjustment**

1. School serves as a formal agent for transmitting societal values to each generation; it is second in importance only to the family as a socializing agent and has a lasting influence on a child's social development.

2. Adapting to school routine, peers, and new authority figures requires much energy.

3. Most children adjust to this new structure with little difficulty.

4. The readiness of the child and parents for separation is an important factor in the adaptation process.

5. In many families both parents work outside the home, and the child is at home alone after school; these "latchkey children" need guidance for safety precautions, productive activities, and telephone use.

IV. Health promotion

A. **Fears**

1. During the school-age years, many fears of earlier childhood resolve or decrease.

2. Common fears may include:
   a. Failure at school
   b. Bullies
   c. Intimidating teachers

3. Parents and other caregivers can help reduce a child's fears by communicating empathy and concern without being overprotective.

B. **Temperament**

1. A child that is slow to warm up needs more time to prepare for events.

2. Parents and teachers should assess the child's temperament and tailor school and responsibility expectations accordingly.

C. **Communication**

1. A school-age child should be given sufficient time before an event

or procedure and allowed to ask questions to validate information.
2. Specific strategies for communicating with school-age children include:
    a. Begin by explaining the details of a procedure or event, then provide a simple rationale for why it is necessary.
    b. Focus on visible realities of the illness or problem.
    c. Use diagrams, models, and other media to make descriptions and explanations more concrete.
    d. Involve the child in procedures as appropriate (e.g., holding equipment, opening packages, monitoring laboratory test results).

D. Discipline
1. School-age children begin to internalize their own controls and need less outside direction.
2. The child does, however, need a parent or other caretaker to answer questions and provide guidance for decisions and responsibilities.
3. Regular household responsibilities help the child feel an important part of the family and increase his or her sense of accomplishment.
4. A weekly allowance, set in accordance with the child's age, needs, and duties, assists in teaching skills, values, and a sense of responsibility.
5. When disciplining a school-age child, parents and other caretakers should set reasonable, concrete limits (and provide plausible explanations) and keep rules to a minimum.

E. Nutrition and feeding
1. A school-age child's daily caloric requirements average 85 kcal.
2. Caregivers should continue to stress the need for a balanced diet from the basic four food groups; resources are being stored for the increased growth needs of adolescence.
3. The child is exposed to broader eating experiences in the school lunchroom; he or she may still be a "picky" eater but should be more willing to try new foods.
4. At home, the child should eat what the family eats; the patterns developed now stay with the child into adulthood.

F. Dental health
1. Beginning around age 6, permanent teeth erupt, and deciduous teeth are gradually lost.
2. Regular dentist visits are important.
3. The child should brush at least twice each day; because of the child's better coordination, parental supervision and assistance usually are not necessary.

G. Sleeping patterns
1. School-age children's individual sleep requirements vary but typically range from 10 to 12 hours a night. Because growth rate has

slowed, the child actually needs less sleep now than he or she will during adolescence.

2. The child's bedtime can be later than during the preschool years but should be firmly established and adhered to on school nights.

3. Reading before bedtime may facilitate sleep and set up a positive bedtime pattern.

H. **Bowel and bladder control**

1. In most cases, a school-age child has gained control over elimination, unless the child has a congenital or acquired problem.

2. The child normally manages elimination without any assistance.

3. Enuresis (urine incontinence with no organic basis after age 4) and encopresis (fecal incontinence after age 4) are rare but major stressors for the child and family.

4. Failure to resolve such a problem interferes with developmental tasks and can lead to feelings of inadequacy and low self-esteem.

I. **Exercise**

1. Regular exercise is important for musculoskeletal development and refinement.

2. The child needs adequate space and proper equipment for enjoyable exercise.

J. **Sex education**

1. A school-age child has acquired much of his or her knowledge of, and many of his or her attitudes toward, sex indirectly at a very early age.

2. During the school-age years, the child refines this knowledge and these attitudes.

3. Questions about sex require honest answers based on the child's level of understanding.

K. **Injury prevention**

1. A school-age child learns to accept more responsibility for personal health care and injury prevention.

2. School-age children who learn safe swimming and diving practices, fire safety, use of seat belts in motor vehicles, and other safety practices are at reduced risk for injury.

3. The child's developing cognitive skills aid in good judgment to avoid many types of injuries.

4. School-age children are still prone to accidents, however, mainly due to increasing motor abilities and independence (e.g., a bicycle can take the child farther from home on his or her own).

5. Major sources of injury include bicycles, skateboards, and team sports. Learning proper techniques, using safe equipment, and, in the case of organized sports, receiving good coaching and playing with children of similar size can help reduce the risk of injury.

6. Parents should continue to provide guidance for new situations and threats to safety.

7. The child should receive education about the use and abuse of alcohol, tobacco, and other drugs.

V. Selected health problems of school-age children

A. School phobia

1. Description: an abnormal, persistent fear of attending school
2. Etiology: related to a dreaded school situation, fear of leaving home, or separation anxiety
3. Assessment findings
   a. Common physiologic manifestations include nausea, vomiting, headache, and stomachache.
   b. These symptoms tend to resolve when the child is allowed to stay home from school.
4. Nursing diagnosis: Fear
5. Planning and implementation
   a. Collaborate with the child's parents, teacher, and school counselor to determine the cause of the problem and identify possible solutions.
   b. Discuss the problem and possible causes and solutions with the child.
   c. Implement plans to return the child to school. (The child should attend school even while the problem is being resolved; keeping him or her out only reinforces feelings of worthlessness, dependency, and inability to cope.)
6. Evaluation
   a. The child attends school regularly.
   b. The child freely discusses any problems with parents, teacher, or school counselor.
   c. The child experiences no related physiologic symptoms.

B. Enuresis

1. Description: repeated, involuntary urination, usually at night, in a child beyond the normal age of gaining bladder control in the absence of an organic or a psychologic cause
2. Etiology
   a. Enuresis may have a familial component; often, a child with enuresis has siblings or a parent who experienced the problem.
   b. A smaller-than-normal functional bladder capacity may be a contributing factor in some cases.
   c. Regardless of the cause, resulting feelings of guilt and shame may contribute to perpetuating the problem.
   d. Incidence approaches 40% of children at age 3, 22% at age 5, 10% at age 10, and 1% to 2% at age 20.
   e. Incidence is greater in boys than in girls.
3. Assessment findings
   a. Common clinical manifestations include nocturnal bed-

wetting, urinary urgency, dysuria, restlessness, and urinary frequency.

    b.   An in-depth physical and psychological evaluation is indicated to rule out physiologic and psychological causes.

  4. Nursing diagnosis: Altered Patterns of Urinary Elimination

  5. Planning and implementation

    a.   Collaborate with the physician, parents, and child to identify causes of the problem and devise strategies to overcome it.

    b.   Set up a feasible therapeutic plan, which may include conditioning devices (e.g., a urine alarm apparatus), drug therapy (e.g., imipramine), bladder training, nighttime fluid and food restrictions, or interrupting the child's sleep for voiding in the bathroom.

    c.   Emphasize the need for patience in overcoming the problem.

    d.   Strive to and encourage parents and other caretakers to make the child feel accepted and to avoid blaming or other attitudes that can foster feelings of worthlessness and hopelessness.

  6. Evaluation

    a.   Enuretic episodes become more infrequent.

    b.   Any related family difficulties are resolved.

    c.   Enuresis ceases.

C. **Appendicitis**

  1. Description: acutely inflamed vermiform appendix

  2. Etiology: commonly results from obstruction of the appendix lumen by a fecalith or from lymphoid hyperplasia

  3. Pathophysiology

    a.   Obstruction leads to compression of blood vessels and subsequent tissue ischemia.

    b.   Ischemia is followed by disruption of the epithelial lining with bacterial invasion.

    c.   Epithelial disruption may progress to perforation and contamination of the peritoneal cavity with fecal matter and bacteria.

  4. Assessment findings

    a.   Typical clinical manifestations include abdominal tenderness in the right lower quadrant, positive McBurney's sign, abdominal rigidity, fever, and vomiting.

    b.   Laboratory tests reveal a mildly elevated WBC count ($>15,000$ cells/mm^3 [μL]), usually with polymorphonuclear leukocytosis; grossly elevated WBC count suggests acute infection or another cause of symptoms.

  5. Nursing diagnoses (preoperative)

    a.   High Risk for Infection

       b.   Altered Comfort: Pain
6. Nursing diagnoses (postoperative)
       a.   Anxiety
       b.   High Risk for Infection
       c.   High Risk for Fluid Volume Deficit
       d.   Altered Nutrition: Less than Body Requirements
       e.   Altered Comfort: Pain
       f.   Knowledge Deficit
       g.   Altered Family Processes
7. Planning and implementation (preoperative)
       a.   Prepare the child for appendectomy.
       b.   Keep the child NPO before surgery; prevent dehydration by administering IV fluids, as ordered.
       c.   Prevent or control fever.
       d.   Assess bowel activity by evaluating for abdominal distention, auscultating bowel sounds, and observing elimination patterns.
       e.   Place the child in low Fowler's position to help localize and prevent the spread of any infection.
       f.   Apply cold packs to the child's abdomen to help relieve discomfort; avoid applying heat and administering laxatives.
8. Planning and implementation (postoperative)
       a.   Monitor vital signs, assess for abdominal distention, and inspect the surgical wound for signs of infection.
       b.   Institute isolation precautions if the wound becomes infected.
       c.   Have the child ambulate within 6 to 8 hours after surgery, if not contraindicated; help the child turn, cough, and deep breathe postoperatively.
       d.   Monitor intake and output; ensure that spontaneous voiding occurs.
       e.   Assess for pain, and administer analgesics as appropriate.
9. Evaluation
       a.   The child is free of infection and fever.
       b.   The surgical wound heals without complications.
       c.   The child ambulates by the first postoperative day.

VI. Hospitalization of school-age children
A. Child's response to hospitalization
1. Common fears include:
       a.   Disability and possibly death
       b.   Unknown events and procedures
       c.   Loss of control and independence
       d.   Interruption of daily routine, separation from peers, inability to participate in usual activities

> 2. A school-age child's reaction to hospitalization depends in large part on his or her experiences and coping abilities.

B. Parents' response to their child's hospitalization

1. Parents exhibit a wide range of responses, including guilt, fear, and uncertainty; their experience with hospitalization contributes to their reaction.
2. Parents need to provide emotional support and reassurance to their child undergoing hospitalization.

C. Nursing considerations

1. Arrange for an age-compatible roommate, if possible.
2. Help the child understand hospital routines and the need for specific procedures.
3. Provide concrete explanations of procedures.
4. Involve the child in his or her own care whenever possible.
5. Provide privacy.
6. Arrange for play and school activities, as appropriate.

Bibliography

Mott, S. R., James, S. R., and Sperhac, A. M. (1990). *Nursing care of children and families* (2nd ed.). Menlo Park, CA: Addison-Wesley.

Pidgeon, V. (1985). Children's concepts of illness: Implications for health teaching. *Maternal-Child Nursing Journal, 14*, 23–35.

Pontious, S. (1982). Practical Piaget: Helping children understand. *American Journal of Maternal/Child Nursing, 7*, 114–117.

Tesler, M., and Savedra, M. (1981). Coping with hospitalization: A study of school-aged children. *Pediatric Nursing, 7*, 35–38.

Whaley, L. F., and Wong, D. L. (1991). *Nursing care of infants and children* (4th ed.). St. Louis: C. V. Mosby.

STUDY QUESTIONS

1. Which of the following best describes typical annual growth during the school-age years?
   a. The child grows an average of 2 inches (5.2 cm) per year.
   b. The child gains an average of 3 pounds (1.4 kg) per year.
   c. Few physical differences are noticeable between agemates throughout this period.
   d. Fat pads increase in number and add to the normal "chubby" appearance of the child.

2. Which of the following statements best describes a child's cognitive ability during Piaget's *concrete operations* stage?
   a. Behavior changes from reflexive to purposeful.
   b. The child is unable to put himself or herself in the place of another.
   c. Thought processes become more systematic and logical.
   d. Abstract thinking and logical conclusions are made more frequently.

3. The peer group is an important socializing medium for the school-age child. What is the major function of the peer group?
   a. helps the child view rules at home as "necessary evils"
   b. provides a forum for conflict resolution
   c. permits bragging and other "ego" needs in front of a "safe" audience
   d. allows the child to learn "bad" behaviors, such as dominance and hostility

4. A bicycle is a common form of transportation for a school-age child. All the following points are important to include when teaching bicycle safety *except*
   a. feet should not touch the ground when seated
   b. wear a safety helmet while riding
   c. ride during daytime hours only
   d. know and follow traffic rules

5. The nurse can provide anticipatory guidance to parents with regard to preventing sports injuries. Which of the following statements is accurate?
   a. Age, not body size, should determine how teams are formed.
   b. Scoring, ranking, and championships often are negative concepts for young children.
   c. A child should not participate in contact sports until adolescence.
   d. Physical mismatches increase the risk of sports injuries.

6. In Piaget's theory of cognitive development, an *operation* is
   a. a mental action that can be reversed
   b. the same as a scheme
   c. a change of intellectual organization to accept new information
   d. the temporary balance of perceptions and experiences that are comfortably organized in the thinking process

7. The moral development of school-age children, as described by Kohlberg, is reflected in all the following statements except one. Which one?
   a. School-age children believe that rules are established by others.
   b. School-age children learn the standards for acceptable behavior, act according to these standards, and feel guilty when they violate these standards.
   c. School-age children judge an act by the intentions that prompted it rather than just by its consequences.
   d. School-age children are likely to interpret accidents and misfortunes as punishment for misdeeds.

8. If a school-age child tells a lie, the best response of the parent or nurse would be to
   a. ignore the behavior
   b. express casual skepticism about the child's statement
   c. demand that the child admit to telling the lie

d. become angry

9. When Owen, age 6, plays a game with his younger brother, he follows the rules strictly. However, if Owen is losing, he may change the rules to his advantage. What developmental concept explains this behavior?
   a. Owen lacks a sense of responsibility for his actions.
   b. Owen has a strong need to win, even if it harms his younger brother.
   c. Owen perceives the rules as flexible standards rather than fixed absolutes.
   d. Owen does not have the ability to develop a personal moral code.

10. Patterns of nutrition established during the school-age years usually persist into adulthood. Which of the following statements associated with a child's eating habits is accurate?
    a. A school-age child should develop impeccable table manners.
    b. A school-age child's food preferences tend to reflect the family's cultural background.
    c. A rigid environment at mealtime, with quiet and strict discipline, is best.
    d. High-energy activities demand high-caloric snacks.

11. Sandy, age 6, is beginning first grade in September. Which of the following descriptions of a 6-year-old child's developing sense of self is most accurate?
    a. dependent on her mother
    b. sensitive to criticism
    c. rebellious to a schedule
    d. boastful and a "tattle-tale"

12. Nursing interventions for health promotion during the school-age years should include

a. stressing increased caloric intake to meet increased metabolic demands
b. instructing parents to obtain orthodontic care for straightening the child's permanent teeth
c. instructing parents to defer answering questions about sex until adolescence
d. advising parents that toward the end of this period, the child will require increasing amounts of rest

13. Which of the following statements about causes of accidents during the school-age years is *inaccurate*?
    a. School-age children are more active and become more adventurous and daring.
    b. School-age children are more susceptible to hazards in the home environment.
    c. School-age children are unable to understand potential dangers.
    d. School-age children are less subject to parental control over their behavior.

14. Michael, age 10, has fallen from his bicycle after accidentally hitting a curb. He is taken to the emergency department of a local hospital with a suspected fractured clavicle and possible head injury. He is conscious and keeps asking what will happen to him. Which of the following nursing diagnoses likely would be most appropriate for Michael?
    a. Anxiety related to separation from support system and unfamiliar environment
    b. High Risk for Hypothermia related to head injury
    c. Altered Family Processes related to maturational crisis
    d. High Risk for Infection related to sepsis

ANSWER KEY

1. *Correct response: a*
   School-age children normally grow about 2 inches (5.2 cm) per year.
   b. School-age children normally gain 4 to 6 lb (1.8 to 2.7 kg) per year.
   c. Children grow at different rates, depending on heredity, nutritional status, and other factors.
   d. Fat pads normally do not increase until adolescence.
   Analysis/Physiologic/Evaluation

2. *Correct response: c*
   During the concrete stage, the child is able to perform mental operations and is more systematic.
   a. This involves cognitive development for the sensorimotor phase of infancy.
   b. The preschool child in the preoperational phase is unable to see another's point of view.
   d. Abstract thinking normally does not occur until adolescence.
   Application/Psychosocial/Assessment

3. *Correct response: b*
   Peers provide conflict resolution on terms that the children can control more easily than in an adult–child authority situation.
   a. Children learn that all homes have rules but that rules and expectations vary.
   c and d. Children have to conform to the rules of the peer group to be accepted; bragging and other obnoxious behaviors may not be acceptable.
   Analysis/Psychosocial/Analysis (Dx)

4. *Correct response: a*
   The child's feet must touch the ground when seated to provide balance and stability when stopping; a too-large bicycle is unsafe.
   b, c, and d. All these promote safety for the child.
   Knowledge/Safe care/Planning

5. *Correct response: d*

Collisions between children of similar size and weight result in fewer and less serious injuries than do collisions between children of widely disparate sizes.
a. Children of similar age commonly are of very different sizes.
b. Children usually can handle scoring and ranking well as they get into competition; parents and coaches may need lessons on losing and winning gracefully.
c. Contact sports with compatibly sized children, safe equipment, and competent coaching can begin earlier.
Application/Safe care/Planning

6. *Correct response: a*
   Before the development of concrete operations, the child in the preoperational phase cannot reverse his or her thinking.
   b. A scheme is the cognitive structure in which a child assimilates information.
   c. This is accommodation.
   d. This is equilibration.
   Comprehension/Psychosocial/Evaluation

7. *Correct response: c*
   This is the exception; children judge an act only by its consequences.
   a, b, and d. All these statements about the school-age child's moral development are true.
   Analysis/Health promotion/Planning

8. *Correct response: b*
   In middle childhood, children commonly lie occasionally because of the difficulty in separating fantasy and reality; parents need to provide guidance and positive role models.
   a. Ignoring the behavior does not help the child understand.
   c. The child may not be able to admit a lie on demand and may feel forced to lie further to defend himself or herself.
   d. Anger does not solve the problem

but rather obscures it and may promote further lying.

Analysis/Health promotion/Analysis (Dx)

9. **Correct response: c**

A school-age child commonly "bends" rules when possible to gain an advantage.

a. Owen may perceive this behavior as responsible.

b. Although a child may feel a need to win, he or she recognizes that purposefully harming another is wrong.

d. Kohlberg's theory of moral development indicates that a child this age is capable of developing a moral code.

Analysis/Psychosocial/Analysis (Dx)

10. **Correct response: b**

The overriding value of nutrition and eating is determined by the family's cultural values.

a. Table manners are important, but peer pressures and society will help mold them later in life.

c. Mealtime should be relaxed with conversation, including the children and their interests.

d. School-age children do need nutritious snacks such as fruit and peanut butter on crackers.

Application/Physiologic/Planning

11. **Correct response: b**

At age 6, the sense of self is precarious; the child tends to overreact to any criticism and feel inferior.

a. By age 6, the child usually has become quite independent of his or her parents for daily tasks.

c. A child this age loves the routine of a schedule.

d. At age 4 and 5, the child had a need to "tattle"; now, he or she wants to make friends and be a friend.

Application/Psychosocial/Assessment

12. **Correct response: d**

As the rapid growth spurt begins at age 11 or 12, the child requires more sleep.

a. Growth slows a little during school-age years, resulting in slightly decreased caloric needs.

b. Not all school-age children require orthodontic braces.

c. A child's questions about sex should be answered at the time they are asked.

Application/Health promotion/Implementation

13. **Correct response: c**

At this age, a child's cognitive level is sufficiently developed to enable good understanding and careful adherence to rules.

a. With greater freedom from home boundaries, this age child becomes adventurous and daring with friends.

b. The home hazards are different for this age; firearms, alcohol, and medicines become tempting.

d. A school-age child is away from home more with less supervision and needs safety education to protect himself or herself from harm.

Comprehension/Safe care/Evaluation

14. **Correct response: a**

The suddenness of the accident, pain, and the unfamiliar experience of hospital admission will produce anxiety.

b. Because Michael is conscious, indicating that the impact to the head was not severe, hypothermia should not develop.

c. An example of a maturational crisis would be the homecoming of a new baby or riding a bicycle for the first time.

d. Infection is not a plausible nursing diagnosis in this situation.

Analysis/Safe care/Analysis (Dx)

Adolescent Growth and Development

6

I. Physical growth and development

A. General characteristics

1. Adolescence encompasses *puberty*, the period when secondary sex characteristics begin to develop.
2. In girls, puberty begins between ages 8 and 14 and is completed

within 3 years; in boys, puberty begins between ages 9 and 16 and is completed by age 18 to 20.

3. During adolescence, hormonal influence causes important developmental changes, including:
   a. Body mass reaches adult size.
   b. Sebaceous glands become active.
   c. Eccrine sweat glands become fully functional.
   d. Apocrine sweat glands develop with hair growth in the axillae, areola of breast, and genital and anal regions.
   e. Body hair assumes characteristic distribution patterns and texture changes.
   f. During puberty, girls experience increases in height, weight, breast development, and pelvic girth with expansion of uterine tissue; menarche (onset of menstrual periods) typically occurs about 2½ years after onset of puberty.
   g. During puberty, boys experience increases in height, weight, muscle mass, and penis and testicle size; facial and body hair growth and voice deepening also occur. Onset of spontaneous nocturnal emissions of seminal fluid is an overt sign of puberty, analogous to menarche in girls.

B. Height and weight changes
1. Normal height changes during puberty include:
   a. Girls gain 2 to 8 inches (5.1 to 20.5 cm) and reach adult height around age 16 or 17.
   b. Boys gain 4 to 12 inches (10.2 to 30.8 cm).
2. Normal weight changes during puberty include:
   a. Girls gain 15 to 55 lb (6.8 to 25 kg) over a 3-year period.
   b. Boys gain 15 to 65 lb (6.8 to 29.5 kg) over a 4-year period.

II. Developmental theories

A. Psychosocial development (Erikson)
1. Erikson terms the psychosocial crisis faced by children aged 13 to 18 *identity vs. role diffusion*.
2. For an adolescent, the radius of significant others is the peer group.
3. The psychosocial theme of this period is "To be oneself; to share or not to share being oneself."
4. To an adolescent, development of who he or she is and where he or she is going becomes the central focus.
5. As rapid physical changes occur, adolescents must reintegrate previous trust in their body, themselves, and how they appear to others.
6. The adolescent continues to redefine his or her self-concept and roles that he or she can play with certainty.
7. The inability to develop a sense of who he or she is and what he

or she can become results in role diffusion and inability to solve core conflicts.

B. **Psychosexual development (Freud)**
1. In the *genital stage* (Oedipus complex revisited), which extends from about age 12 to 20, an adolescent focuses on the genitals as an erogenous zone and engages in masturbation and sexual relations with others.
2. During this period of renewed sexual drive, an adolescent experiences conflict between his or her own needs for sexual satisfaction and society's expectations for control of sexual expression.
3. Core concerns of adolescents include body image development and acceptance by the opposite sex.

C. **Cognitive development (Piaget)**
1. In the development of *formal operations*, which commonly occurs from age 11 to 15, the adolescent moves from deductive to abstract reasoning.
2. This period consists of three substages:
    a. In substage 1, the adolescent sees relationships involving the inverse of the reciprocal.
    b. In substage 2, the adolescent develops the ability to order triads of propositions or relationships.
    c. In substage 3, the adolescent develops the capacity for true formal thought.
3. In true formal thought, the adolescent thinks beyond the present and forms theories about everything, delighting especially in considerations of "that which is not."
4. Relationships are hypothesized as casual and are analyzed for effects that they bring.
5. Random cognitive behavior is replaced by a systematic approach to problems.

D. **Moral development (Kohlberg)**
1. Development of the *postconventional level of morality* occurs at about age 13, marked by the development of an individual conscience and a defined set of moral values.
2. For the first time, the adolescent can acknowledge a conflict between two socially accepted standards and try to decide between them.
3. Control of conduct is now internal, both in standards observed and in reasoning about right and wrong.

III. **Social development**
A. **Identity**
1. To free himself or herself from family domination, an adolescent must define an identity separate from parental authority.
2. This period of rebellion and uncertainty—the final separation–individuation process of childhood—can resemble the toddler period in certain respects.

3. Requisites for this emancipation from home include acceptance by peers, a few close friends, and secure love of a supportive family.
4. Relationships with parents change as the adolescent achieves competence and autonomy.
5. Peer relationships become all important for advice and support.
6. Being found attractive by members of the opposite sex is important to an adolescent's self-esteem.

B. Social activities
1. Group parties and dates typically occupy much of an adolescent's social time.
2. Heterosexual relationships begin with groups of teens, followed by group dating, paired dating in groups, and then a couple on a double-date or alone.
3. The degree of sexual intimacy that an adolescent experiences depends in large part on peer group codes and the adolescent's expectations and value system.
4. Movies and music provide enjoyable diversions for most adolescents.
5. Generally, boys are involved in more sports activities than girls, who tend to be more interested in self-improvement and hobbies.
6. Older adolescents of both sexes commonly are interested in the independence and status represented by owning an automobile.

C. Job responsibilities
1. Common early jobs for adolescents include babysitting and lawn mowing.
2. Starting at age 16, an adolescent can obtain a more formal job, earning money and learning responsibility.
3. The adolescent typically spends money earned on dates, clothes, and other items important to him or her.

IV. Health promotion
A. Fears
1. Common fears of adolescents include:
   a. Relationships with persons of the opposite sex
   b. Homosexual tendencies
   c. Ability to assume adult roles
2. Listening to an adolescent's concerns and encouraging open communication help the adolescent develop increased confidence in his or her ability to cope with fearful situations.

B. Communication
1. An adolescent has the capacity for hypothetical thinking and logical reasoning and can understand factors related to health status, illness, and other situations.
2. An adolescent typically is interested in discussing his or her health problems and scheduled procedures.

3. Of particular concern is how a health problem will affect body image, social activities, school and work, popularity, relationships with the opposite sex, marriage, and reproduction.
4. Patient teaching for an adolescent can begin with the rationale for and importance of a procedure and proceed to concrete details of how the procedure is performed.
5. Because of their ability to think vertically, adolescents may experiment with their treatment plan (e.g., changing time or amount of insulin dosage to see whether it makes a difference).
6. The essence of all patient teaching is to involve the adolescent in planning and implementation with the aim of improving compliance with the treatment plan.

C. **Discipline**
1. Firm but reasonable limit setting is still necessary and appreciated by most adolescents.
2. A supportive, yet noninterfering, family is essential.
3. An adolescent's privileges and responsibilities should be balanced in accordance with his or her maturity.

D. **Nutrition**
1. An adolescent's daily intake should be balanced among the basic four food groups; average daily caloric requirements vary with sex and age, as follows:
   a. Girls aged 11 to 14—48 kcal/kg/d
   b. Girls aged 15 to 18—38 kcal/kg/d
   c. Boys aged 11 to 14—60 kcal/kg/d
   d. Boys aged 15 to 18—42 kcal/kg/d
2. Adolescents typically eat whenever the have a break in activities; readily available nutritious snacks provide good insurance for a balanced diet.
3. Milk (calcium) and protein are needed in quantity to aid bone and muscle growth.
4. Maintaining adequate quality and quantity of daily intake may be difficult because of such factors as busy schedule, influence of peers, and easy availability of fast foods.
5. Family eating patterns established during school-age years continue to influence an adolescent's food selection.

E. **Sleep and rest**
1. During adolescence, rapid growth, overexertion in activities, and a tendency to stay up late commonly interfere with sleep and rest requirements.
2. In an attempt to "catch up" on missed sleep, many adolescents sleep late at every opportunity.

F. **Dental health**
1. Regular preventive check-ups should continue during adolescence.

    2. Many adolescents must wear orthodontic braces, which may be a source of embarrassment (unless many peers also wear braces).

    3. An adolescent must pay special attention to careful brushing and care of teeth.

G. **Personal care**

    1. Because of increased sebaceous gland and apocrine gland secretions (and, for girls, menstruation), an adolescent must pay careful attention to body cleanliness; a daily shower should be encouraged.

    2. Ear piercing is popular; it should be done by a nurse or physician using sterile equipment.

    3. Regular vision and hearing screening should be conducted. An adolescent needing vision correction may be able to choose between eyeglasses and contact lenses.

H. **Sex education**

    1. Teaching about sexual function, begun during the school-age years, should expand to cover more in-depth information on the physical, hormonal, and emotional changes of puberty.

    2. An adolescent needs accurate, complete information on sexuality and cultural and moral values; information must include:

        a. How pregnancy occurs

        b. Methods of preventing pregnancy, stressing that male and female partners both are responsible for contraception

        c. Transmission of and protection against sexually transmitted diseases, especially acquired immunodeficiency syndrome (AIDS)

    3. Ideally, a well-informed parent who communicates well with the adolescent will provide information; a nurse or teacher also can provide information, with parents' knowledge.

I. **Injury prevention**

    1. When providing safety teaching to an adolescent, keep in mind that adolescents commonly are risk-takers and often do not consider safety before acting.

    2. Adolescents contribute substantially to motor vehicle accidents through:

        a. Inexperience and poor judgment

        b. Reckless driving or speeding

        c. Driving under the influence of alcohol or other drugs

        d. Failure to use safety belts

        e. Peer pressure for unsafe driving practices

    3. Adolescents also are prone to accidents from unsafe use of bicycles, skateboards, motorcycles, boats, all-terrain vehicles, and snowmobiles.

    4. Accidental injury can result from improper use of firearms; safety instruction on proper use and storage of firearms and other non-powder arms (e.g., BB guns) should be provided.

5. An adolescent is particularly prone to swimming and diving accidents; swimming and diving safety must be taught.
6. Safety teaching also should reinforce the need for proper respect for gasoline, electricity, and fire.
7. An adolescent needs instruction on avoiding sports injuries (e.g., avoiding overexertion, using proper equipment, using proper techniques for making plays).
8. Use of sunscreen during periods of prolonged sun exposure should be encouraged.
9. Smoking and use of alcohol and other drugs should be discouraged.

V. Selected health problems of adolescents
A. Teenage pregnancy
1. Description: pregnancy before age 19, usually unplanned and out of wedlock
2. Incidence and pathophysiology
   a. In the United States, about 1 million girls under age 20 become pregnant each year, representing 1 in 10 female adolescents.
   b. Although teenage pregnancy no longer is considered hazardous to the fetus, it still is viewed as socially, economically, psychologically, and educationally disadvantageous to the mother.
   c. Mortality for teenage pregnancies is declining, but morbidity remains high.
   d. Complications of pregnancy associated with teenage pregnancy include preeclampsia, iron-deficiency anemia, prolonged labor, and increased incidence of premature birth.
   e. A pregnant adolescent commonly faces many crises.
   f. Early crises include recognizing the pregnancy, informing the partner, and informing the parents.
   g. Prenatal crises include deciding whether to carry the fetus to term or seek an abortion; providing for financial, medical, and nutritional needs; and dealing with interpersonal relationships at home and in school.
   h. Intrapartal crises revolve around environmental control and depersonalization issues.
   i. Common postpartum crises include whether to keep the infant or put it up for adoption, dealing with body image changes, and bonding and parenting difficulties.
3. Assessment findings
   a. Because an adolescent commonly denies pregnancy, early recognition by a parent or health care provider may be crucial to timely initiation of prenatal care.
   b. Initial signs include cessation of menstruation and breast enlargement.

    4. Nursing diagnoses
      a. Knowledge Deficit
      b. Altered Sexuality Patterns
      c. High Risk for Altered Parenting

    5. Planning and implementation
      a. In collaboration with the pregnant adolescent and her support persons, implement a plan of care that includes prenatal visits; proper nutritional intake; exercise program; avoidance of alcohol, nonprescribed drugs, and cigarettes; emotional support; plans for delivery; plans for infant care; and anticipatory guidance about birth control and future sexual conduct.
      b. Assess for complications of pregnancy.

    6. Evaluation
      a. The adolescent understands and follows the plan of care.
      b. The adolescent who decides to carry the fetus to term delivers a healthy infant.
      c. The adolescent is comfortable with the decisions she has made.

B. Suicide

    1. Description
      a. Suicidal behavior refers to destructive, self-inflicted behaviors that result in harm.
      b. Suicide is the intentional taking of one's own life.

    2. Etiology
      a. Suicide is second only to accidents as a leading cause of death in adolescents.
      b. The common stresses of adolescence, compounded by limited problem-solving abilities, sometimes result in harmful, even life-threatening, behavior.
      c. Common contributing factors include family dysfunction and low self-esteem.
      d. An adolescent who attempts or successfully commits suicide often has a family history of suicide or suicidal behavior.

    3. Assessment findings
      a. Depression usually precedes suicide; signs of depression may be overt or subtle.
      b. Danger signs include lethargy, malaise, inability to sleep or early morning waking, loss of appetite or overeating, excessive crying, giving away of cherished possessions, preoccupation with death, and statement of intentions to commit suicide.

    4. Nursing diagnoses
      a. Altered Thought Processes
      b. Social Isolation

        c.   Chronic Low Self-Esteem

        d.   Ineffective Individual Coping

  5.   Planning and implementation

        a.   Provide information for teachers, parents, and adolescents about risk factors, counseling available to adolescents, and stress reduction and problem-solving strategies.

        b.   Provide crisis intervention for an adolescent who gestures or attempts suicide and plan for family follow-up care. Ensure that the adolescent understands that he or she must cease or not implement this destructive behavior.

        c.   Arrange for counseling and hospitalization if necessary; refer the adolescent and family to a professional therapist who will work with them through this crisis.

        d.   After a successful suicide, counsel the adolescent's family and friends to help them understand and work through their grief.

  6.   Evaluation

        a.   An adolescent who made suicide attempts or gestures displays improved self-esteem, positive behaviors, and more effective coping and problem-solving strategies.

        b.   Family and friends of an adolescent who successfully committed suicide work through their grief and resolve the loss over time.

C. **Obesity**

  1.   Description: excessive accumulation of adipose tissue in the body

  2.   Etiology and pathophysiology

        a.   An estimated 10% to 30% of all adolescents in the United States are obese.

        b.   Obesity most commonly results from overeating in combination with underactivity, a pattern that often begins in infancy and persists throughout childhood and into adolescence.

        c.   Obesity not specifically related to overeating and underactivity may be associated with endocrine or metabolic disorders, such as Cushing's syndrome, hypogonadism, hypothyroidism, and hypothalmic tumors, or long-term drug therapy with agents such as phenothiazines and corticosteroids.

        d.   Social and psychological factors also may contribute to obesity.

        e.   Homeostatic mechanisms support the maintenance of obesity once it is established.

        f.   Family influences on eating patterns, attitudes toward food, and activity patterns are significant in the development of childhood obesity.

        g.   Obesity assumes particular significance during adolescence because of its effects on developmental tasks such as identity and self-esteem.

3. Assessment findings

    a.   Weight more than 20% above the norm for height and body build

    b.   Excessive accumulation of adipose tissue, as evidenced by triceps skin-fold measurements

4. Nursing diagnoses

    a.   Altered Nutrition: More than Body Requirements

    b.   Chronic Low Self-Esteem

    c.   Body Image Disturbance

5. Planning and implementation

    a.   In collaboration with the adolescent and parents, develop a diet plan that provides for weight loss with no metabolic complications or excessive hunger, preservation of lean body mass, absence of psychiatric reactions, normal activity, and normal growth and development.

    b.   Encourage regular exercise that the adolescent enjoys, such as swimming or walking.

    c.   Use behavior modification techniques focusing on social and behavioral aspects that accompany eating and not on food itself; changing the adolescent's perception to a positive self-image is crucial.

    d.   Discourage use of medications such as amphetamines because of the risk of addiction.

    e.   Explain that surgical bypass procedures to treat obesity are controversial in adolescents.

    f.   Encourage the adolescent to seek a support group of other adolescents in similar circumstances.

    g.   Emphasize the need for emotional support and encouragement from family members and friends; as necessary, discuss the need to alter certain family eating habits.

    h.   Suggest nonfood rewards for weight loss achievements (e.g., a movie or a shopping trip with friends).

6. Evaluation

    a.   The adolescent achieves steady weight loss.

    b.   The adolescent expresses a more positive self-image.

    c.   Family and friends provide emotional support and positive reinforcement.

    d.   The adolescent begins to establish positive eating and exercise habits for effective lifelong weight control.

VI. Hospitalization of adolescents

A. Adolescent's response to hospitalization

    1. Common fears of hospitalized adolescents include:

        a.   Loss of control—enforced dependency and loss of identity

        b.   Bodily injury and pain—mutilation, sexual changes

      c.   Separation from peer group
2. Behaviors may include:
      a.   Rejection, uncooperativeness, withdrawal
      b.   Self-assertion, self-control, cooperation
      c.   Anxiety
      d.   Overconfidence, manipulation
      e.   Depression, loneliness, boredom

B. **Parents' response to their adolescent's hospitalization**
1. Parents' emotional response to hospitalization of their adolescent may be less intense than for a younger child but still involve similar elements.
2. Although the adolescent has less need for his or her parents' constant presence, parents should plan to be present to provide support before, during, and after stressful procedures.

C. **Nursing considerations**
1. Arrange for an age-compatible roommate, if possible.
2. Involve the adolescent in planning and scheduling care measures.
3. Involve the adolescent and family in home care routines when follow-up care is necessary.

Bibliography

Erikson, E. (1968). *Identity: Youth and crisis*. New York: W. W. Norton.

Mott, S. R., Fazekas, N. F., and James, S. R. (1985). *Nursing care of children and families: A holistic approach*. Menlo Park, CA: Addison-Wesley.

Nelms, B. C. (1981). What is a normal adolescent? *American Journal of Maternal/Child Nursing*, 6, 402–406.

Whaley, L. F., and Wong, D. L. (1991). *Nursing care of infants and children* (4th ed.). St. Louis: C. V. Mosby.

STUDY QUESTIONS

1. Daniel, aged 14, asks the nurse why he needs to use underarm deodorant daily. What related physiologic change should the nurse explain to Daniel?
   a. Increased sweat production results from an increase in adipose tissue distribution, which better insulates the body.
   b. Apocrine sweat glands reach secretory capacity during adolescence.
   c. Eccrine sweat glands become fully functional during puberty.
   d. Sebaceous glands become very active during puberty.

2. According to Erikson, why may an adolescent may have difficulty mastering appropriate psychosocial tasks?
   a. The basic focus is on mastery of sexual relationships.
   b. Only limited interaction occurs between the culture and the basic pattern of individual development.
   c. Modern culture tends to make identity crisis the most challenging to resolve.
   d. The adolescent commonly lacks positive role models.

3. Maturity, as a developmental concept, is defined as
   a. the ability to wait for needs gratification
   b. the social behavior an adolescent displays in the company of peers
   c. an adolescent's growing independence from his or her parents
   d. the internal processes controlled by genetic makeup

4. Which of the following is *not* a common behavioral characteristic of adolescents?
   a. tendency toward idealism
   b. daydreaming
   c. predictability
   d. moodiness

5. Peer relationships during the adolescent years are important for all the following reasons *except*
   a. encouraging a sense of belonging
   b. providing a setting in which to move from autonomy to dependency
   c. providing opportunities to learn about themselves and others
   d. strongly influencing self-evaluation and behavior

6. Parent–adolescent conflicts are inevitable. What is the primary reason for most of these conflicts?
   a. Adolescents are basically rude and without manners.
   b. An adolescent does not "feel right" unless arguing with his or her parents.
   c. The adolescent is searching for how his or her needs and identity fit with parental expectations.
   d. Parents become worried that they were too lenient in earlier years, so they tighten up the rules.

7. What is menarche?
   a. a girl's first menstruation
   b. the first year of menstruation, which usually occurs without ovulation
   c. the entire span of the menstrual cycle from onset to menopause
   d. the onset of uterine maturation

8. Aaron, aged 14, has some facial acne. According to his parents, he spends an inordinate amount of time in front of the bathroom mirror, tying up the bathroom. They ask the nurse why he does so and what they should do about it. When the nurse talks with Aaron and his parents, which of the following remarks would be the *least* helpful?
   a. "This is probably the only concern Aaron has about his body, so I wouldn't bother him about it."
   b. "Both boys and girls are anxious about how they will be perceived by their peers, and so spend much time in grooming."
   c. "An adolescent may develop a poor self-image when experiencing acne

problems. Do you feel this way sometimes, Aaron?''

d. "Aaron appears to be keeping his face well-washed in an effort to reduce the acne. Would you feel comfortable sharing your cleansing method, Aaron?''

9. Ann, aged 15, confides in the nurse that she became sexually active about 6 months ago with her boyfriend. She worries that her parents would "kill her" if they found out—especially if she were to get pregnant. Based this assessment data, which of the following nursing diagnoses would be most appropriate?

a. Altered Growth and Development Patterns related to sexual activity

b. Impaired Social Interaction Patterns related to parental limits

c. Altered Sexuality Patterns related to parental expectations

d. Fear related to expectations of boyfriend

10. Which of the following would be an appropriate approach for further assessment of Ann?

a. "You seem frightened that you could become pregnant; why don't you stop seeing this boyfriend?"

b. "You are expressing concern about becoming pregnant; would you like more information on methods of contraception or on waiting for sexual gratification with your boyfriend?"

c. "You obviously have exceeded your parents' limits; how can we work this out?"

d. "Have you discussed this with your girlfriends? Perhaps they can help you figure a way out of this dilemma."

11. Kathryn, aged 16, has been overweight for as long as she can remember. During her annual health assessment, she expresses a desire "to do something about it." When developing a plan for Kathryn in collaboration with a dietitian,

the nurse should include all the following *except*

a. selecting low-calorie foods in small servings from the basic four food groups

b. providing nutritious foods as a reward for achieving weight loss goals

c. developing a schedule of walking for 20 minutes three times or more each week

d. discussing a menu plan and more healthful food preparation methods with Kathryn's mother

12. Kathryn returns to the clinic in 3 months and states that she lost 10 lb during the first 8 weeks but now has hit a plateau. She seems discouraged and says all she wants to do is "fill up on junk food." Her weight loss goal is 25 lb. Which of the following would be the nurse's most appropriate first suggestion?

a. Discuss changing the weight loss goal.

b. Congratulate her on the 10-lb loss, and encourage her to keep at it.

c. Help her identify changes in the original plan that can help remotivate her.

d. Point out that plateaus are common, and encourage her not to become discouraged.

13. One of the changes in Kathryn's diet plan that emerges is to keep a food diary. The primary purpose of this activity is to

a. keep Kathryn busy and more focused on weight loss

b. analyze the amount of actual intake and where most of the eating occurs

c. identify whether Kathryn is cheating on the diet plan

d. provide documentation to aid nursing assessment at the next visit

14. Which of the following commonly poses a major threat to a hospitalized adolescent?

a. restricted activity

b. fear of pain

c. fear of altered body image

d. separation from home and family

ANSWER KEY

1. **Correct response: b**
   Apocrine glands are larger than eccrine glands and grow in conjunction with hair follicles in the underarms, genital area, and other locations.
   a. Although adipose tissue does increase, it is not linked to increased sweat production.
   c. Eccrine sweat glands are distributed over the entire body.
   d. Sebaceous glands contribute to acne, not sweating.
   Application/Physiologic/Planning

2. **Correct response: c**
   An adolescent must resolve many choices and demands to master the task of identity.
   a. Mastery of sexual relationships is part of the young adult (age 18 to 40) task of intimacy.
   b. An adolescent has much interaction with the culture, through peers, school, family, and the mass media.
   d. Peers, teachers, parents, and extended family all serve as role models; peers have the most influence.
   Analysis/Psychosocial/Evaluation

3. **Correct response: a**
   The ability to wait demonstrates that internal controls have developed and provide guidance for decisions.
   b. Usually this behavior reflects one-upmanship and is quite immature.
   c. Adolescents must free themselves from parental dominance, establish their own identity, and become independent to achieve maturity.
   d. This is a description of physiologic maturation.
   Comprehension/Psychosocial/Evaluation

4. **Correct response: c**
   Hormonal influences and uncertainty about self-identity make for very unpredictable behavior.
   a and b. Adolescents enjoy daydream-
   ing and thinking about ideal situations for themselves; would make "life" easier for them.
   d. Adolescents commonly experience moodiness when faced with conflicts such as rejection in relationships or difficulty with school or parents.
   Application/Physiologic/Assessment

5. **Correct response: b**
   The goal of an adolescent is to move from dependency to self-reliance or increased autonomy.
   a. Peer group relationships provide the adolescent with a sense of acceptance and belonging.
   c. Discussions with peers enable expression of feelings and concerns.
   d. The opinions of the peer group have a profound influence on an adolescent's self-concept.
   Analysis/Psychosocial/Evaluation

6. **Correct response: c**
   The change in their relationship from protection and dependency to mutual affection and equality involves role changes for both and creates tension.
   a. Adolescents normally have developed acceptable manners but may not consistently put them into practice.
   b. Adolescents prefer that their life run smoothly and enjoy periods of mature discussion with their parents.
   d. As the adolescent assumes increased responsibility, rules usually loosen.
   Application/Psychosocial/Assessment

7. **Correct response: a**
   Menarche refers to the onset of the first menstrual cycle.
   b and c. Menarche refers to the first cycle only.
   d. Uterine growth and broadening of the pelvic girdle occurs before menarche.

Knowledge/Physiologic/Assessment

8. *Correct response: a*
   This response shuts off further investigation and likely will make Aaron and his parents feel defensive.
   b. Time spent in front of the mirror is important to the adolescent's developing self-image.
   c. This response will encourage Aaron to share his feelings.
   d. This response can help identify any patient teaching needs for Aaron regarding cleansing.

Application/Physiologic/Implementation

9. *Correct response: c*
   Ann is expressing concern about the conflict between parental expectations and her own desires.
   a and b. This is a normal experimental pattern for many adolescents, but Ann verbalizes parental expectations against this behavior.
   d. Ann is not expressing any conflict with her boyfriend.

Application/Safe care/Analysis (Dx)

10. *Correct response: b*
    This response can help open up other possibilities for discussion and problem solving.
    a. Ann needs help with preventing pregnancy and resolving conflicts with her parents, not with choosing a suitable boyfriend.
    c. This response makes the nurse a "co-conspirator" against Ann's parents, which is not helpful in problem solving.
    d. Ann should be able to count on a skilled professional nurse for guidance.

Analysis/Physiologic/Implementation

11. *Correct response: b*
    The nurse should suggest a reward other than food for losing weight (e.g., a movie or a shopping trip with her friends).
    a and d. Kathryn needs to develop lifelong habits for nutritious, low-calorie food selection and preparation in order to improve her own health and the health of others around her.
    c. Exercise is an excellent adjunct to reduced caloric intake in weight loss; it also promotes improved physiologic function.

Application/Physiologic/Planning

12. *Correct response: c*
    This is the best first approach because a change in the exercise or eating plan may identify problems with the original plan and spark renewed commitment.
    a. This approach is a possibility, but an evaluation of the original plan and its implementation would be better.
    b and d. These approaches may sound good, but they do not provide the evaluation needed at this stage; plateaus are common, but do not last forever.

Comprehension/Physiologic/Evaluation

13. *Correct response: b*
    Kathryn's cognitive level of formal operations will help her identify and evaluate eating behaviors that she may now be unaware of.
    a. Kathryn needs other activities besides a focus only on the diet plan.
    c. This represents a punishment approach that will not be as helpful.
    d. The documentation is more for Kathryn's benefit than for the nurse although the nurse can use it as well.

Analysis/Safe care/Implementation

14. *Correct response: c*
    Body image is important to the developing adolescent; any threat to this is a priority.
    a. The adolescent adapts well to restricted motor activity because of his or her increased cognitive ability.
    b. An adolescent commonly has a high pain tolerance.
    d. An adolescent typically is more concerned with separation from peers than from family.

Application/Psychosocial/Evaluation

Fluid and Electrolyte Imbalance and Renal Dysfunction

I. Essential concepts: fluid and electrolyte balance

A. Body fluid composition

1. Body fluid is expressed as a percentage of body weight; this percentage varies with age.

   a. In infants, total body water constitutes 80% of body weight.

   b. By age 3 years, total body water constitutes about 65% of body weight.

   c. By age 15 years, total body water constitutes 60% of body weight.

2. Age-specific fluid-intake requirements include:

   a. Newborn: 80 to 100 mL/kg/24 h

   b. Infant: 120 to 130 mL/kg/24 h

   c. Age 2 years: 115 to 125 mL/kg/24 h

   d. Age 6 years: 90 to 100 mL/kg/24 h

   e. Age 15 years: 70 to 85 mL/kg/24 h

   f. Age 18 years: 40 to 50 mL/kg/24 h

3. Fluid and electrolyte disturbances (e.g., diarrhea, vomiting, and fever) occur more frequently and develop more rapidly in infants and young children than in older children and adults.

4. Infants and young children are more vulnerable to alterations in fluid and electrolyte balance due to:

   a. A relatively larger percentage of fluid volume as a percentage of body weight

   b. A greater body surface area in proportion to body mass

   c. Higher metabolic rates, which increase the body's fluid demands

   d. Immature kidney function

B. Acid–base disturbances

1. Acid–base imbalances are common complications of diarrhea, vomiting, and febrile conditions in infants and young children, as well as possible complications of respiratory, endocrine, renal and metabolic disorders.

2. Acid–base disturbances include *acidosis*, resulting from either accumulation of acid or loss of base, and *alkalosis*, resulting from either accumulation of base or loss of acid (Table 7–1).

   a. *Respiratory acidosis* results from diminished or inadequate pulmonary ventilation, leading to an elevated PCO_2 level and a decreased plasma pH.

   b. *Metabolic acidosis* results from a gain of nonvolatile acids or the loss of base and leads to decreased plasma pH and decreased plasma HCO_3 concentration.

   c. *Respiratory alkalosis* results from an increase in the rate and depth of pulmonary ventilation leading to a decreased PCO_2 level and an elevated plasma pH.

d. *Metabolic alkalosis*, produced by a gain in base or a loss of acid, results in elevated urine pH, elevated plasma pH, and elevated plasma HCO_3 concentration.

3. Compensatory mechanisms refer to the body's attempts to correct an acid–base imbalance through compensatory changes in the component of the acid–base equation not primarily affected.

4. Interventions that can sustain a child with an acid–base imbalance until the primary disorder has resolved include:
   a. Providing adequate hydration
   b. Replacing electrolytes
   c. Correcting the acid–base imbalance

II. Fluid imbalance: dehydration

A. Description: excessive loss of fluid from body tissues that exceeds the total intake

B. Etiology

1. Dehydration most commonly results from abnormal fluid losses, such as from excessive vomiting or diarrhea.

2. Other possible causes include insufficient fluid intake, diabetic ketoacidosis, severe burns, prolonged high fever, and hyperventilation.

C. Pathophysiology

1. Depending on the cause and nature of fluid loss, a child will lose water and various electrolytes.

2. Dehydration is classified as isotonic, hypertonic, or hypotonic.

3. In *isotonic dehydration*, electrolyte and water deficits occur in approximately balanced proportions.
   a. This is the most common type, accounting for about 70% of dehydration cases linked to diarrhea in infants.
   b. The major loss involves extracellular components and circulating blood volume, making the child susceptible to hypovolemic shock.

TABLE 7–1.
Acid–Base Disturbances

DISTURBANCE	INITIAL METABOLIC CHANGE	EFFECT ON BLOOD PH	COMPENSATORY REACTION
Metabolic alkalosis	Decreased H, increased HCO_3	Increased	Increased PCO_2
Metabolic acidosis	Decreased HCO_3	Decreased	Decreased PCO_2
Respiratory alkalosis	Decreased PCO_3	Increased	Decreased HCO_3
Respiratory acidosis	Increased PCO_2	Decreased	Increased HCO_3

      c.   Serum sodium (Na^+) is decreased or within the normal range; chloride (Cl^-) is decreased; and potassium (K^+) is normal to increased.

      d.   Deficits should be corrected over a 24-hour period.

  4.   In *hypertonic dehydration*, water loss exceeds electrolyte loss.

      a.   This type accounts for about 20% of cases resulting from severe diarrhea in infants.

      b.   It results in fluid shifts from the intracellular compartment to the extracellular compartment, which can lead to neurologic disturbances such as seizures.

      c. Na^+ is increased; K^+, varied; Cl^-, increased.

  5.   In *hypotonic dehydration*, electrolyte deficit exceeds water deficit.

      a.   It may be caused by excessive perspiration, severe diarrhea, or administration of oral or IV fluids without electrolytes added; it accounts for 10% of cases in infants resulting from severe diarrhea.

      b.   In response to hypotonic dehydration, water shifts from the extracellular to the intracellular compartments in an attempt to establish osmotic equilibrium, which further increases extracellular fluid loss and commonly results in *hypovolemic shock*.

      c. Na^+ is decreased; Cl^-, decreased; K^+, variable.

      d.   Volume and Na^+ should be replaced within 24 to 36 hours.

  6.   The degree of dehydration can be estimated by comparing the child's current weight with his or her preillness weight.

  7.   Dehydration can be classified by severity:

      a.   Mild: Loss of up to 5% of preillness body weight

      b.   Moderate: Loss of up to 10% of preillness body weight

      c.   Severe: Loss of up to 15% of preillness body weight

D. **Assessment findings**

  1.   Common clinical manifestations include:

      a.   Weight loss

      b.   Dry mucous membranes

      c.   Decreased tear production

      d.   Poor skin turgor

      e.   Sunken eyeballs

      f.   Depressed fontanels (in infants)

      g.   Decreased urine output

      h.   Tachycardia

      i.   Tachypnea

      j.   Decreased blood pressure

      k.   Excessive thirst

  2.   Laboratory study results may reveal:

      a.   Concentrated urine with high specific gravity (> 1.03) and high osmolarity

    b.   Elevated hematocrit

    c.   Elevated blood urea nitrogen (BUN)

    d.   Decreased urine sodium concentration

    e.   Altered serum electrolyte values (Na^+; K^+; Cl^-)

    f.   Low serum pH if the child is acidotic

E. Nursing diagnoses

1. Altered Family Processes
2. Fluid Volume Deficit
3. Hyperthermia
4. High Risk for Infection
5. Knowledge Deficit
6. Altered Nutrition: Less than Body Requirements
7. Imapaired Tissue Integrity

F. Planning and implementation

1. Obtain an accurate initial weight, and monitor for changes indicating fluid gains and losses.
2. Evaluate the child's health history, physical assessment findings, and laboratory study results to help identify the underlying cause of dehydration.
3. Administer clear liquids orally, as ordered, to correct fluid imbalance.
4. Offer oral fluids in small quantities (e.g., 1 to 2 oz every hour); withhold a full diet until the child is well hydrated and the underlying problem is under control.
5. If the child is unable to ingest sufficient fluid orally, start an IV line and administer appropriate replacement solution, as ordered.
6. Monitor IV replacement therapy, checking the IV site frequently.
7. Instruct parents of a child with an IV on positioning, moving, and care.
8. Evaluate the child's hydration status by assessing for signs and symptoms of dehydration.
9. Monitor and record intake and output, and note urine specific gravity.
10. Help maintain skin integrity by providing good hygiene and skin care, turning frequently, changing damp or soiled linen as indicated, carefully washing and drying the diaper area with every change, using aseptic technique when inserting IV catheters, and monitoring the IV infusion site for signs of infiltration.
11. Prevent infection by maintaining good hygiene and handwashing and instituting necessary isolation techniques appropriate to the cause of dehydration.
12. Reintroduce the child to a regular diet gradually, as ordered;

monitor the child's response to diet changes by noting his or her ability to retain orally ingested food and fluids.

13. Provide support to the family and explain all tests and therapeutic measures.
14. Encourage family members to participate in the child's care as appropriate.
15. Provide patient and family teaching, covering:
    a. Diet and oral fluid instructions
    b. Causes of dehydration, and signs and symptoms of dehydration to watch for and report
    c. Handwashing and hygiene instructions as indicated.
    d. Follow-up appointments

G. Evaluation
1. The child displays no signs of dehydration and tolerates a regular diet.
2. The family verbalizes knowledge of home diet and fluid intake instructions, causes of dehydration, signs and symptoms of dehydration, the importance of handwashing and good hygiene, and scheduled follow-up appointments.

III. Essential concepts: renal system anatomy and physiology

A. Development
1. Kidney development begins during the first few weeks of gestation but is not complete until the end of the first year after birth.
2. Infants are unable to excrete a water load at the same rate as older children and adults; glomerular filtration and absorption do not reach adult capabilities until age 1 to 2 years.
3. Newborns are more prone to developing severe acidosis.
4. Sodium excretion also is reduced during infancy, and the kidneys are less adaptable to sodium deficiency or excess.

B. Function
1. The kidney's functional unit, the *nephron*, comprises:
   a. Glomeruli, which filter water and solutes from blood
   b. Tubules, which reabsorb needed substances (water, proteins, electrolytes, glucose, amino acids) from filtrate and allow unneeded substances to leave body in urine
2. Kidney functions include:
   a. Maintain body fluid volume and composition by responding appropriately to alterations in internal environment caused by variations in dietary intake and extrarenal losses of water and solutes
   b. Secrete hormones: erythropoietic stimulating factor (ESF), which stimulates production of red blood cells, and renin, which stimulates production of angiotensin, causing arteriolar constriction and blood pressure elevation, and aldosterone

3. Urine is formed in the nephron, then passes into the renal pelvis, through the ureter into the bladder, and out of the body through the urethra.

IV. Renal system overview

A. Assessment

1. Health history findings possibly pointing to renal dysfunction include:
   a. Neonate: poor feeding, failure to thrive, frequent urination and crying on urination, dehydration, convulsions
   b. Infant: same findings as in a neonate, plus persistent diaper rash, foul-smelling urine, straining on urination
   c. Older child: poor appetite; vomiting; excessive thirst; enuresis; incontinence; frequent urination; painful urination; bloody urine; fatigue; abdominal, flank, or back pain
   d. Family history of renal disease, hypertension, and other problems related to renal dysfunction

2. Physical assessment may uncover signs and symptoms of renal dysfunction, such as:
   a. Abnormal rate and depth of respirations
   b. Hypertension
   c. Fever
   d. Growth retardation
   e. Signs of circulatory congestion, such as peripheral cyanosis, slow capillary refill time, pallor, and peripheral edema
   f. Abdominal distention
   g. Early signs of uremic encephalopathy: lethargy, poor concentration, confusion
   h. Signs of congenital anomalies, such as phimosis, hypospadias, ear abnormalities (floppy, low-set, malformed), prominent epicanthal folds, beaklike nose, small chin

B. Laboratory studies and diagnostic tests

1. Urinalysis is the most valuable laboratory test for renal function (Table 7–2).
2. BUN and creatinine are common blood tests of renal function.
   a. BUN represents a gross index of glomerular filtration rate; impaired renal function and rapid protein catabolism result in elevated BUN.
   b. Creatinine is a by-product of energy metabolism; as long as muscle mass remains constant, creatinine levels are constant; renal disorders reducing creatinine excretion result in increased serum creatinine levels.
   c. Creatinine generally is a more sensitive indicator of acute renal failure than is BUN.

    3. Tests performed to identify anatomic abnormalities contributing to the development of infection may include:
- a. Ultrasonography
- b. Voiding cystourethrography
- c. Intravenous pyelography
- d. Cystoscopy

C. **Psychosocial implications**

    1. Infants: Comforting the infant following threatening procedures and acceptance by parents and family members is vital to the development of a positive body image.

    2. Toddlers: Problems of immobilization frustrate the toddler's drive for independence; allowing the toddler to participate in care, as appropriate, may be helpful.

TABLE 7–2.
Normal Urine Values in Children

PARAMETER	AGE	NORMAL RANGE
Color		Pale yellow to dark amber
Clarity		Clear
Volume (mL/day)	Newborn	50–300
	Child	500–1000
	Thereafter	800–2000
Addis count		
Leukocytes		<10
Erythrocytes		<5
Casts		Occasional hyaline
Colony count (midstream clean catch; colonies/mL)	Infant/child	<100
Fresh specimen	Thereafter	<10,000
Microscopic (per high-power field)		
Leukocytes		0–1
Erythrocytes		Rare
Casts		Rare
Osmolarity (mOsm/L)	Premature/newborn	50–600
	Thereafter	50–1400
	Thereafter	>850 after fluid restriction
pH	Premature/newborn	5.0–7.0
	Thereafter	4.8–7.8
Protein		
Qualitative		Negative
Quantitative		10–100 mg/day
Specific gravity (random)	Newborn/infant	1.001–1.020
	Thereafter	1.001–1.030
	Thereafter	>1.025 after fluid restriction
Sugar		Negative
Ketones		0

(Fischbach, R.A. (1988). A manual of laboratory diagnostic tests (3rd ed.). Philadelphia: J.B. Lippincott)

3. Preschoolers: At this age, body image awareness is heightened, and the child's natural curiosity about the body may be stimulated by physical examinations. The child's active fantasy life can contribute to fear of the simplest procedures.
4. School-age children: Appearing different from peers is extremely anxiety producing, as are prohibitions on diet, sports, and other activities that focus on the child's differences from agemates.
5. Adolescents: Because of an adolescent's increased need for independence, the enforced dependence imposed by rigorous therapeutic regimens can increase feelings of resentment and rebelliousness.

V. Urinary tract infections (UTIs)

A. **Description: inflammation, usually bacterial in origin, of the urethra (urethritis), bladder (cystitis), ureters (ureteritis), or kidneys (pyelonephritis)**

B. **Etiology and incidence**

1. Most common causative organisms are gram negative, including *Escherichia coli* (accounting for up to 85% of UTIs), *Klebsiella*, enteric streptococci, and *Staphylococcus epidermis*.
2. Other possible contributing factors to UTI include:
   a. Urine stasis
   b. Urine reflux
   c. Poor perineal hygiene
   d. Constipation
   e. Pregnancy
   f. Noncircumcision (in males)
   g. Indwelling catheter placement
   h. Antimicrobial agents that alter normal urinary tract flora
   i. Tight clothing or diapers
   j. Bubble baths or shampoo in bath water
   k. Local inflammation, such as from vaginitis, which increases the risk of ascending infection
   l. Sexual intercourse
3. Peak incidence occurs between ages 2 and 6 years, with increased incidence also noted in adolescents who are sexually active.
4. Females have a 10 to 30 times greater risk of developing UTIs than males (except in neonates) because of their shorter urethral structure, which provides a ready pathway for ascendance of organisms.

C. **Pathophysiology**

1. Inflammation usually is confined to the lower urinary tract in uncomplicated UTI. Recurrent cystitis, however, may produce anatomic changes in the ureter that leads to vesicoureteral

valve incompetence and resulting reflux of urine, which can result in access of organisms to the upper urinary tract.

2. Pyelonephritis usually results from an ascending infection from the lower urinary tract and can lead to acute and chronic inflammatory changes in the pelvis and medulla, with scarring and loss of renal tissue.

3. Recurrent or chronic infection results in increased fibrotic tissue and kidney contraction.

D. Assessment findings

1. Clinical manifestations vary with age; common signs and symptoms according to age group include:
   a. Newborns: fever or hypothermia, sepsis
   b. Infants: frequent or infrequent urination, constant squirming and irritability, strong-smelling urine, persistent diaper rash, failure to thrive, feeding problems, vomiting, diarrhea, abdominal distention, jaundice
   c. Toddlers, preschoolers, and school-age children: enuresis or daytime incontinence in a child who has been toilet-trained, fever, strong- or foul-smelling urine, frequent urination, dysuria, urinary urgency, abdominal or flank pain, hematuria, vomiting, change in urinary stream, fever and chills
   d. Adolescents: frequent and painful urination, hematuria

2. Urinalysis may demonstrate hematuria, proteinuria, and pyuria. Urine may have a foul odor and appear cloudy with strands of mucous or pus.

3. Diagnosis is confirmed by detection of bacteria in urine culture.

E. Nursing diagnoses

1. High Risk for Altered Body Temperature
2. Altered Family Processes
3. Altered Growth and Development
4. High Risk for Infection
5. Knowledge Deficit
6. Pain
7. Impaired Tissue Integrity
8. Altered Patterns of Urinary Elimination

F. Planning and implementation

1. Administer prescribed medications as ordered, which may include:
   a. Antibiotic agents such as sulfisoxazole, ampicillin, and cephalexin
   b. Urinary antiseptic agents such as nitrofurantoin
   c. Aminoglycoside antibiotics such as gentamicin or tobramycin to treat nosocomial infection

      d.   Cefaclor to treat resistant UTIs

      e.   Prophylactic regimen of co-trimoxazole

2. Help prevent infection by maintaining sterile technique when performing urinary catheterization.

3. Assess urinary status by observing the appearance and odor of urine and noting signs and symptoms such as frequency, burning, enuresis, urinary retention, or flank pain.

4. Provide comfort measures: Maintain bed rest, administer prn analgesics and antipyretics as indicated, and encourage increased fluid intake to reduce fever and dilute urine.

5. Provide emotional support to family members and explain all tests and treatments.

6. Provide patient and family teaching, covering:

    a.   Medication dosage schedule and administration techniques

    b.   Surgical correction of anatomic abnormalities, if necessary to prevent recurrence

    c.   Follow-up urine cultures, typically done at monthly intervals for 3 months, then at 3-month intervals for the next 6 months

    d.   Preventive measures, such as good perineal hygiene (e.g., cleansing a girl from the urethra back toward the anus); avoiding irritants such as bubble baths and tight-fitting clothing; wearing cotton underwear rather than synthetic fabrics such as nylon; maintaining adequate fluid intake; voiding regularly and completely emptying the bladder with each urination; maintaining acidic urine by drinking cranberry juice or apple juice and taking ascorbic acid

    e.   The importance of voiding both before and immediately after intercourse (for a sexually active adolescent)

G. **Evaluation**

1. The child voids in a normal pattern and is asymptomatic.

2. Parents verbalize knowledge of rest, fluid intake, medications, prevention of recurrence, and follow-up care, including the scheduled intervals for obtaining urine specimens.

VI. Vesicoureteral reflux (VUR)

A. **Description: retrograde flow of bladder urine up the ureters during voiding**

B. **Etiology and incidence**

1. Primary reflux results from congenital abnormalities in insertion of ureters into the bladder.

2. Secondary reflux results from infection and ureterovesicular junction incompetency related to edema; it also may be related to neurogenic bladder or result from progressive dilation of ureters following surgical urinary diversion.

3. Familial factors apparently contribute to development of VUR.
4. Up to 40% of cases may be associated with UTIs.
5. Incidence is about 10 times greater in girls than in boys.
6. Black children have a much lower incidence than white children.

C. **Pathophysiology**
1. VUR occurs when the pressure of a full bladder forces urine into the upper urethra.
2. As pressure is decreased, urine refluxes into the bladder, predisposing the child to UTI.
3. VUR is classified according to the degree of reflux of urine from the bladder into upper genitourinary tract structures:
   a. Grade I: reflux into lower ureter only
   b. Grade II: ureteral and pelvic filling without calyceal dilation
   c. Grade III: ureteral and pelvic filling with mild calyceal blunting
   d. Grade IV: marked distention of pelvis, calyces, and ureter
   e. Grade V: massive reflux associated with severe hydronephrosis
4. VUR is an important cause of renal damage; refluxed urine ascending into the collecting tubules of nephrons gives microorganisms access to the renal parenchyma, initiating renal scarring.
5. If the amount of refluxed urine is large, the child feels an urge to void shortly after voiding previously. If the amount is small, it may remain in the bladder, causing urine stasis and predisposing the child to infection.

D. **Assessment findings**
1. Clinical manifestations may include:
   a. Dysuria
   b. Urinary frequency, urgency, and hesitancy
   c. Urine retention
   d. Cloudy, dark, or blood-tinged urine
2. Urinalysis may reveal RBCs in urine or pyuria.
3. Structural abnormalities may be detected on intravenous pyelography, voiding cystourethrography, and cystoscopy.

E. **Nursing diagnoses**
1. Altered Family Processes
2. Potential for Infection
3. Knowledge Deficit
4. Pain
5. Altered Patterns of Urinary Elimination
6. Urinary Retention

F. **Planning and implementation**
1. Administer or teach parents to administer prescribed medications, such as continuous low-dose antibacterial therapy, usually given as nightly dose of nitrofurantoin, trimethoprim, or sulfisoxazole.
2. Instruct the child to use a double-voiding technique in which voiding is followed by a 5-minute interval and then another attempt to void. Encourage parents to observe for complete voiding.
3. Provide support to the family by answering questions and providing information about diagnosis, tests, and treatments. As appropriate, explain that antireflux surgery, involving reimplantation of ureters, is indicated for prevention of renal damage secondary to recurrent infections.
4. Provide preoperative and postoperative care following antireflux surgery:
   a. Monitor quantity and quality of urine output.
   b. Observe and protect urinary drainage tubes (e.g., indwelling catheter, suprapubic catheter, ureteral stents).
   c. Administer analgesics for pain and antispasmodics for bladder spasms, as ordered.
   d. Provide routine postoperative care (e.g., dressing changes, vital sign monitoring, progressive diet, ambulation).
5. Provide patient and family teaching, covering:
   a. Medication dosage schedule and administration techniques
   b. Measures to help prevent UTIs, such as good perineal hygiene (e.g., cleansing a girl from the urethra back toward the anus); avoiding irritants such as bubble baths and tight-fitting clothing; wearing cotton underwear rather than synthetic fabrics such as nylon; maintaining adequate fluid intake; voiding regularly and completely emptying the bladder with each urination; maintaining acidic urine by drinking cranberry juice or apple juice and taking ascorbic acid
   c. The importance of voiding both before and immediately after intercourse (for a sexually active adolescent)

G. **Evaluation**
1. The child voids in a normal pattern and is asymptomatic.
2. Parents verbalize knowledge of rest, fluid intake, medications, prevention of recurrence, and follow-up care, including scheduled intervals for obtaining urine specimens.

VII. Nephrotic syndrome

A. Description: a symptom complex commonly accompanying glomerular disease and characterized by severe proteinuria leading to edema, hypoalbuminemia, and hypercholesterolemia

B. Etiology and incidence

1. Congenital nephrotic syndrome is caused by an autosomal recessive gene. The disorder does not respond to usual therapy, and the infant usually dies within the first year or two after birth.

2. Secondary nephrotic syndrome occurs after glomerular damage of known or presumed etiology (e.g., acute or chronic glomerulonephritis).

3. Minimal change disease, so named because the histologic changes seen on electron microscopy are limited to effacement of epithelial foot processes, accounts for 80% of cases of nephrotic syndrome in children aged 2 to 5 years. Onset often is preceded by a nonspecific viral illness occurring 4 to 8 days before onset.

4. Nephrotic syndrome occurs in 2 of 100,000 children per year.

5. It primarily affects preschoolers, with the most common age of onset between $1\frac{1}{2}$ and 3 years.

6. Incidence in boys is double that in girls.

C. Pathophysiology

1. Disturbance in the glomerular basement membrane leads to increased permeability to protein.

2. Proteins leak through glomerular membrane resulting in:

   a. Protein, especially albumin, in urine (hyperalbuminuria or proteinuria)

   b. Decreased serum albumin level (hypoalbuminemia)

3. Decreased colloidal osmotic pressure in capillaries leads to fluid shifting, causing fluid to accumulate in interstitial spaces and body cavities, particularly the abdomen (ascites).

4. Massive fluid shift leads to hypovolemia, which stimulates the renin-angiotensin system to increase secretion of ADH and aldosterone, leading to sodium and water reabsorption and further increased edema.

5. Hyperlipidemia occurs for as yet poorly understood reasons.

D. Assessment findings

1. Common clinical manifestations include:

   a. Weight gain

   b. Periorbital edema, ascites, peripheral edema, and edema in the labia or scrotum

   c. Respiratory difficulty secondary to pleural effusion

   d. Anorexia and diarrhea secondary to edema of the intestinal mucosa

        e.   Signs of malnourishment (may be masked by edema)
        f.   Dark, frothy urine
        g.   Oliguria
        h.   Pallor
        i.   Irritability
        j.   Fatigue, lethargy
        k.   Increased susceptibility to infection
    2.   Laboratory studies and diagnostic tests may reveal:
        a.   Massive proteinuria
        b.   Proteinemia
        c.   Elevated serum cholesterol
        d.   Effacement of epithelial cell foot processes seen on elec-
             tron microscopy
E.   **Nursing diagnoses**
    1.   Activity Intolerance
    2.   Body Image Disturbance
    3.   Altered Family Processes
    4.   High Risk for Fluid Volume Deficit
    5.   Altered Growth and Development
    6.   High Risk for Infection
    7.   Knowledge Deficit
    8.   Altered Nutrition: Less than Body Requirements
    9.   Impaired Tissue Integrity
F.   **Planning and implementation**
    1.   Administer prescribed medications as ordered, which may in-
         clude:
        a.   Prednisone at a dose of 2 mg/kg/day to reduce protein-
             uria
        b.   Immunosuppressant therapy (usually cyclophospha-
             mide) for a child failing to respond to steroid therapy
        c.   Spironolactone in combination with hydrochlorothia-
             zide to treat severe edema
        d.   A broad-spectrum antimicrobial agent to reduce the risk
             of infection
    2.   Assess for fluid volume deficit by monitoring for increased
         edema and taking daily measurements of abdominal girth,
         weight, intake and output, blood pressure, and pulse.
    3.   Prevent skin breakdown by checking areas of edema for skin
         breakdown, ensuring frequent position changes, using scrotal
         supports in boys, and providing good skin care.
    4.   Maintain or improve nutritional status by providing a high-
         protein, high-calorie diet. Offer small frequent meals of pre-
         ferred foods in a pleasant atmosphere.
    5.   Monitor for signs of infection, and take precautions to prevent
         infection. (The child is susceptible to secondary infections be-
         cause of the loss of immunoglobulin [a protein] in urine.)

6. Conserve the child's energy by enforcing bedrest and encouraging quiet activities.
7. Help improve the child's self-concept by providing positive feedback, emphasizing strengths, and encouraging social interaction and pursuit of interests.
8. Support the family by answering questions and providing information on diagnosis, tests, and treatments.
9. Provide patient and family teaching, covering:
   a. Signs and symptoms of relapse to watch for and report
   b. Urine testing for albumin
   c. Medication dosage schedule, administration techniques, and side effects
   d. Special dietary instructions
   e. Infection prevention measures
   f. Skin care

G. Evaluation
1. The child exhibits reduced edema and ascites, absence of skin breakdown and infection, and urine output within acceptable range.
2. Parents verbalize knowledge of the disorder, treatments, medications, home monitoring, diet instructions, and follow-up care.
3. The child resumes or maintains age-appropriate development and participates in age-appropriate activities as tolerated.

VIII. Acute poststreptococcal glomerulonephritis (APSGN)

A. Description: an acute, self-limiting autoimmune disease that follows group A beta-hemolytic streptococcal infection (e.g., pharyngitis, impetigo); the most common type of acute glomerulonephritis

B. Etiology and incidence
1. The precipitating streptococcal infection commonly occurs in the upper respiratory tract or skin.
2. Incidence varies with the particular environmental prevalence of specific streptococcal strains.
3. APSGN primarily affects early school-age children.
4. Incidence in boys is double that in girls.

C. Pathophysiology
1. Onset commonly occurs within 7 to 14 days after antecedent infection.
2. Some theorize that streptococcal infection is followed by release of a membranelike substance from the specific organism, which is antigenic in nature.
3. Antibody forms in response, and an immune-complex reaction occurs.
4. Immune complexes lodge in glomeruli, leading to inflamma-

tion and obstruction; subsequent decreased glomerular filtration and tissue injury results in excretion of red blood cells and casts.

5. Kidneys enlarge, and sodium and water are retained, leading to edema. Protein is excreted in urine.

6. Most children with APSGN recover completely; some, however, develop chronic disease.

7. Although rare, complications are associated with APSGN; the most serious include hypertensive encephalopathy, pulmonary edema, and acute renal failure.

D. **Assessment findings**

1. Common clinical manifestations include:
   a. Hematuria resembling tea or cola
   b. Oliguria
   c. Weight gain
   d. Periorbital and generalized edema
   e. Pallor
   f. Irritability
   g. Fatigue, lethargy
   h. Mild to moderately elevated blood pressure

2. Onset of complications can lead to serious sequelae if not detected and treated early; signs and symptoms of complications include:
   a. Markedly elevated blood pressure, headache, dizziness, abdominal discomfort and vomiting, and altered level of consciousness possibly progressing to seizures (hypertensive encephalopathy)
   b. Coughing, restlessness, paroxysmal nocturnal dyspnea (pulmonary edema)
   c. Severe oliguria or anuria (acute renal failure)

3. Urinalysis indicates the presence of protein, red blood cells, white blood cells, and casts with associated increase in urine specific gravity.

4. Other laboratory study data may reveal:
   a. Mild anemia and leukocytosis
   b. Positive antistreptolysin-O titers, indicating a recent streptococcal infection
   c. Elevated erythrocyte sedimentation rate
   d. Elevated BUN and creatinine levels

5. Renal biopsy, if done, shows an increased number of cells in each glomerulus.

E. **Nursing diagnoses**

1. Diversional Activity Deficit
2. Altered Family Processes
3. Fluid Volume Deficit

    4. Fluid Volume Excess
    5. High Risk for Infection
    6. Knowledge Deficit
    7. Altered Nutrition: Less than Body Requirements

F. Planning and implementation

1. Ensure early detection of complications by closely monitoring blood pressure and respiratory rate.
2. Assess fluid status by monitoring intake and output, taking and recording daily weights, and observing for edema.
3. Administer prescribed medications as ordered, which may include:
   a. IV diazoxide and furosemide to treat severe hypertension
   b. Methyldopa or hydralazine, usually in conjunction with reserpine or furosemide, to treat moderate hypertension
   c. Oral hydrochlorothiazide to treat mild hypertension
   d. Antibiotics to treat existing streptococcal infection
   e. Digitalis to combat circulatory overload
   f. Diuretic therapy, such as hydrochlorothiazide or furosemide, for severe edema
4. Stimulate the child by providing quiet, ambulatory play activities.
5. Maintain adequate caloric intake and good nutrition by planning meals around the child's dietary preferences and serving meals in a pleasant atmosphere.
6. Impose sodium, potassium, or fluid restrictions, as ordered.
7. Support the child and parents by explaining and answering questions about diagnosis, treatment, and home care.
8. Refer the child and family to a community health nurse for home visits, as needed, to help them adjust to home management.
9. Provide patient and family teaching, covering:
   a. The need for medical evaluation and culture of all sore throats
   b. Home care measures, including urinary testing, blood pressure monitoring, activity and diet instructions, infection-prevention measures, and signs and symptoms of potential complications to watch for and report (The child will require monitoring of urinalysis and blood pressure monthly for 6 months and then every 3 to 6 months until he or she has been symptom-free for 1 year.)
   c. Medication dosage schedule, administration techniques, and side effects
   d. The possible need for peritoneal dialysis or hemodialysis if renal failure occurs

G. **Evaluation**
  1. The child demonstrates improved urine output, maintains weight, adheres to diet restrictions, and is free from life-threatening complications.
  2. Parents verbalize knowledge of treatment, home care, and follow-up.

Bibliography

Brunner, L. S., and Suddarth, D. S. (1986). *Lippincott manual of nursing practice* (4th ed.). Philadelphia: J. B. Lippincott.

Mott, S. R., Fazekas, N. F., and James, S. R. (1990). *Nursing care of children and families* (2nd ed.). Menlo Park, CA: Addison-Wesley.

Waechter, E. H., Phillips, J., and Holaday, B. (1985). *Nursing care of children*. Philadelphia: J. B. Lippincott.

Whaley, L. F., and Wong, D. L. (1991). *Nursing care of infants and children* (4th ed.). St. Louis: C. V. Mosby.

Wilson, D., and Killion, D. (1989). Urinary tract infections in the pediatric patient. *Nurse Practitioner: Primary Health Care, 14* (7), 38, 41–42.

STUDY QUESTIONS

1. Why is maintenance of fluid and electrolyte balance is more critical in infants than in adults?
   a. Renal function is immature in infants.
   b. Cellular metabolism is less stable than in adults.
   c. The proportion of water in infants' bodies is less than that in adults.
   d. The daily fluid requirement per unit of body weight is less than that in adults.

2. The mother of an infant who is dehydrated and receiving parenteral fluid therapy asks if she is allowed to hold her baby. Which of the following would be the nurse's best response?
   a. "It's better not to move him to prevent dislodging the IV."
   b. "Dehydration promotes skin breakdown, so it's better to let him lie quietly in bed."
   c. "Only the nurses should hold him because of the IV."
   d. "Certainly. Let me show you how to lift him so that the IV isn't disturbed."

3. When caring for a child with nephrotic syndrome, the nurse's primary goal is to
   a. reduce excretion of urinary protein
   b. minimize edema and hypertension through bedrest and fluid restriction
   c. carefully assess for urinary alterations by monitoring intake and output and observing for hematuria
   d. reduce the risk of cardiac or renal failure by carefully monitoring fluid and electrolyte balance

4. Which of the following phrases best describes acute glomerulonephritis?
   a. a syndrome involving a gain in nonvolatile acids or a loss of base
   b. a disorder occurring after an antecedent streptococcal infection
   c. a disorder resulting in massive urinary protein loss
   d. a disorder involving a defect in the kidneys' ability to concentrate urine

5. After the physician directs the nurse to add potassium to a child's IV fluid, the nurse should first
   a. monitor apical pulse rate
   b. monitor blood pressure hourly
   c. monitor intake and output to assess kidney function
   d. monitor respiratory rate and depth

6. Sarah, aged 4 months, has had vomiting and diarrhea for the last day and a half. She is diagnosed as being dehydrated and is hospitalized for fluid replacement therapy. Her mother is upset and tells the nurse that Sara's illness is all her fault. Which of the following would be the nurse's most appropriate response?
   a. "Don't be so upset. Sara will be just fine."
   b. "Try not to cry in front of Sara, it may upset her."
   c. "Tell me why you think that Sara's illness is your fault."
   d. "Maybe next time you'll bring the baby to the doctor sooner."

7. Which of the following interventions would be most appropriate in evaluating total fluid losses and gains while Sarah is receiving parenteral fluid therapy?
   a. weighing the infant daily
   b. measuring the infant's height
   c. determining the infant's birth weight
   d. asking the mother how much weight the infant has lost since the onset of vomiting and diarrhea

8. The most common type of dehydration in children is
   a. isotonic
   b. hypertonic
   c. hypotonic
   d. nonspecific

9. Which of the following organisms is the most common cause of UTI in children?
   a. *Staphylococcus*
   b. *Klebsiella*
   c. *Pseudomonas*
   d. *Escherichia coli*

10. Which of the following instructions would *not* be included in a teaching plan for a child with UTI?
    a. the importance of avoiding irritants such as bubble bath, tight-fitting clothing, and nylon underwear
    b. the importance of completing the prescribed antibiotic regimen even though symptoms of UTI subside
    c. the need to return to the hospital for monthly intravenous pyelography
    d. the need to have the child void regularly and drink plenty of fluids

11. UTI in a child often is closely associated with
    a. toilet training
    b. increased fluid intake
    c. antecedent streptococcal infection
    d. vesicoureteral reflux

12. Which of the following signs and symptoms are characteristic of minimal change nephrotic syndrome?
    a. gross hematuria, proteinuria, fever
    b. hypertension, edema, hematuria
    c. poor appetite, proteinuria, edema
    d. hypertension, edema, proteinuria

13. For a child with recurring nephrotic syndrome, which of the following areas of potential disturbance should be a prime consideration when planning ongoing nursing care?
    a. muscle coordination
    b. sexual maturation
    c. intellectual development
    d. body image

14. When teaching parents about known antecedent infections in acute glomerulonephritis, which of the following should the nurse cover?
    a. herpes simplex
    b. scabies
    c. varicella (chickenpox)
    d. impetigo

ANSWER KEY

1. *Correct response: a*
   Immature renal function makes infants prone to overhydration and dehydration.
   - b. The metabolic rate is significantly higher in infants than in adults, but metabolism is not less stable.
   - c. Fluid volume is proportionately greater in infants than in adults.
   - d. Water requirements in terms of kilograms per day are proportionately greater in infants and children than in adults.

   Analysis/Physiologic/Analysis (Dx)

2. *Correct response: d*
   The nurse should encourage parents to hold their children and instruct them on IV care measures to enhance their confidence and comfort.
   - a and b. Infants with IVs should be held with care taken to watch IV.
   - c. Parents should be encouraged to participate in their child's care whenever appropriate.

   Application/Psychosocial/Evaluation

3. *Correct response: a*
   The primary objective of medical management is to reduce excretion of urinary protein and maintain a protein-free urine.
   - b. Hypertension does not occur in nephrotic syndrome, and fluid restrictions are not applicable.
   - c. Hematuria is not associated with nephrotic syndrome.
   - d. Cardiac failure is not a common complication of nephrotic syndrome.

   Analysis/Health promotion/Planning

4. *Correct response: b*
   Acute glomerulonephritis usually is preceded by an antecedent streptococcal infection occurring about 10 days before onset of symptoms.
   - a. This phrase describes metabolic acidosis.

   - c. This phrase describes nephrotic syndrome.
   - d. The kidneys' inability to concentrate urine is not the major etiologic factor in acute glomerulonephritis.

   Comprehension/Physiologic/Assessment

5. *Correct response: c*
   Potassium should not be added to IV fluid until adequate kidney function is restored.
   - a, b, and d. These measures are not related to potassium administration.

   Application/Safe care/Implementation

6. *Correct response: c*
   Often, parents feel responsible for their child's illness and may need teaching regarding the actual causes of dehydration.
   - a and b. These responses do not allow recognition of the mother's feelings.
   - d. This response is inappropriate and may increase the mother's feelings of guilt.

   Application/Psychosocial/Evaluation

7. *Correct response: a*
   Weight measurements accurately reflect total fluid losses and gains.
   - b. Height is not a significant measurement in evaluating dehydration.
   - c. The child's birth weight is not indicative of present fluid alterations.
   - d. This assessment may not provide accurate information.

   Analysis/Safe care/Implementation

8. *Correct response: a*
   Isotonic dehydration, the most common type of dehydration in children, involves balanced electrolyte and water deficits.
   - b and c. Hypertonic dehydration, occurring when water loss exceeds electrolyte loss, and hypotonic dehydration, occurring when electrolyte deficit

exceeds water loss, occur less often in children.

d. This is not applicable.

Comprehension/Physiologic/Analysis (Dx)

9. *Correct response: d*

This is the most common causative organism associated with UTI.

a, b, and c. Each of these organisms may cause UTI, but none is the most common causative agent.

Knowledge/Physiologic/Assessment

10. *Correct response: c*

Continued surveillance of urine cultures will be maintained, but monthly intravenous pyelographic testing is not necessary.

a, b, and d. These are appropriate aspects of the care plan.

Application/Health promotion/Evaluation

11. *Correct response: d*

An estimated 40% of children have vesicoureteral reflux associated with UTI.

a. Toilet training is not associated with UTI.

b. Decreased fluid intake is associated with UTI.

c. This type of infection is associated with acute glomerulonephritis, not UTI.

Analysis/Physiologic/Analysis (Dx)

12. *Correct response: c*

Clinical manifestations of nephrotic syndrome include loss of appetite due to edema of intestinal mucosa, proteinuria, and edema.

a. Gross hematuria is not associated with nephrotic syndrome. Fever would occur only if a concurrent infection existed.

b. Hypertension and hematuria are not associated with nephrotic syndrome.

d. Hypertension is not a symptom of nephrotic syndrome.

Analysis/Physiologic/Assessment

13. *Correct response: d*

Potential self-concept and body image disturbances related to changes in appearance and social isolation should be considered.

a. Muscle coordination is not affected.

b. Sexual maturation is not affected.

c. Intellectual development is not affected.

Application/Psychosocial/Planning

14. *Correct response: d*

Impetigo, a bacterial skin infection caused by streptococci, is known to commonly precede acute glomerulonephritis.

a. This is a viral condition not associated with acute glomerulonephritis.

b. This skin condition results from mite infestation and is not associated with acute glomerulonephritis.

c. This communicable disease is not associated with acute glomerulonephritis.

Knowledge/Physiologic/Planning

Respiratory Dysfunction

I. Essential concepts: respiratory anatomy and physiology

A. Development

1. Appearance of the laryngotracheal groove around the fourth week of gestation is closely followed by development of the larynx and trachea.

2. Development of the bronchial tree occurs predominantly between weeks 5 and 16 of gestation.

3. In weeks 16 through 24 of gestation, luminal and blood vessel growth occurs in bronchi and bronchioles.

4. Production of surfactant (a phospholipid protein complex that reduces surface tension of the alveoli, thereby decreasing tendency of alveoli to collapse during expiration) begins at about 24 weeks of gestation.

5. Two surface tension–reducing substances—lecithin and sphingomyelin—can be detected in amniotic fluid and are useful predictors of lung maturity; a lecithin/sphingomyelin ratio of 2:1 or greater indicates fetal lung maturity.

6. The presence of phosphatidylglycerol in amniotic fluid also indicates fetal lung maturity.

7. At birth, the lungs contain fluid; this is replaced by air as the infant begins respiration.

8. Lungs continue to develop after birth, and new alveoli are formed until about age 8 years. Thus, a child with pulmonary damage or disease at birth may regenerate new pulmonary tissue and eventually attain normal respiratory function.

B. Function

1. The major respiratory system function is to oxygenate arterial blood and remove carbon dioxide (CO_2) from venous blood, a process known as *gas exchange*.

2. Normal gas exchange depends on three processes:
   a. Ventilation: movement of gases from the atmosphere to the alveoli
   b. Diffusion: transfer of inhaled gases across the alveolar membrane to the lung
   c. Perfusion: movement of oxygenated blood from the lungs to body tissues

3. Control of respiration involves neural and chemical processes.

4. The neural system, comprising four parts located in the pons, medulla, and spinal cord, coordinates respiratory rhythm and regulates depth of respirations.

5. Chemical processes perform several vital functions, including:
   a. Regulate alveolar ventilation and maintain normal blood gas tension
   b. Guard against hypercapnia (excessive CO_2 in the blood) as well as hypoxia (reduced tissue oxygenation caused by

decreased arterial O_2 [PaO_2]). An increase in arterial CO_2 (PCO_2) stimulates ventilation; conversely, a decrease in PCO_2 inhibits ventilation

    c.   Help maintain respiration (through peripheral chemoreceptors) when hypoxia occurs

6. The normal functions of gas exchange, O_2 and CO_2 tension, and chemoreceptors are similar in children and adults. However, children respond differently from adults to respiratory disturbances; major areas of difference include:

    a.   Poor tolerance of nasal congestion—especially in infants, who are obligatory nose breathers until age 2 to 4 months

    b.   Increased susceptibility to ear infection due to shorter, broader, and more horizontally positioned eustachian tubes

    c.   Increased severity of respiratory symptoms due to smaller airway diameters

    d.   A total-body response to respiratory infection, with such symptoms as fever, vomiting, and diarrhea

II. Respiratory system overview

A. Assessment

1. Health history should determine whether the problem is acute or chronic, self-limiting, recurrent, or life threatening. Other important points include alleviating or exacerbating factors, effects of prior treatments, and family history of respiratory problems.

2. Physical assessment should focus on the following:

    a.   Alertness, changes in mental status

    b.   Activity level and complaints of fatigue

    c.   Skin color changes, particularly cyanosis

    d.   Respiratory rate and pattern, presence of apnea (Table 8–1)

    e.   Intracostal retractions: presence, severity, location

    f.   Adventitious lung sounds (wheezes, crackles, rhonchi)

    g.   Cough (productive or nonproductive)

TABLE 8–1.
Normal Respiratory Rates by Age

AGE	BREATHS/MIN
Birth to 6 months	30 to 50
6 months to 2 years	20 to 30
3 to 10 years	20 to 28
10 to 18 years	12 to 20

    h. Dyspnea, stridor, grunting, nasal flaring

B. **Laboratory studies and diagnostic tests**

  1. Radiologic evaluation may include:

    a. Chest radiograph, to visualize internal structures

    b. Lung scan, to visualize pulmonary blood flow

  2. Thoracentesis involves puncturing the chest wall with a needle to obtain a pleural fluid specimen for analysis.

  3. Pulmonary function tests include a series of measurements to evaluate ventilatory function.

  4. Blood gas analysis involves measuring PaO_2 and PCO_2 and blood pH.

C. **Psychosocial implications**

  1. Acute respiratory illness is frightening to both the child and parents, calling for effective crisis intervention by the nurse.

  2. Chronic respiratory illness in children often is accompanied by a history of acute crisis episodes and chronic stress.

  3. The respiratory-impaired child's developmental needs can best be met by maintaining optimal exercise and activity levels.

III. **Acute otitis media**

  A. **Description: inflammation of the middle ear**

  B. **Etiology and incidence**

    1. The most common causative organisms are *Haemophilus influenzae* and *Streptococcus pneumoniae*.

    2. Factors predisposing infants and young children to otitis media include:

      a. Anatomic features: short, horizontally positioned eustachian tubes

      b. Poorly developed cartilage lining, which makes eustachian tubes more likely to open prematurely

      c. Enlarged lymphoid tissue, which obstructs eustachian tube openings

      d. Immature humoral defense mechanisms, which increase the risk of infection

      e. Bottle-feeding an infant in the supine position, which promotes pooling of formula in the pharyngeal cavity

    3. Otitis media is one of most prevalent diseases of early childhood, with peak incidence occurring between ages 6 months and 2 years.

    4. Boys are affected more frequently than girls.

    5. Breast-fed infants have a lower incidence than formula-fed infants.

  C. **Pathophysiology**

    1. Eustachian tube dysfunction enables bacterial invasion of the middle ear and obstructs drainage of secretions.

    2. In most cases, antibiotic therapy resolves infection.

3. Myringotomy (an incision in the posterior inferior aspect of the tympanic membrane) may be necessary to promote drainage of exudate and release pressure.

4. Tympanoplasty ventilating tubes, or pressure-equalizing tubes, may be inserted into the middle ear to create an artificial auditory canal that equalizes pressure on both sides of the tympanic membrane.

D. Assessment findings

1. Otoscopy typically reveals:
   a. Tympanic membrane injection (sometimes bright red)
   b. Bulging tympanic membrane with no visible landmarks or light reflex
   c. Diminished tympanic membrane mobility
   d. Purulent discharge; culture and sensitivity testing is indicated

2. Audiometric testing establishes a baseline or detects any hearing loss secondary to recurring infection.

3. Health history and physical assessment may reveal one or more of following:
   a. Ear pain, pulling at ears
   b. Fever
   c. Irritability
   d. Loss of appetite
   e. Purulent drainage in external ear canal
   f. Nasal congestion
   g. Cough
   h. Vomiting and diarrhea

E. Nursing diagnoses

1. High Risk for Altered Body Temperature
2. Ineffective Breathing Patterns
3. High Risk for Fluid Volume Deficit
4. Altered Growth and Development
5. Knowledge Deficit
6. Pain
7. Impaired Tissue Integrity

F. Planning and implementation

1. Reduce fever by administering antipyretics, as prescribed, and by having the child remove extra clothing.

2. Relieve pain by administering analgesics, as prescribed, by helping the child limit chewing by offering liquid or soft foods, and by applying local heat or a cool compress over the affected ear.

3. Facilitate drainage by having the child lie with the affected ear in a dependent position.

4. Help prevent skin breakdown by keeping the external ear clean and dry. Apply zinc oxide or petrolatum to protect skin, if needed.

5. Assess for hearing loss and refer for audiology testing, if necessary.

6. Administer prescribed medications as ordered, which may include:
   a. Amoxicillin or ampicillin for 10 to 14 days
   b. Prophylactic antibiotic treatment with a combination of amoxicillin and sulfisoxazole, in a child with recurrent infection
   c. Analgesic or antipyretic drugs, such as acetaminophen
   d. Oral decongestants, such as pseudoephedrine hydrochloride, to relieve nasal congestion

7. Provide patient and family teaching, covering:
   a. Dosage, administration techniques, and possible side effects of all prescribed medications
   b. The importance of completing the entire prescribed regimen of antibiotics, even though symptoms may subside earlier
   c. Signs of hearing loss and the importance of audiology testing, if needed
   d. Preventive measures, such as holding the child upright for feedings, gentle nose blowing, blowing games, and chewing sugarless gum
   e. The need for follow-up care to check for persistent infection after completing the medication regimen (typically 10 to 14 days after initiation of treatment)

8. If the child requires surgical intervention, provide appropriate preoperative and postoperative teaching.

G. Evaluation

1. The child is afebrile and without pain, hears adequately, and takes antibiotics as prescribed.

2. Parents verbalize knowledge of diagnosis, treatment, home care, preventive measures, and follow-up measures.

3. Following tympanoplasty with ventilating tubes, parents verbalize the necessity of preventing water from entering the child's ear to reduce the risk of infection.

IV. Acute laryngotracheobronchitis (LTB)

A. Description: severe inflammation and obstruction of the upper airway; the most common form of croup

B. Etiology and incidence

1. LTB usually results from viral infection; common causative organisms include parainfluenza viruses, adenoviruses, respiratory syncytial virus, and influenza and measles viruses.

2. It also may be of bacterial origin (diphtheria or pertussis).

3. LTB affects boys more than girls, typically between ages 6 months and 3 years.

    4.   Incidence peaks in the winter months.

C. **Pathophysiology**
1. LTB usually is preceded by an upper respiratory infection, which proceeds to laryngitis and then descends into the trachea and sometimes the bronchi.
2. The flexible larynx of a young child is particularly susceptible to spasm, which may cause complete airway obstruction.
3. Profound airway edema may lead to obstruction and seriously compromised ventilation.

D. **Assessment findings**
1. Health history and physical examination typically reveal one or more of the following:
   a. Upper respiratory infection
   b. Inspiratory stridor
   c. Substernal and suprasternal retractions
   d. Barking cough, hoarseness
   e. Pallor or cyanosis
   f. Restlessness, irritability
   g. Low-grade fever
   h. Crackles, rhonchi, expiratory wheezing, and localized areas of diminished or absent breath sounds
2. Diagnosis is based on symptoms; LTB is differentiated from epiglottitis by a lateral neck radiograph showing a normal epiglottis.

E. **Nursing diagnoses**
1. Ineffective Airway Clearance
2. Anxiety
3. Ineffective Breathing Pattern
4. Family Coping: Potential for Growth
5. Altered Family Processes
6. High Risk for Fluid Volume Deficit
7. High Risk for Injury
8. Knowledge Deficit

F. **Planning and implementation**
1. Assess for airway obstruction by evaluating respiratory status: color, respiratory effort, evidence of fatigue, and vital signs. Keep emergency equipment at the bedside.
2. Increase the atmospheric humidity with either a mist tent or a cool mist vaporizer.
3. Administer oxygen therapy, as ordered, to alleviate hypoxia.
4. Administer IV fluids, as ordered, to ensure adequate hydration.
5. Administer prescribed medications as ordered, which may include:
   a. Racemic epinephrine via nebulizer

          b.   Antibiotics, if LTB is bacterial in origin

          c.   Corticosteroids to reduce inflammation (*Note:* This therapy is controversial.)

6. Help reduce the child's anxiety by maintaining a quiet environment, promoting rest and relaxation, and minimizing intrusive procedures. Encourage parents to bring a favorite toy for the child.

7. Support parents by answering questions and explaining all treatments and procedures. Encourage them to be present and participate in their child's care, as appropriate.

8. Provide patient and family teaching, covering:

    a.   Medication dosages, administration techniques, and possible side effects

    b.   Symptoms of croup to watch for and report

    c.   How to manage home vaporizer or mist treatments (e.g., when the child awakens with barking cough and other symptoms of croup, put him or her in the bathroom and run hot water to produce steam, which may help reduce symptoms)

G. **Evaluation**

1. The child exhibits no signs of respiratory distress and is afebrile and well hydrated.

2. Parents verbalize understanding of diagnosis, treatment, home care, and follow-up.

V. Epiglottitis

A. **Description: acute inflammation of the epiglottis that obstructs the airway**

B. **Etiology and incidence**

1. Epiglottitis most commonly results from infection with *H influenzae* type B; other possible causative organisms include pneumococci and group A streptococci.

2. Peak incidence occurs between ages 3 and 6 years.

C. **Pathophysiology**

1. Acute epiglottitis often is preceded by a minor upper respiratory infection of several days' duration.

2. Untreated, it may rapidly progress to complete upper airway obstruction.

3. Progressive obstruction results in hypoxia, hypercapnia, and acidosis, closely followed by decreased muscle tone, altered level of consciousness, and, if obstruction becomes complete, sudden death.

4. After diagnosis is confirmed, endotracheal intubation or tracheostomy typically is performed to maintain a patent airway. Swelling usually decreases after 24 hours, and the child generally is extubated by the third day.

5. Infection usually is treated with antibiotics for 7 to 10 days, and an IV line is started to maintain adequate hydration and enable antibiotic administration.

D. Assessment findings

1. Health history and physical assessment typically reveal one or more of the following:
   a. Sudden onset of symptoms, often preceded by upper respiratory infection
   b. Sore throat, pain on swallowing, refusal to eat or drink due to dysphagia
   c. High fever
   d. Characteristic positioning: sitting upright, leaning forward, with chin outthrust, mouth open, and tongue protruding (tripod position)
   e. Drooling
   f. Irritability, restlessness
   g. Wheezy inspiratory stridor and snoring expiratory sound; froglike croaking sound on inspiration (not hoarseness)
   h. Suprasternal and substernal retractions
   i. Tachycardia, thready pulse
   j. Late signs of hypoxia: listlessness, cyanosis, bradycardia, decreased respiratory rate with decreased aeration
2. On inspection, the child's throat appears red and inflamed, with a large, cherry-red, edematous epiglottis. (*Note:* When symptoms of epiglottitis occur, throat inspection should be done only by an otolaryngologist or other properly trained personnel, and equipment should be readily available for performing emergency endotracheal intubation or tracheostomy since examination may precipitate complete airway obstruction.)
3. Laboratory study and diagnostic test results may include:
   a. Lateral neck film showing epiglottal enlargement, which confirms diagnosis
   b. Elevated white blood cell count and increased bands and neutrophils on differential count
   c. Identification of causative bacteria through blood cultures

E. Nursing diagnoses

1. Ineffective Airway Clearance
2. Anxiety
3. High Risk for Altered Body Temperature
4. Altered Family Processes
5. High Risk for Fluid Volume Deficit
6. High Risk for Infection
7. High Risk for Injury

8. Knowledge Deficit
9. Pain
F. Planning and implementation
1. Closely monitor respiratory status to ensure airway patency. If the child presents with symptoms of epiglottitis, ensure that throat examination is performed by a trained professional with emergency equipment on hand.
2. After the child is intubated, monitor closely and maintain a patent airway. Suction as needed, and provide oxygen therapy as ordered.
3. Observe closely for signs of respiratory distress after extubation.
4. Monitor for signs and symptoms of infection.
5. Ensure adequate hydration by monitoring IV fluid administration and keeping strict intake and output records.
6. Help relieve anxiety by maintaining a calm relaxing atmosphere, limiting intrusive procedures, encouraging parents to bring in a security object from home, providing age-appropriate play activities, assisting the child to the most comfortable position for breathing before intubation, and administering a sedative agent, as ordered, while the child is intubated.
7. Support the family by answering their questions and providing information about diagnosis and treatment. Allow parents to be present and to participate in their child's care, as appropriate.
8. Administer prescribed medication as ordered, which may include:
   a. Ampicillin and chloramphenicol IV for the first few days, followed by PO for 3 to 7 days.
   b. Sedation with diazepam, pentobarbital, or chloral hydrate while the child is being intubated
   c. Corticosteroids to reduce edema (*Note:* This therapy is controversial.).
9. Provide patient and family teaching, covering:
   a. Home care and follow-up
   b. Recommendations that all children over age 2 years receive haemophilus type B polysaccharide vaccine, to reduce the incidence of epiglottitis
G. Evaluation
1. The child displays no signs of respiratory distress and is afebrile and well hydrated.
2. Parents verbalize understanding of diagnosis, treatment, home care, and follow-up.

VI. Pneumonia
A. Description
1. Acute inflammation of the lung parenchyma (the respiratory

bronchioles, alveolar ducts and sacs, and alveoli) that impairs gas exchange.

2. Pneumonia is classified according to etiologic agent (see section VI.B).

3. Pneumonia also may be classified according to location and extent of involvement as:

   a. *Lobar pneumonia*, involving a large segment of one or more lung lobes

   b. *Bronchopneumonia*, beginning in the terminal bronchioles and involving nearby lobules

   c. *Interstitial pneumonia*, confined to the alveolar walls and peribronchial and interlobular tissues

B. Etiology and incidence

1. Pneumonia most commonly results from infection with viruses, bacteria, or mycoplasmas, or from aspiration of foreign substances. (This entry deals primarily with viral and bacterial pneumonia.)

2. Viral pneumonia is the most common type, with respiratory syncytial virus the most common causative organism. Others include influenza and parainfluenza viruses, psittacosis, rhinovirus, and adenovirus.

3. Major causative organisms in bacterial pneumonia include pneumococci, streptococci, and staphylococci.

   a. Pneumococci: the most common cause of lobar pneumonia; most often affects children age 1 to 4, with highest incidence in late winter or early spring

   b. Streptococci: infection usually results in lobular pneumonia; commonly occurs as complication of influenza or measles

   c. Staphylococci: the most common cause of bronchopneumonia; most often affects children under age 2 years, with highest incidence in winter

4. Pneumonia occurs in about 4% of children under age 4; incidence decreases with advancing age.

C. Pathophysiology

1. Pneumonia typically begins as a mild upper respiratory infection.

2. As the disorder progresses, parenchymal inflammation occurs.

3. Bacterial pneumonia most often causes lobular involvement and sometimes consolidation; viral pneumonia, inflammation of interstitial tissue.

D. Assessment findings

1. Common clinical manifestations of *viral pneumonia* include:

   a. Signs and symptoms varying from mild fever, slight cough, and malaise to high fever, severe cough, and prostration

      b.   Cough nonproductive or productive of whitish sputum

      c.   Rhonchi or fine crackles

2.   In *pneumococcal pneumonia*, clinical manifestations vary with age and commonly include:

      a.   Infants: vomiting, seizures, poor feeding, fretfulness, fever, stiff neck, bulging anterior fontanel, circumoral cyanosis, respiratory distress, diminished breath sounds and rales, pleural friction rub

      b.   Older children: headache, abdominal or chest pain, high fever with chills, intermittent drowsiness and restlessness, tachycardia, tachypnea, hacking nonproductive cough, expiratory grunting, circumoral cyanosis, diminished breath sounds, tactile and vocal fremitus, tubular breath sounds and disappearance of crackles (indicating consolidation), moist crackles and cough productive of copious blood-tinged mucus (as the disease resolves)

3.   Clinical findings in *streptococcal pneumonia* are similar to those of pneumococcal pneumonia, with sudden onset of:

      a.   Fever and chills

      b.   Signs of respiratory distress

      c.   Listlessness or extreme prostration

      d.   Rales

4.   Clinical findings in *staphylococcal pneumonia* may include:

      a.   High fever

      b.   Cough

      c.   Tachypnea

      d.   Cyanosis

      e.   Anorexia

      f.   Dyspnea

      g.   Subcostal and sternal retractions

      h.   Grunting respirations

      i.   Nasal discharge

      j.   Lethargy

      k.   Abdominal distention

      l.   Diminished breath sounds, crackles, and rhonchi

      m.   As the child's condition deteriorates, signs of empyema (purulent fluid in the pleural cavity) or pneumothorax

5.   Radiologic findings may include:

      a.   Viral pneumonia: diffuse or patchy infiltration with peribronchial distribution

      b.   Pneumococcal pneumonia: areas of consolidation (usually patchy) in one or more lobes

      c.   Streptococcal pneumonia: disseminated infiltration

      d.   Staphylococcal pneumonia: patchy clouding in one or more lobes

6.   Laboratory study results commonly include:

a. Elevated white blood cell count
b. Identification of the causative organism through blood cultures
c. In streptococcal pneumonia, positive antistreptolysin-O titer

7. Diagnostic thoracentesis may be performed if fluid in the pleural cavity is suspected.

E. **Nursing diagnoses**
1. Activity Intolerance
2. Ineffective Airway Clearance
3. High Risk for Altered Body Temperature
4. Ineffective Breathing Pattern
5. Altered Family Processes
6. Potential Fluid Volume Deficit
7. Knowledge Deficit
8. Altered Nutrition: Less than Body Requirements
9. Pain

F. **Planning and implementation**
1. Assess for respiratory distress by monitoring vital signs and respiratory status.
2. Ease respiratory effort by:
   a. Administering oxygen therapy as ordered
   b. Creating a high humidity atmosphere using a humidifier or mist tent
   c. Performing chest physiotherapy and postural drainage
   d. Using incentive spirometry
   e. Suctioning as needed
   f. Changing position frequently and elevating the head of the bed
3. Help prevent dehydration by ensuring adequate oral or IV fluid intake; evaluate fluid status by monitoring intake and output and weighing the child daily.
4. Promote rest by maintaining bedrest and organizing nursing care to minimize disturbances.
5. Ensure adequate nutrition by providing desirable high-calorie foods served in a pleasant, relaxed atmosphere.
6. Support the child's family by answering questions and explaining all treatments and procedures. Encourage parents to participate in their child's care, as appropriate.
7. Administer prescribed medications as ordered, which may include:
   a. Penicillin G to treat pneumococcal and streptococcal pneumonia
   b. Synthetic penicillin to treat staphylococcal pneumonia
   c. Antipyretics to reduce fever

8. Provide patient and family teaching, covering:
   a. Recommendations for the pneumococcal polysaccharide vaccine for children over age 2 years who are at risk for acquiring pneumococcal infection
   b. Home care and follow-up measures

G. Evaluation

1. The child exhibits no signs of respiratory distress and is afebrile and well hydrated.
2. Parents verbalize understanding of diagnosis, treatment, home care, and follow-up measures.

VII. Asthma

A. Description: a chronic, episodic, reversible obstructive disorder characterized by airway narrowing due to bronchospasms, increased mucous secretion, and mucosal edema

B. Etiology and incidence

1. Asthma most commonly results from allergic hyperresponsiveness of the trachea and bronchi to irritants.
2. Common precipitants include respiratory viral infection, air pollution, animal danders, dust, molds, pollens, certain foods, exercise, rapid changes in environmental temperature, and physical or psychological stress.
3. A familial tendency has been observed.
4. The most common chronic lung disease in children, asthma, affects between 2.5% and 5% of all children.
5. Before puberty, asthma affects twice as many boys as girls; at puberty, the incidence in girls increases.
6. Asthma tends to be more severe in younger children; improvement often occurs in adolescence.
7. Incidence is greater in urban dwellers.

C. Pathophysiology

1. Obstruction due to edema of the respiratory mucosa causes bronchiolar narrowing, secretion accumulation, and bronchial and bronchiolar smooth muscle spasm. This leads to air trapping, characteristic wheezing, and respiratory distress.
2. If not treated promptly, status asthmaticus—acute, severe, prolonged asthma attack that does not respond to usual treatment—may result, requiring hospitalization.

D. Assessment findings

1. Health history and physical examination will reveal one or more of the following:
   a. Dyspnea, air hunger
   b. Anxiety
   c. Coughing
   d. Wheezing, particularly expiratory
   e. Fatigue

      f.   Tachypnea

      g.   Complaints of chest tightness

      h.   Costal retractions

      i.   Cyanosis

      j.   Diaphoresis

  2. Improvement in respiratory function following use of a bronchodilator points to a diagnosis of asthma.

  3. Skin sensitivity tests may identify the causative allergen.

E. **Nursing diagnoses**

  1. Activity Intolerance

  2. Ineffective Airway Clearance

  3. Anxiety

  4. Body Image Disturbance

  5. Ineffective Breathing Pattern

  6. Altered Family Processes

  7. High Risk for Fluid Volume Deficit

  8. Altered Health Maintenance

  9. Health-Seeking Behaviors

  10. High Risk for Infection

  11. High Risk for Injury

  12. Knowledge Deficit

  13. Noncompliance

  14. Self-Esteem Disturbance

F. **Planning and implementation**

  1. Increase respiratory effectiveness by:

      a.   Administering medications as ordered (see section VII.F.6)

      b.   Elevating the head of the patient's bed

      c.   Administering oxygen therapy as needed

      d.   Performing chest physiotherapy and suctioning as needed

  2. Assess respiratory status, closely evaluating breathing patterns and monitoring vital signs.

  3. In an acute attack:

      a.   Administer prescribed medication, as ordered, which may include inhaled bronchodilators, epinephrine or terbutaline SC, or aminophylline IV.

      b.   Assess respiratory and cardiovascular status closely.

      c.   Monitor arterial blood gas results for Pco_2 and Pao_2 (Table 8–2).

      d.   Administer oxygen—or, in severe cases, provide ventilatory assistance—as needed.

      e.   Administer IV fluid therapy, as ordered, to prevent dehydration.

  4. Promote rest by scheduling nursing activities to allow for pe-

TABLE 8–2.
Normal Arterial Blood Gas Values by Age

PARAMETER	NORMAL VALUE
PO_2	At birth: 8–24 mmHg Age 1 day: 45–95 mmHg Thereafter: 83–108 mmHg (decreases with age)
PCO_2	Neonate: 27–40 mmHg Infant: 27–41 mmHg Thereafter: Male: 35–48 mmHg Female: 32–45 mmHg
pH	Premature neonate (48 hours after birth): 7.35–7.5 Term neonate (at birth): 7.11–7.36 Age 1 day: 7.29–7.45 Thereafter: 7.35–7.45

riods of rest and encouraging activities appropriate to the child's tolerance level.

5. Prevent dehydration by encouraging oral fluid intake or monitoring IV fluid therapy, carefully monitoring intake and output, recording daily weights, and assessing for signs of dehydration.

6. Administer prescribed medications as ordered, which may include:

   a. Methylxanthines, especially theophylline and aminophylline, to provide bronchodilation for both daily maintenance and acute attacks

   b. Sympathomimetics (beta-adrenergics), to promote bronchodilation in acute attacks: epinephrine, isoetharine, isoproterenol, metaproterenol, albuterol, terbutaline

   c. Cromolyn sodium, administered via inhaler four times per day as a prophylactic agent

   d. Corticosteroids, to reduce airway inflammation during acute attacks or as prophylactic therapy

   e. Antihistamines, to decrease postnasal drip-induced cough that may lead to bronchospasm

   f. Antibiotics, if respiratory tract infection is present

7. Monitor for effectiveness and side effects of medication therapy.

8. Help the child and family identify possible precipitating factors in asthma attacks, and discuss possible ways to limit exposure to these factors.

9. Explain the possible use of hyposensitization injections to prevent allergic reactions to known precipitants.

10. Teach the child and family to prevent respiratory infection by avoiding exposure to persons with infection and maintaining good hygiene and sound health practices.

11. Encourage physical activity based on the child's tolerance level. Explain that the child may require pretreatment with bronchodilator inhalation before exercising.

12. Encourage chest physiotherapy, breathing exercises, and inhalation therapy to help strengthen respiratory musculature and develop more efficient breathing patterns.

13. Help the child cope with poor self-esteem by encouraging him or her to ventilate feelings and concerns, listening actively as the child does so, focusing on his or her personal strengths and helping him or her assume an active role in identifying both the positive and negative aspects of his or her situation.

14. Help alleviate the child's anxiety by remaining calm and staying with him or her in emergency and anxiety-producing situations. Provide explanations of and preparation for all treatments and procedures.

15. Support the family by answering questions, providing reassurance, explaining treatments and procedures, and apprising them of their child's condition.

16. Encourage family members to participate in the child's care when hospitalized, as appropriate.

17. Encourage family members to express their feelings and concerns in acute situations and related to asthma's chronic nature and its effects on family functioning. Assess the family to identify maladaptive behaviors or undue stress; refer for counseling, as needed.

18. Discuss the need for periodic pulmonary function tests to evaluate and guide therapy and monitor the course of the disease.

19. Provide patient and family teaching, covering:
    a. Diagnosis
    b. Ways to identify and prevent contact with known precipitants of asthma attacks
    c. The importance of promoting overall physical and psychological well-being in the child
    d. The need for adequate hydration to keep secretions from thickening
    e. Physical activities commensurate with the child's capabilities
    f. Breathing exercises, inhalation therapy, and chest physiotherapy
    g. Dosage, administration, and side effects of all prescribed medications
    h. Signs and symptoms of acute asthma attack and appropriate treatments

20. Refer the family to the Asthma and Allergy Foundation of America or the American Lung Association for further information about home management.

G. **Evaluation**
1. The child exhibits a normal breathing pattern with lungs clear on auscultation and is afebrile and well hydrated.
2. Parents verbalize knowledge of the above-listed aspects of patient and family teaching (see section VII.F.19), as well as knowledge of follow-up care.

VIII. Cystic fibrosis

A. **Description: a chronic inherited disorder of the exocrine glands characterized by abnormally thick respiratory secretions and other multisystem affects**

B. **Etiology and incidence**
1. Cystic fibrosis is inherited as an autosomal recessive trait.
2. The most common lethal inherited disease affecting whites, cystic fibrosis occurs in about 1 in 1,600 live births; incidence drops to 1 in 17,000 live births in American blacks, Native Americans, and Asians.
3. Incidence is equal in both sexes.
4. About half of affected children die by age 16 years; mean life expectancy is 20 years.

C. **Pathophysiology**
1. The underlying defect in cystic fibrosis likely is related to protein or enzyme alteration.
2. Generalized exocrine gland dysfunction results in increased viscosity of mucous secretions.
3. Abnormally viscous secretions affect the normal function of multiple organ systems, including:
   a. Bronchi, manifested by chronic bronchial pneumonia and generalized obstructive emphysema
   b. Small intestine, manifested by intestinal obstruction and failure of a newborn to pass meconium
   c. Pancreatic ducts, manifested by malabsorption syndrome
   d. Bile ducts, manifested by biliary cirrhosis and portal hypertension
   e. Salivary and sweat glands, resulting in increased sodium and chloride excretion; parents sometimes report that their child "tastes salty" when kissed
   f. Autonomic nervous system, marked by hyperactivity

D. **Assessment findings**
1. Clinical manifestations vary in severity and time of emergence; they may be apparent at birth or may take years to develop.
2. Respiratory manifestations commonly include:
   a. Wheezing, dyspnea, and dry nonproductive cough

b.   As the disease progresses, atelectasis and generalized obstructive emphysema due to mucoid obstruction in
small airways, producing the characteristic features of
barrel-shaped chest, cyanosis, and clubbing of fingers
and toes

c.   Chronic sinusitis; bronchitis; bronchopneumonia; or
ear, nose, and throat problems

3.   Gastrointestinal effects may include:

a.   Meconium ileus in a newborn

b.   Later, obstruction of pancreatic ducts and absence of
pancreatic enzymes (trypsin, amylase, and lipase) leading
to malabsorption syndrome, marked by chronic diarrhea
with large, frothy, foul-smelling stools; abdominal cram-
ping and abdominal distention; foul-smelling flatus;
weight loss despite increased appetite; and an overall
malnourished and vitamin-deficient state

c.   Cirrhosis, possibly leading to portal hypertension with
resultant splenomegaly and esophageal varices

4.   Reproductive system effects may include:

a.   Females: decreased fertility apparently due to increased
viscosity of cervical mucous, which blocks the entry of
sperm

b.   Males: sterility, due to blockage of the vas deferens with
abnormal secretions, which prevents sperm formation

5.   Cardiovascular system manifestations may include:

a.   Cor pulmonale, right-sided heart enlargement and congestive heart failure resulting from obstruction of pulmonary blood flow

b.   Signs and symptoms of hyponatremia, necessitating
rapid IV replacement to prevent circulatory collapse

6.   Laboratory study and diagnostic tests results may include:

a.   Elevated sodium and chloride levels detected on the
sweat test

b.   Absence of pancreatic enzyme activity, helping to confirm diagnosis

c.   Steatorrhea detected on stool analysis

d.   Evidence of generalized obstructive emphysema on
chest radiograph

7.   Early identification of family history may be helpful in initiating early diagnosis and treatment.

E.   Nursing diagnoses

1.   High Risk for Activity Intolerance
2.   Ineffective Airway Clearance
3.   Ineffective Breathing Pattern
4.   Altered Family Processes
5.   Impaired Gas Exchange

      6. Anticipatory Grieving
      7. High Risk for Infection
      8. Knowledge Deficit
      9. Altered Nutrition: Less than Body Requirements
    10. Sleep Pattern Disturbance
    11. Self-Esteem Disturbance

F. Planning and implementation

1. Encourage pulmonary hygiene measures to aid sputum expectoration, such as chest physiotherapy, postural drainage, aerosol treatments with bronchodilators, and breathing exercises.
2. Monitor respiratory status by evaluating breathing patterns and vital signs.
3. Encourage adequate nutrition; serve desired foods in a pleasant, relaxed atmosphere. (The prescribed diet typically is high in calories and protein, with fats as tolerated and increased salt intake during hot weather or febrile periods.)
4. Assess nutritional status by maintaining calorie counts, monitoring intake and output, and recording daily weights.
5. Provide support for the child's family at diagnosis and throughout the course of the disorder.
6. Administer prescribed medications as ordered, which may include:
   a. Aminoglycosides such as amikacin sulfate, gentamicin, and tobramycin, and penicillins such as carbenicillin, ticarcillin, and piperacillin to prevent or treat infection
   b. Isoproterenol to produce bronchodilation
   c. Pancreatic enzymes in the form of pancrease and Cotazym-S
   d. Vitamin supplements and iron
   e. Medium-chain triglycerides as diet supplements
7. Administer pancreatic enzymes with food. Be sure to carefully wipe the child's lips and face after administration because of the substance's caustic nature.
8. Provide and encourage activities according to the child's developmental level and physical capabilities.
9. Monitor for signs of infection; prevent infection by promoting good health and hygiene practices as well as limiting exposure to persons with respiratory infections.
10. Promote adequate rest by clustering nursing activities and scheduling regular rest periods.
11. Help the child maintain a positive self-concept by actively listening, encouraging him or her to ventilate feelings, emphasizing his or her personal strengths, and helping him or her identify both the positive and negative aspects of his or her situation.
12. As necessary, assist in arranging for a tutor or other help with schoolwork while the child is hospitalized.

13. Support the family by encouraging ventilation of feelings concerning the child's disease and long-term implications. Refer to counseling, support groups, and other resources such as a dietitian, social worker, physical therapist, tutor, or chaplain as needed.
14. Provide patient and family teaching, covering:
    a. Diagnosis, disease process, long-term implications, and chronic nature
    b. The importance of good pulmonary hygiene, including instruction on postural drainage, chest percussion, breathing exercises, and inhalation treatments
    c. Dosage, administration, and side effects of prescribed medications
    d. Special dietary instructions

G. Evaluation
1. The child exhibits improved respiratory status, is afebrile and expresses no pain or discomfort, and tolerates the prescribed diet and gains weight.
2. Parents verbalize knowledge of the above-listed aspects of patient and family teaching (see section VIII.F.14), as well as follow-up instructions.

IX. Bronchopulmonary dysplasia (BPD)
A. Description: a chronic pulmonary disease of infancy marked by the need for oxygen therapy beyond 28 days after birth
B. Etiology and incidence
1. The cause of BPD is unknown although several risk factors have been identified, and it has been attributed to iatrogenic causes—therapies used to treat lung disease.
2. BPD most commonly affects very low birth weight infants with lung disorders (e.g., hyaline membrane disease, meconium aspiration, persistent pulmonary hypertension). For instance, it occurs in 10% to 15% of very low birth weight infants treated for hyaline membrane disease.
3. A premature infant who is mechanically ventilated and receives high concentrations of oxygen is at greatest risk.

C. Pathophysiology
1. Positive inspiratory pressures and high concentrations of oxygen can injure the alveolar sacules and small airway epithelium, leading to fibrosis of these structures.
2. Areas of cystic foci and atelectasis appear in the lung parenchyma.
3. Airway smooth muscle hypertrophy results in bronchospasm, and endothelial cell damage causes interstitial edema.
4. These changes further aggravate airway obstruction and necessitate long-term oxygen therapy.
5. Cor pulmonale is the leading cause of death in infants with BPD.

D. Assessment findings

1. BPD occurs in four stages, each with distinctive clinical manifestations.

2. Stage I, acute respiratory distress, occurs in infants age 2 to 3 days and is manifested by:
   a. Tachypnea
   b. Grunting
   c. Retractions
   d. Cyanosis

3. Stage II, pulmonary regeneration, occurs between ages 4 and 10 days and is characterized by:
   a. Slow improvement of symptoms
   b. Ability to be weaned from peak inspiratory pressures, sometimes even to hood oxygen, followed by a drop in lung compliance and increased difficulty in ventilation

4. Stage III, transition to chronic disease, occurs between ages 10 and 30 days in an infant surviving stage II. Clinical manifestations include:
   a. Stable oxygen and ventilator requirements
   b. Improvement or deterioration in condition

5. Stage IV, chronic lung disease, develops in infants after age 1 month. Characteristics include:
   a. Oxygen dependence for several months
   b. Gradual improvement in condition or development of complications such as right-sided congestive heart failure, pulmonary hypertension, and eventually cor pulmonale

E. Nursing diagnoses

1. Activity Intolerance
2. Ineffective Airway Clearance
3. High Risk for Altered Body Temperature
4. Ineffective Breathing Pattern
5. Altered Family Processes
6. High Risk for Fluid Volume Deficit
7. Knowledge Deficit
8. Altered Nutrition: Less than Body Requirements
9. Pain

F. Planning and Implementation

1. Provide respiratory support through continuous mechanical ventilation and administration of oxygen via hood, nasal catheter, or cannula.

2. Support safe weaning from oxygen as indicated by the infant's clinical manifestations:
   a. Maintenance of normal arterial blood gases or PaO_2 and PCO_2 levels

    b.   No increase in the work of breathing

    c.   Normal growth and development

3. Provide chest physiotherapy (postural drainage with percussion and vibration) consistent with the infant's tolerance level, as monitored by transcutaneous oxygen levels with each position change and a determination of the time it takes for the infant to return to pretreatment oxygen saturation levels.

4. Periodically change the infant's position from side to side and front to back to improve bronchial drainage and promote expansion and ventilation of all lung fields.

5. Protect the compromised infant from infection by maintaining strict asepsis.

6. Promote optimal nutrition without overhydration by spacing feedings and closely monitoring fluid intake.

7. Teach parents and other family members about the disease process, complications, and treatments, providing answers to their questions and reinforcing information provided by the physician and other members of the health care team.

8. As part of the preparation for home care, encourage parents to become involved in their infant's care in the hospital, as appropriate.

9. Provide the opportunity for parents to express their feelings and concerns.

10. Participate with other health care team members in preparing the family for home care.

G. **Evaluation**

1. The infant's supplemental oxygen requirements are stabilized, or supplemental oxygen no longer is required.

2. Parents verbalize an understanding of diagnosis, treatments, home care, and follow-up measures.

3. The infant is adequately incorporated into the family unit.

Bibliography

Fischbach, F. (1988). *Manual of laboratory and diagnostic tests* (3rd ed.). Philadelphia: J. B. Lippincott.

Mott, S. R., Fazekas, N. F., and James, S. R. (1985). *Nursing care of children and families*. Menlo Park, CA: Addison-Wesley.

Waechter, E. H., Phillips, J., and Holaday, B. (1985). *Nursing care of children*. Philadelphia: J. B. Lippincott.

Whaley, L. F. and Wong, D. L. (1991). *Nursing care of infants and children* (4th ed.). St. Louis: C. V. Mosby.

STUDY QUESTIONS

1. One factor that predisposes infants and young children to the development of otitis media is the unique anatomic features of the
   a. nasopharynx
   b. eustachian tubes
   c. external ear canals
   d. tympanic membranes

2. Which of the following nursing interventions for initial contact with a child with suspected epiglottitis would be *most* appropriate?
   a. Perform an in-depth assessment of the child's physiologic status, including rectal temperature measurement since high fever is a common indication of epiglottitis.
   b. Examine the child's throat with a tongue depressor and flashlight to check for redness and swelling.
   c. Prepare to administer aerosol racemic epinephrine to decrease airway resistance.
   d. Maintain the child in the most comfortable position for breathing, and prepare for a lateral neck radiograph.

3. Which of the following drug groups is most important in treating an acute asthma attack in a young child?
   a. beta-adrenergics, such as epinephrine
   b. corticosteroids, such as methylprednisolone
   c. antihistamines
   d. antibiotics, such as ampicillin

4. After a parent teaching session about proper medication administration for a child with cystic fibrosis, which of the following statements made by a parent would indicate that the teaching session was effective?
   a. "Pancrease should be given with all meals and snacks."
   b. "Pancrease is an antibiotic."
   c. "A pancrease dose should never be skipped even if the child is not eating."

d. "A pancrease dose should be skipped if the child is passing frequent, bulky stools."

5. Raymond, aged 2 years, is brought to the ambulatory care clinic by his mother, who states he has been irritable and febrile throughout the night. Physical assessment reveals a bright red, bulging tympanic membrane with diminished mobility and no visible landmarks or light reflex. Which of the following medical approaches would be most appropriate for Raymond?
   a. Forgo treatment because his middle ear is only mildly infected.
   b. Administer a decongestant because the tympanic membrane is bulging.
   c. Administer antibiotic therapy for 10 to 14 days.
   d. Refer Raymond to an otolaryngologist for a myringotomy.

6. A surgical myringotomy with placement of pressure-equalizer tubes is indicated to treat otitis media when
   a. there is evidence of severe pain requiring immediate relief
   b. medical intervention proves unsuccessful in preventing recurrent infections
   c. the child is critically ill
   d. the child is immunocompromised

7. A nurse developing a care plan for a toddler hospitalized with croup understands that an important psychosocial consideration involves encouraging the child's mother to be present and to participate in the child's care as much as possible. Which of the following is the most appropriate rationale for including this nursing intervention in the child's care plan?
   a. The mother might experience guilt if she is not allowed to be present.
   b. The mother's presence will reduce the child's anxiety, which can help ease his respiratory effort.
   c. The mother can assist the nurse in

providing close observation of the child's respiratory effort.

d. The mother can assist the nurse in keeping track of the child's many activities.

8. When planning nursing care for a child with epiglottitis, which of the following interventions would be of highest priority?
   a. providing adequate psychological support
   b. preventing respiratory obstruction
   c. preventing cross-contamination of other patients
   d. administering antibiotics as ordered

9. Which of the following respiratory conditions is always considered a medical emergency?
   a. acute LTB
   b. epiglottitis
   c. asthma
   d. cystic fibrosis

10. Immunization of children over 24 months with the haemophilus type B polysaccharide vaccine will decrease incidence of which of the following respiratory conditions?
    a. acute LTB
    b. epiglottitis
    c. bacterial pneumonia
    d. cystic fibrosis

11. Which of the following best describes the characteristic clinical manifestations of viral pneumonia?
    a. signs and symptoms ranging from mild fever, slight cough, and malaise to high fever, severe cough, and prostration
    b. stiff neck, bulging anterior fontanel, circumoral cyanosis, diminished breath sounds, and rales on auscultation

c. prodromal streptococcal respiratory infection
d. rapidly deteriorating condition with empyema and pneumothorax typically developing

12. In a child with asthma, methylxanthines such as theophylline and aminophylline are administered primarily to
    a. decrease postnasal drip–induced cough
    b. dilate the bronchioles
    c. reduce airway inflammation
    d. reduce infection

13. Which of the following statements about cystic fibrosis is correct?
    a. It is inherited as an autosomal dominant trait.
    b. It is characterized by a decreased concentration of electrolytes in the sweat.
    c. Clinical manifestations are caused by obstruction resulting from increased viscosity of mucous gland secretions.
    d. Increased fat metabolism occurs.

14. The mother of an adolescent male with cystic fibrosis asks the nurse whether her son can become a biologic father. Which of the following would be the nurse's most appropriate response?
    a. "Don't worry about that now. If for some reason he can't be a biologic father, he could still adopt a child."
    b. "Yes, your son has just as much chance to be a biologic father as any other male his age."
    c. "It will be difficult for him to be a biologic father since he will probably be incapable of having an erection."
    d. "Most males with cystic fibrosis are sterile."

ANSWER KEY

1. **Correct response: b**
   The eustachian tubes are short and lie in a horizontal plane, predisposing a child to otitis media due to secretions from the nasopharynx entering the tubes.
   a, c, and d. No unusual features of these structures predispose to otitis media.
   Knowledge/Physiologic/Analysis (Dx)

2. **Correct response: d**
   Before intubation, the child should be maintained in the most comfortable position for breathing. An abnormal lateral neck radiograph confirms diagnosis of epiglottitis.
   a. The nurse should perform as few intrusive procedures as possible to minimize the child's anxiety.
   b. Physical examination of the throat should be performed only by an otolaryngologist or anesthesiologist.
   c. Racemic epinephrine is used to treat croup not epiglottitis.
   Application/Safe care/Implementation

3. **Correct response: a**
   Beta-adrenergics such as epinephrine are administered for acute attacks of asthma.
   b. Corticosteroids are used as adjunct therapy during an acute attack, as well as for chronic oral administration.
   c. Antihistamines are sometimes given to decrease postnasal drip-induced cough, but not as therapy in an acute attack.
   d. Antibiotics may be administered if infection is present but are not an important therapy for an acute attack.
   Application/Safe care/Evaluation

4. **Correct response: a**
   Pancrease is given with all meals and snacks to minimize malabsorption.
   b. Pancrease is a form of pancreatic enzyme.

   c. Pancrease should be omitted if the child is not eating.
   d. Pancrease should not be omitted if the child is passing frequent, bulky stools; rather, dosage may be increased.
   Analysis/Health promotion/Evaluation

5. **Correct response: c**
   Otitis media calls for treatment with an appropriate antibiotic for a course of 10 to 14 days.
   a. Even mild infection necessitates antibiotic therapy.
   b. Although decongestants can be used to treat nasal congestion, antibiotics are the drugs of choice for otitis media.
   d. A child with concurrent infections may be referred for a myringotomy but must first be treated with an antibiotic.
   Application/Health promotion/Evaluation

6. **Correct response: b**
   Myringotomy is indicated when medical treatment with antibiotics alone proves unsuccessful in preventing recurrent infections.
   a. Pain is not an indication for myringotomy. An analgesic may be administered.
   c. A child with simple otitis media is not critically ill.
   d. Compromised defenses are not an issue in otitis media.
   Comprehension/Safe care/Evaluation

7. **Correct response: b**
   The mother should be encouraged to be present to help reduce the child's anxiety.
   a. The mother may or may not experience guilt, but this is not the main consideration in this nursing intervention.
   c. Appropriate measures should be taken to prevent cross-contamination of other patients, but this is not of highest priority.

d. Antibiotics are administered to treat the infection, but this is not of highest priority.

Analysis/Safe care/Planning

8. **Correct response: b**

Respiratory obstruction is a potential life-threatening complication of epiglottitis and therefore represents the highest priority.

a. Adequate psychological support is important but not life threatening when setting priorities.

c. Appropriate measures should be taken to prevent cross-contamination of other patients, but this is not of highest priority.

d. Antibiotics are administered to treat the infection, but this is not of highest priority.

Analysis/Safe care/Planning

9. **Correct response: b**

Epiglottis is always considered a medical emergency because of its life-threatening nature.

a. Acute LTB requires close observation for complications of obstruction, but it is not always considered a medical emergency.

c. Asthma is a chronic disease although patients with status asthmaticus require prompt treatment and close observation.

d. Cystic fibrosis is a chronic respiratory condition in children and is not considered a medical emergency.

Analysis/Safe care/Analysis (Dx)

10. **Correct response: b**

Epiglottis is a bacterial infection of the epiglottitis; the causative organism is usually Hemophilus influenza type B. Administration of the haemophilus type B polysaccharide vaccine should decrease the incidence of epiglottis.

a. Acute LTB usually has a viral etiology.

c. The most common bacterial organisms causing pneumonia in children are pneumococci, streptococci, and staphylococci.

d. Cystic fibrosis is inherited as an autosomal recessive trait.

Application/Health promotion/ Implementation

11. **Correct response: a**

These signs and symptoms are characteristic of viral pneumonia.

b. These signs and symptoms are characteristic of bacterial pneumonia caused by pneumococcal infection.

c. This is characteristic of bacterial pneumonia caused by streptococcal infection.

d. These manifestations are characteristic of bacterial pneumonia caused by staphylococcal infection.

Knowledge/Physiologic/Assessment

12. **Correct response: b**

Methylxanthines are highly effective bronchodilators.

a. Antihistamines may be given for this reason.

c. Corticosteroids may be given for this reason.

d. Antibiotics may be given for this reason.

Application/Physiologic/Assessment

13. **Correct response: c**

Generalized dysfunction of the exocrine gland resulting in increased viscosity of mucous gland secretions leads to obstruction in various body organs.

a. It is inherited as an autosomal recessive trait.

b. There is an increase in sodium and chloride in both saliva and sweat.

d. Obstruction of pancreatic ducts and absence of pancreatic enzymes leads to malabsorption of fats.

Analysis/Physiologic/Analysis (Dx)

14. **Correct response: d**

Most males are sterile due to blockage of vas deferens with abnormal secretions, which prevents sperm formation.

a. This answer is inappropriate because it does not really answer the mother's question.

b. Most males with cystic fibrosis are sterile.

    c. The ability or inability to achieve an erection is not the etiology of the sterility.

Comprehension/Health promotion/ Evaluation

Gastrointestinal Dysfunction

I. Essential concepts: gastrointestinal (GI) anatomy and physiology

A. Development

1. Development of a primitive digestive system begins during the fourth week of gestation, with the most extensive development occurring in the last few weeks before birth.
2. A newborn's stomach capacity is only 10 to 20 mL at birth, and peristalsis is rapid, resulting in frequent regurgitation.
3. Normal newborns pass one to six stools a day.

B. Function

1. *Digestion* involves physical and chemical breakdown of food into absorbable substances.
2. *Absorption* involves transfer of the end products of digestion across the intestinal wall into the circulation for use by cells.

II. Gastrointestinal system overview

A. Assessment

1. Assessing a child's GI system involves obtaining a complete health history and performing a physical assessment, particularly of the abdomen.
2. Abnormal findings indicating possible GI dysfunction include:
   a. Growth and development: height and weight below standard age-related norms
   b. Skin: pallor, jaundice, carotenemia
   c. Hair: abnormal texture and sparseness
   d. Head: microcephaly, craniotabes
   e. Mouth: caries, periodontal disease
   f. Abdomen: distention or depression; umbilical herniation; visible peristaltic waves; tenderness; masses; splenomegaly; hepatomegaly; and increased, decreased, or absent bowel sounds
   g. Anus: rectal bleeding, nonpatency

B. Laboratory studies and diagnostic tests performed to evaluate GI function include:

1. Stool cultures
2. Stool sample evaluation for the presence of ova and parasites
3. Stool sample evaluation for the presence of blood, mucus, fat, urobilinogen, trypsin, leukocytes (Table 9–1)
4. Stool-reducing substances and pH tests
5. Complete blood count with differential, hemoglobin, and hematocrit
6. Urine specific gravity
7. Bowel studies: upper GI series, barium enema, biopsy, rectosigmoidoscopy
8. Liver and endocrine function tests
9. Abdominal radiographs

C. **Psychosocial implications**
1. Infants: Oral gratification may be compromised by an infant's inability to suck well due to cleft lip or palate, surgery, and alternate feeding methods; the child may develop inappropriate ways to meet his or her oral needs (e.g., sucking on a blanket, hand, or other object).
2. Toddlers: Locomotion is compromised in a child receiving long-term hyperalimentation or IV drug therapy.
3. Preschoolers: Malnourishment may interfere with development of normal motor skills (e.g., running, skipping).
4. School-age children and adolescents: Body image and self-concept development may be challenged by a child's altered body function and health maintenance needs.

III. Cleft lip and palate
A. **Description**
1. Cleft lip: a congenital anomaly involving one or more clefts in the upper lip ranging from a slight dimple to a large cleft involving nasal structures

TABLE 9–1.
Stool Analysis

PARAMETER	NORMAL FINDINGS	IMPLICATIONS OF ABNORMAL FINDINGS
Color	Brown; shade varies with diet	Black: upper GI bleeding Tan or clay-colored: blockage of common bile duct, pancreatic insufficiency Red-streaked: lower GI bleeding
Blood	Negative	GI bleeding, ulcerative colitis
Mucus	Negative	Ulcerative colitis, bacillary dysentary
Fat	Fatty acids: Age 0–6 yr: <2 g/24 hours Over 6 yr: 2–6 g/24 hours	Increase: malabsorption syndromes
Urobilinogen	30–200 mg/100g of feces	Increase: hemolytic anemia Decrease: biliary obstruction, severe liver disease, oral antibiotic therapy that alters interstinal flora, disorders causing decreased hemoglobin turnover (e.g., aplastic anemia)
Trypsin	Positive for small amounts in 95% of children	Absence: pancreatic insufficiency
Ph	7.0–7.5	Acid: carbohydrate fermentation Alkaline: protein breakdown
Nitrogen	1–2 g/24 hours	Increase (along with high fecal fat): chronic progressive pancreatitis

2. Cleft palate: a congenital anomaly consisting of a cleft ranging from soft palate involvement alone to a defect including the hard palate and portions of the maxilla in severe cases

B. Etiology and incidence

1. Causes include genetic, hereditary, environmental, and teratogenic factors.
2. Cleft lip occurs in approximately 1 in every 1,000 births, most commonly in boys. Cleft palate occurs in 1 in 2,500 births; incidence in girls is double that in boys.

C. Pathophysiology

1. These defects occur during embryonic development. Cleft lip results from failure of fusion of lateral and medial tissues forming the upper lip; cleft palate, from failure of fusion of tissues forming the palate.
2. These defects may occur separately or in combination to produce complete unilateral or bilateral cleft from the lip through the soft palate.
3. Depending on the defect's severity and the child's general health, surgical correction of cleft lip typically is done at age 1 to 2 months; of cleft palate, between ages 6 and 18 months. Cleft palate repair may require several operations performed in stages.
4. Early correction of cleft palate enables development of more normal speech patterns. Delayed closure or large defects may require the use of orthodontic devices.

D. Assessment findings

1. These defects are readily apparent at birth.
2. Careful physical assessment should be performed to rule out other midline birth defects.

E. Nursing diagnoses

1. Ineffective Airway Clearance
2. Altered Family Processes
3. High Risk for Infection
4. High Risk for Injury
5. Knowledge Deficit
6. Altered Nutrition: Less than Body Requirements
7. Pain

F. Planning and implementation

1. Take steps to ensure adequate nutrition and prevent aspiration of secretions:
   a. Provide special nipples or feeding devices for a child unable to suck adequately on a standard nipple.
   b. Hold the child in a semi-upright position, and direct formula to the side and back of the mouth to prevent aspiration.

      c.   Feed the infant slowly and burp him or her often to prevent excessive air swallowing and regurgitation.

2. Support the infant's and parents' emotional and social adjustment. Help facilitate the family's acceptance of the infant by encouraging the parents to express their feelings and concerns and by conveying an attitude of acceptance toward the infant. Reassure parents that reparative surgery usually is successful.

3. Preoperatively, reinforce the physician's explanations of the surgical procedure, anticipated outcome, and postoperative care to the parents and other family members.

4. Postoperatively, prevent infection by cleaning the suture line and applying antibacterial ointment after each feeding. Monitor the suture area for signs of infection.

5. Help maintain suture line integrity by placing the infant in elbow restraints. Remove the restraints every 2 hours for skin care and range-of-motion exercises.

6. In a child who underwent surgery to correct cleft lip, ensure that the Logan bow remains in place to protect the suture line.

7. Feed the infant with a rubber-tipped medicine dropper or bulb syringe or Breck feeder with a rubber tip, to help preserve the integrity of suture line.

8. Alleviate pain by administering analgesics, as ordered.

9. Monitor for signs of respiratory distress after surgery and during feedings. After feedings, place the infant on his or her side with the head elevated; suction as necessary.

10. Provide patient and family teaching, covering:
    a.   Surgical wound care
    b.   Proper feeding and positioning techniques
    c.   The importance of long-term follow-up, including speech therapy and prevention or correction of dental abnormalities
    d.   The need for annual hearing evaluations because of the child's increased susceptibility to recurrent ear infections. The child may require myringotomy and surgical placement of drainage tubes

G. Evaluation

1. The child gains weight and is free from infection and signs of respiratory distress.

2. Parents demonstrate acceptance of the child and verbalize an understanding of preoperative and postoperative aspects of care.

3. The family is referred for follow-up care from a multidisciplinary health care team that may include a pediatrician, nurse, plastic surgeon, orthodontist, prosthodontist, otolaryngologist, speech therapist, psychiatrist, and social worker.

4. The family is referred to a cleft palate support group.

5. Parents receive genetic counseling, if desired.

IV. Pyloric stenosis

A. **Description: narrowing of the pyloric sphincter at the outlet of the stomach**

B. **Etiology and incidence**

1. Although the exact cause remains unknown, heredity may play an important role.
2. Incidence is 1 in 500 live births; highest in boys, firstborns, and whites.

C. **Pathophysiology**

1. The pylorus narrows because of progressive hypertrophy and hyperplasia of the circular pyloric muscle. (The muscle may grow to twice its normal size.)
2. This leads to obstruction of the pyloric sphincter, with subsequent gastric distention, dilatation, and hypertrophy (Fig. 9–1).
3. Pyloromyotomy (creation of an incision along the anterior pylorus to split the muscle) is commonly performed to relieve the obstruction.

D. **Assessment findings**

1. Clinical manifestations of pyloric stenosis commonly include:
   a. No abnormal signs in the first week or two after birth
   b. Regurgitation or nonprojectile vomiting beginning by age 3 weeks; emesis is not bile stained and contains only gastric contents but may be blood tinged
   c. Vomiting increasing in frequency and force over next 1 to 2 weeks until most of ingested food is expelled through projectile vomiting
   d. Good appetite and feeding habits
   e. No evidence of pain
   f. Weight loss
   g. Decreased frequency and quantity of stools
   h. Signs of malnutrition and dehydration
   i. Upper abdominal distention
   j. Palpable olive-shaped mass in the epigastrium just to the right of the umbilicus
   k. Visible gastric peristaltic waves moving from left to right across the epigastrium
2. Ultrasonography and upper GI series may reveal delayed gastric emptying and an elongated, thin pylorus.
3. Laboratory findings may include:
   a. Increased pH and bicarbonate, indicating metabolic alkalosis
   b. Decreased serum chloride, sodium, and potassium levels
   c. Increased hematocrit and hemoglobin values, reflecting hemoconcentration

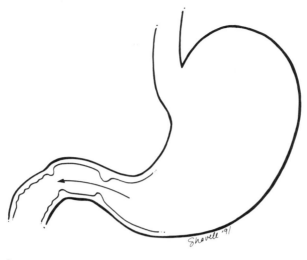

A

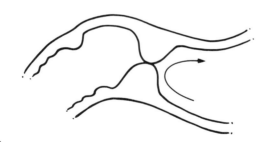

B

FIGURE 9–1.
Pyloric stenosis. (**A**) Normal passage through pyloric sphincter. (**B**) Stoppage of flow due to stenotic sphincter.

E.   Nursing diagnoses
   1.   High Risk for Aspiration
   2.   Ineffective Breathing Patterns
   3.   Family Coping: Potential for Growth
   4.   Altered Family Processes
   5.   High Risk for Fluid Volume Deficit
   6.   Knowledge Deficit
   7.   Altered Nutrition: Less than Body Requirements
   8.   Pain
   9.   High Risk for Altered Parenting
  10.   Impaired Skin Integrity

F. **Planning and implementation**
1. Administer parenteral fluids as ordered to replenish potassium and correct alkalosis.
2. Monitor hydration status: Record intake and output hourly, evaluate urine specific gravity, and monitor daily weights.
3. Assess the amount, frequency, and characteristics of emesis.
4. Provide postoperative nutrition as ordered; typically, clear liquids 4 to 6 hours postoperatively, advancing to formula and regular diet as tolerated.
5. Feed the infant slowly, burp frequently, and position in high-Fowler's position on the right side after feedings.
6. Promote comfort by providing good oral care and offering a pacifier while the infant is NPO, by rocking and cuddling the infant, and by encouraging the parents to hold the infant and participate in care when appropriate.
7. Provide patient and family teaching, covering:
   a. All procedures, scheduled surgical procedure, and preoperative and postoperative care measures
   b. Feeding and positioning techniques
   c. Surgical wound care

G. **Evaluation**
1. The child appears well hydrated, retains feedings, gains weight, and appears comfortable and satisfied after feedings.
2. The child exhibits no signs of excessive peristalsis or abdominal distention and experiences fewer vomiting episodes.
3. Parents verbalize understanding of feeding techniques, wound care, and follow-up appointments.

V. **Gastroesophageal reflux (GER)**

A. **Description: backflow of gastric contents into the esophagus resulting from relaxation or incompetence of the lower esophageal (cardiac) sphincter**

B. **Etiology and incidence**
1. The exact cause is unknown, but GER may result from delayed maturation of lower esophageal neuromuscular function or impaired local hormonal control mechanisms.
2. GER is the most common esophageal problem in infancy. Some reflux of gastric contents normally occurs in infants, children, and adults. GER is deemed pathologic when it is unusually severe, persists into late infancy, or is associated with complications.

C. **Pathophysiology**
1. Inappropriate relaxation or failure of lower esophageal sphincter contraction leads to increased gastric or abdominal pressure and resultant reflux of gastric contents.
2. Delayed gastric emptying may be a contributing factor in GER.

3. Repeated reflux of acidic gastric contents can damage delicate esophageal mucosa.
4. GER commonly is self-limiting, usually resolving by age 1 year. In more severe cases, the child may require hospitalization and possibly surgery, such as Nissen fundoplication, in which the gastric fundus is wrapped around the distal esophagus.

D. Assessment findings

1. Health history and physical assessment may reveal:
   a. Forceful vomiting, possibly with hematemesis
   b. Weight loss, failure to thrive
   c. Aspiration and recurrent respiratory infections
   d. Near-miss sudden infant death syndrome and cyanotic episodes
   e. Esophagitis and bleeding due to repeated irritation of esophageal lining with gastric acid
   f. Melena
   g. Heartburn, abdominal pain, and bitter taste in older children
2. Laboratory study and diagnostic test results may include:
   a. Absence of gastric or duodenal obstruction on barium swallow and upper GI radiograph
   b. Low resting lower esophageal sphincter pressure on esophageal manometry
   c. Anemia secondary to blood loss
3. Other useful studies may include:
   a. The acid reflux (Tuttle) test
   b. Gastroesophageal scintigraphy
   c. Esophagoscopy

E. Nursing diagnoses

1. Ineffective Airway Clearance
2. Diversional Activity Deficit
3. Altered Family Processes
4. Fluid Volume Deficit
5. High Risk for Infection
6. Knowledge Deficit
7. Altered Nutrition: Less than Body Requirements
8. Pain
9. Impaired Tissue Integrity

F. Planning and implementation

1. Ensure adequate hydration by assessing for signs and symptoms of dehydration, monitoring intake and output, and administering IV fluids as ordered.
2. Assess the amount, frequency, and characteristics of emesis.
3. Assess the relation of vomiting to the time of feedings and the infant's activity level.

4. Improve nutritional status through feeding techniques such as thickening formula with cereal, enlarging nipple openings, and burping the infant frequently.
5. Help prevent respiratory complications by positioning the infant upright, as ordered.
6. Assess breath sounds before and after feedings; keep suctioning equipment at the bedside.
7. Place the infant on a cardiac/apnea monitor, as ordered.
8. Administer prescribed medications, as ordered, which may include:
    a. Drugs that promote gastric emptying or pyloric sphincter relaxation, such as bethanechol, metoclopramide, and domperidone
    b. Antacids, to neutralize the acidity of refluxed contents and help prevent esophageal tissue damage
9. Provide family teaching, covering:
    a. Proper feeding techniques (i.e., how to thicken the formula and position the infant upright for feeding)
    b. All treatments and procedures
    c. Minor problems that may follow surgery (e.g., flatulence, inability to vomit, poor feeding habits, and choking on solid foods)

G. Evaluation
1. The child gains weight and eats normally.
2. The child maintains balanced fluid and electrolyte status and exhibits decreased vomiting, clear lungs on auscultation, and no signs of respiratory distress.
3. Parents verbalize understanding of and demonstrate proper technique for feedings.
4. Parents plan follow-up care to monitor weight gain and nutritional status.

VI. Celiac disease
A. Description: a chronic inability to tolerate foods containing gluten
B. Etiology and incidence
1. Celiac disease is believed to result from either an inborn error of metabolism or an abnormal immunologic response. Most likely, it is inherited through a dominant gene with incomplete penetrance.
2. Incidence is about 21 per 100,000 live births.
3. Celiac disease occurs more frequently in Europe than in the United States; it is rarely reported in Asians or blacks.
C. Pathophysiology
1. Intolerance for and inability to digest gluten (malabsorption of gluten)—specifically, the gliadin fraction of gluten found in

wheat, barley, rye, and oats—results in accumulation of the amino acid glutamine, which is toxic to intestinal mucosal cells.

2. As a result, intestinal villi eventually atrophy, which reduces the absorptive surface of the small intestine and affects absorption of ingested nutrients.

3. The disorder is characterized by episodes of *celiac crisis*, precipitated by infections, prolonged fasting, ingestion of gluten, or exposure to anticholinergic drugs and characterized by a general flare-up of symptoms.

4. Celiac crisis may lead to electrolyte imbalance, rapid dehydration, and severe acidosis.

D. Assessment findings

1. Symptoms typically appear within 3 to 6 months after introduction of gluten (usually in the form of grains) into the child's diet and include:

   a. Frequent bulky, greasy, malodorous stools with frothy appearance due to fat in stool (steatorrhea); in some cases, constipation

   b. Growth failure, weight loss, and muscle wasting resulting from fecal loss of fat, protein, and carbohydrates as well as loss of appetite

   c. Abdominal distention due to weakened musculature, accumulation of intestinal secretions and gas, altered peristaltic activity, and fluid from altered osmotic pressure resulting from protein loss

   d. Vomiting and abdominal pain

   e. Peripheral edema, usually of the lower extremities, due to hypoproteinemia

   f. Epistaxis, ecchymosis, or intestinal hemorrhage resulting from disturbed blood coagulation due to inadequate vitamin K

   g. Rickets or tetany, reflecting impaired calcium absorption related to low levels of vitamin D

   h. Behavioral changes such as irritability and apathy

2. For unknown reasons, some children do not exhibit symptoms until after age 5 years; in these cases, growth retardation and delayed sexual maturation are the predominant manifestations.

3. Laboratory studies and diagnostic tests may reveal:

   a. Flat mucosal surface, absence or atrophy of villi, and deep crypts visible on biopsy specimen of the small intestine. (These characteristic lesions return to normal after dietary restriction of gluten, which helps confirm diagnosis.)

   b. Steatorrhea on analysis of 72-hour quantitative fecal fat level

> c. Anemia caused by low serum iron and inadequate vitamin B_{12} and folic acid
> d. Osteoporosis (reduction of bone mass) and osteomalacia (softening of the bone as a result of demineraliztion) due to impaired calcium absorption related to low levels of vitamin D

E. **Nursing diagnoses**
1. Diarrhea
2. Altered Family Processes
3. Altered Health Maintenance
4. High Risk for Infection
5. High Risk for Injury
6. Knowledge Deficit
7. Altered Nutrition: Less than Body Requirements
8. Self-Esteem Disturbance

F. **Planning and implementation**
1. Promote optimal nutrition through education and support regarding dietary restrictions, which typically include:
   a. Gluten-free diet (Table 9–2)
   b. Supplemental vitamin calcium, iron, folate
   c. Temporary parenteral hyperalimentation if the child is seriously malnourished
2. Refer the parents and child for nutritional counseling; ensure that the child's food preferences are taken into account in diet planning.
3. Prevent infection through good general hygiene and avoiding exposure to persons with infection.

TABLE 9–2.
Basics of Gluten-Free Diet

Foods Allowed

Meats: beef, pork, poultry, fish

Eggs

Milk and dairy products: milk, cream, cheese

Vegetables: all

Fruits: all

Grains: rice, corn, gluten-free wheat flour, puffed rice, corn flakes, corn meal, precooked gluten-free cereals

Foods Prohibited

Milk: commercially prepared ice cream, malted milk, prepared puddings

Grains: anything made from wheat, rye, oats, or barley (e.g., bread, rolls, cookies, cakes, crackers, cereal, spaghetti, macaroni, noodles)

Beer and ale

---

4. If celiac crisis occurs, prepare the child for gastric decompression and fluid and electrolyte replacement therapy, as ordered.
5. Support the parents by encouraging them to express their feelings and concerns. Refer them to the American Celiac Society for additional information and support.
6. Promote a positive self-concept in an older child by allowing the child to express feelings about the disease and dietary restrictions and by emphasizing positive changes that will result from adherence to these restrictions.
7. Provide patient and family teaching, covering:
   a. Information about celiac disease and diet restrictions
   b. The importance of adhering to a gluten-free diet after symptoms subside to prevent recurrence. (Ensure that parents and child understand that these restrictions are lifelong.)
   c. Measures to prevent celiac crisis
   d. The need for infection prevention

G. Evaluation
1. The child maintains adequate nutritional status and avoids celiac crisis.
2. The child or parents verbalize an understanding of the disease and its treatment.
3. Parents are referred to the American Celiac Society.

VII. Hirschsprung's disease (congenital aganglionic megacolon)

A. Description: a congenital anomaly resulting in mechanical intestinal obstruction due to inadequate motility in an intestinal segment

B. Etiology and incidence
1. Hirschsprung's disease is believed to be a familial, congenital defect.
2. Incidence is about 1 in 5,000 live births.
3. The disorder is at least four times more common in males than females and is most prevalent in whites.
4. It has been associated with other anomalies, such as Down syndrome and genitourinary abnormalities.

C. Pathophysiology
1. Absence of autonomic parasympathetic ganglion cells in one segment of colon causes lack of innervation in that segment.
2. This leads to absence of propulsive movements, causing accumulation of intestinal contents and distention of the bowel proximal to the defect (megacolon) (Fig. 9–2).

D. Assessment findings
1. Clinical manifestations vary according to the child's age at diagnosis and commonly include:
   a. Newborns: failure to pass meconium, reluctance to ingest fluids, abdominal distention, bile-stained emesis

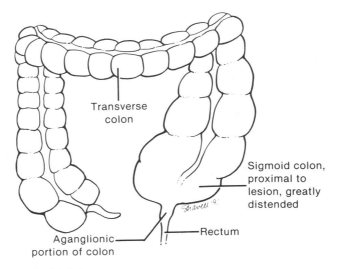

Transverse colon

Sigmoid colon, proximal to lesion, greatly distended

Rectum

Aganglionic portion of colon

FIGURE 9–2.
Hirschsprung's disease. Note dilated colon proximal to bowel.

b. Infants: failure to thrive, constipation, abdominal distention, vomiting, episodic diarrhea
c. Toddlers and older children: chronic constipation, foul-smelling stools, abdominal distention, visible peristalsis, palpable fecal mass, malnourishment, signs of anemia and hypoproteinemia
2. Rectal examination typically reveals a rectum empty of stool, tight internal sphincter, and stool leakage.
3. Explosive, watery diarrhea; fever; and severe prostration signal inflammation of the small bowel and colon (enterocolitis), a potentially life-threatening situation.
4. Laboratory studies and diagnostic tests commonly reveal:
  a. Megacolon detected on barium enema
  b. Absence of ganglion cells on rectal biopsy, which confirms diagnosis

E. Nursing diagnoses
  1. Constipation
  2. Altered Family Processes
  3. High Risk for Fluid Volume Deficit
  4. Altered Health Maintenance
  5. Knowledge Deficit
  6. Altered Nutrition: Less than Body Requirements
  7. Pain

F. Planning and implementation
  1. Improve nutritional status by providing smaller and more frequent feedings.

2. Assess hydration status by monitoring intake and output and daily weights.
3. Note and record the frequency and characteristics of stools.
4. Administer enemas as necessary to relieve constipation.
5. Avoid taking temperatures by the rectal route because of the potential for damaging fragile rectal mucosa.
6. Assess for and promptly report signs of enterocolitis.
7. Administer prescribed medications as ordered, which may include:
   a. Systemic antibiotics given with enemas to reduce intestinal flora
   b. Stool softeners to reduce constipation
8. Carefully assess for altered fluid status in a child who is NPO and receiving frequent enemas. Administer IV fluids as ordered.
9. Periodically measure abdominal girth to assess for increasing distention.
10. Decrease discomfort due to abdominal distention by elevating the head of the bed and changing the child's position frequently. Assess for any respiratory difficulty associated with distention.
11. Support the child and parents, and encourage them to express their feelings and concerns. Encourage parents to visit and participate in the care of their hospitalized child, as appropriate.
12. Prepare the child and parents for procedures and treatments, which may include:
   a. Manual dilatation of the anus, dietary management, and cleansing enemas until the child is able to tolerate surgery
   b. Surgery to remove the aganglionic, nonfunctioning segment of the colon, followed by anastomosis in a three-stage approach, which involves a temporary colostomy before definitive surgery to allow the bowel to rest and the child to gain weight; reanastomosis by means of an abdominoperineal pull-through about 9 to 12 months later; and closure of the colostomy about 3 months following the pull-through procedure
   c. In a small percentage of children diagnosed later in childhood with mild symptoms, possibly conservative management with enemas, stool softeners, and a low-residue diet
13. Provide patient and family teaching, covering:
   a. Enemas, stool softeners, and a low-residue diet
   b. Diagnosis, surgery, preoperative and postoperative care, and colostomy care, if applicable
14. Arrange for consultation with an ostomy nurse to assist with teaching, as indicated.

G. Evaluation

1. The child exhibits improved nutritional and hydration status, gains weight, has no signs of abdominal distention or respiratory discomfort and exhibits appropriate elimination patterns after surgery or other treatment.
2. Parents verbalize an understanding of the treatment regimen.
3. Parents demonstrate knowledge of colostomy care, if appropriate.
4. Parents verbalize an understanding of the need for medical and surgical follow-up.

VIII. Intussusception

A. Description: invagination of one portion of the intestine into an adjacent distal portion, causing obstruction

B. Etiology and incidence

1. In most cases, the cause of intussusception is unknown. It may be linked to viral infections, intestinal polyps, Meckel's diverticulum, lymphoma, foreign body obstruction, or other predisposing factors.
2. One of the most common causes of intestinal obstruction in infancy, it typically affects previously healthy infants between ages 3 and 12 months but also may affect toddlers and older children.
3. Incidence is about three times higher in males than in females.

C. Pathophysiology

1. Invagination commonly begins with hyperactive peristalsis in an intestinal segment—most often, at or near the ileocecal valve.
2. Peristalsis continues to pull the invaginated segment along the bowel; intestinal edema and obstruction occur, and blood supply to the area is cut off (Fig. 9–3).
3. Intussusception rarely reduces spontaneously. Initial treatment focuses on reduction through barium enema (hydrostatic reduction); if this proves unsuccessful, surgical reduction is required.
4. If treatment is delayed for longer than 24 hours, bowel strangulation may occur, leading to necrosis, hemorrhage, perforation, peritonitis, and shock.

D. Assessment findings

1. Health history and physical assessment may reveal:
   a. Severe paroxysmal abdominal pain, causing the child to scream and draw his or her knees to the abdomen
   b. Vomiting of gastric contents
   c. Tender, distended abdomen, possibly with a palpable mass
   d. With continued obstruction, lethargy, "currant jelly"

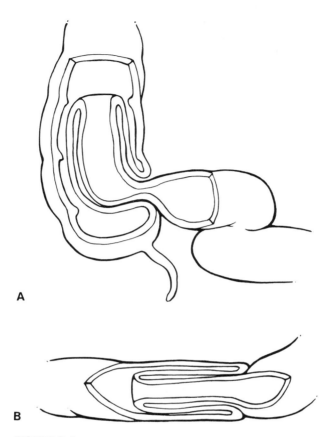

FIGURE 9–3.
Intussusception. **(A)** Ileocolic variety **(B)** Ileoileal variety. *(Redrawn from Ciba Collection of Medical Illustrations)*

stools (containing blood and mucus), bile-stained or fecal emesis, and shocklike syndrome, which may progress to death

2. Barium enema indicating intestinal invagination confirms diagnosis.

E. Nursing diagnoses

1. Altered Family Processes
2. High Risk for Fluid Volume Deficit
3. High Risk for Injury
4. High Risk for Infection
5. Knowledge Deficit
6. Pain
7. Impaired Tissue Integrity

F. Planning and implementation

1. Assess hydration status; evaluate for signs of dehydration and

monitor intake and output, including IV fluid therapy when the patient is NPO and nasogastric tube drainage following surgery.

2. Encourage intake of clear liquids after surgery and advance as tolerated.

3. Monitor bowel elimination status for return to normal function; assess stool amount and characteristics, guaiac test all stools, observe for abdominal distention, and auscultate for bowel sounds.

4. Postoperatively, monitor for infection; assess the surgical wound for redness, swelling, and drainage, and monitor temperature.

5. Support the child's parents by allowing them to express their anxieties and concerns and encouraging them to participate in their child's care, as appropriate.

6. Provide patient and family teaching, covering:
   a. Diagnosis
   b. Treatment
   c. Preoperative and postoperative care measures

G. **Evaluation**

1. The child appears comfortable, attains normal hydration status, and demonstrates normal bowel activity.

2. Parents verbalize knowledge of follow-up care.

IX. Abdominal wall defects: umbilical and inguinal hernias and hydrocele

A. **Description**

1. Hernia: protrusion of the bowel through an abnormal opening in the abdominal wall—in children, most commonly at the umbilicus and through the inguinal canals

2. Hydrocele: presence of abdominal fluid in the scrotal sac

B. **Etiology and incidence**

1. These defects most commonly arise from congenital anomalies.

2. Inguinal hernias occur most often in males (90%) and account for about 80% of all hernias in general; umbilical hernias are most common in black children.

C. **Pathophysiology**

1. In an umbilical hernia, incomplete closure of the umbilical ring results in protrusion of portions of the omentum and intestine through the opening. The defect usually closes spontaneously by age 3 or 4 years; surgical correction is necessary if closure does not occur or if incarceration of herniated bowel occurs.

2. Inguinal hernia results from incomplete closure of the tube (processus vaginalis) between the abdomen and the scrotum (or uterus in females), leading to descent of an intestinal portion. Incarceration results when the descended portion be-

comes tightly caught in the hernial sac, compromising its blood supply. An incarcerated hernia is considered a medical emergency requiring immediate surgical repair; a nonincarcerated hernia also necessitates surgery.

    3.   Hydrocele may be communicating or noncommunicating.

        a.   In a noncommunicating hydrocele, most commonly seen at birth, residual peritoneal fluid is trapped within the lower segment of the processus vaginalis (the tunica vaginalis), with no communication with the peritoneal cavity. The fluid usually is absorbed during the first months after birth and requires no treatment.

        b.   A communicating hydrocele is commonly associated with a hernia since the processus vaginalis remains open from the scrotum to the abdominal cavity. In most cases, hydrocelectomy is performed if spontaneous resolution does not occur by age 1 year.

D. **Assessment findings**

    1.   Clinical manifestations of umbilical hernia typically include a soft swelling or protrusion around the umbilicus, usually reducible with the finger.

    2.   Inguinal hernia commonly produces painless inguinal swelling that is reducible. The swelling may disappear during periods of rest and is most noticeable when the infant coughs or cries.

    3.   An incarcerated hernia produces such symptoms as irritability, tenderness at the site, anorexia, abdominal distention, and difficulty in defecating and may lead to complete intestinal obstruction and gangrene.

    4.   A noncommunicating hydrocele is usually asymptomatic; a communicating hydrocele may produce a bulge in the inguinal area or scrotum that is smaller in the morning—not more noticeable with coughing or straining (as in an inguinal hernia)—and nonreducible.

E. **Nursing diagnoses**

    1.   Altered Family Processes

    2.   High Risk for Fluid Volume Deficit

    3.   High Risk for Injury

    4.   Knowledge Deficit

    5.   Pain

F. **Planning and implementation**

    1.   Postoperatively, assess for wound infection by observing the incision for redness or drainage and monitoring temperature.

    2.   Maintain good hydration status by administering IV fluids, as ordered, monitoring intake and output, and advancing the child's diet as tolerated after surgery.

    3.   Promote comfort by administering prn analgesics as needed and, in a child who has undergone hydrocelectomy, applying ice bags and using a scrotal support to help relieve pain and swelling.

4. Support the child's parents by encouraging them to express their feelings and concerns and allowing them to participate in their child's care, as appropriate.

5. Provide patient and family teaching, covering:
   a. Signs and symptoms of incarceration to watch for and report
   b. The need to avoid ineffective and potentially harmful home remedies (e.g., taping a hernia)
   c. Surgical procedure, preoperative and postoperative care, and home care
   d. Signs and symptoms of wound infection
   e. Precautions and restrictions (e.g., not tub-bathing an infant until the incision heals, having an older child avoid strenuous physical activity for about 3 weeks)

G. Evaluation

1. The child resumes a regular diet and exhibits no signs of infection.

2. Parents verbalize knowledge of signs of infection, home care, and follow-up.

Bibliography

Fischbach, F. (1988). *Manual of laboratory diagnostic tests* (3rd ed.). Philadelphia: J. B. Lippincott.

Mott, S. R., Fazekas, N. F., and James, S. R. (1990). *Nursing care of children and families* (2nd ed.). Menlo Park, CA: Addison-Wesley.

Waechter, E. H., Phillips, J., and Holaday, B. (1985). *Nursing care of children*. Philadelphia: J. B. Lippincott.

Whaley, L. F., and Wong, D. L. (1991). *Nursing care of infants and children* (4th ed.). St. Louis: C. V. Mosby.

STUDY QUESTIONS

1. Which of the following best describes the cause of Hirschsprung's disease?
   a. overuse of laxatives, resulting in frequent evacuation of solids, liquids, and gas
   b. congenital absence of parasympathetic ganglion cells in a segment of the colon
   c. viral infection resulting in excessive peristaltic movements within the GI tract
   d. a congenital anomaly often diagnosed in newborns because of failure to pass the transitional stool within 24 hours after birth

2. Invagination of a bowel segment into a distal segment is associated with
   a. stenosis
   b. herniation
   c. intussusception
   d. atresia

3. When planning a teaching program for the parents of a child with celiac disease, the nurse should emphasize that the child must comply with dietary restrictions
   a. until symptoms disappear
   b. until the child reaches adulthood
   c. throughout life
   d. until the child achieves all major growth and development milestones

4. Feeding precautions for an infant who has undergone cleft lip repair commonly include
   a. positioning on the abdomen after feeding
   b. burping less frequently
   c. removing the Logan bow during feeding
   d. holding the infant semi-upright while feeding

5. When caring for an infant with bilateral cleft lip and palate and intervening with his or her parents, which of the following nursing interventions would be most appropriate?

   a. telling the parents not to worry because the defect can be repaired
   b. keeping the baby and mother apart until the lip has been repaired
   c. verbally minimizing the defect by discussing more serious congenital defects that affect other children
   d. encouraging the parents to express their feelings and concerns and conveying an attitude of acceptance toward the child

6. Which of the following methods is commonly used to feed an infant with cleft lip?
   a. gastric gavage
   b. IV fluid infusion
   c. asepto syringe with a rubber tip
   d. thickened formula

7. Andrew, a 4-week-old white boy, is admitted to the hospital with a history of "spitting up" since age 3 weeks. Andrew's vomiting has become more projectile in nature during the last 24 hours, and he is showing signs of mild dehydration. After vomiting, he sucks eagerly. Physical assessment reveals a readily palpable olive-shaped mass in the epigastrium just to the right of the umbilicus. The most likely medical diagnosis for Andrew would be
   a. intussusception
   b. GER
   c. hernia
   d. pyloric stenosis

8. Conservative management of GER commonly includes
   a. positioning the infant on the right side after feeding
   b. feeding a formula consisting of a 1:2 ratio of water to formula
   c. providing frequent low-volume feedings
   d. surgical correction through Nissen fundoplication

9. When planning a teaching program regarding dietary restrictions for a child with celiac disease, the nurse might in-

clude which of the following foods as a suggested lunch entree?

a. spaghetti
b. soup
c. chicken
d. macaroni and cheese

10. A newborn's failure to pass meconium within the first 24 hours after birth could indicate
    a. hirschsprung's disease
    b. celiac disease
    c. intussusception
    d. an abdominal wall defect

11. Nursing assessment measures that contribute to a diagnosis of intussusception include all the following *except*
    a. description of stools
    b. pattern of pain
    c. family history
    d. abdominal palpation

12. When intervening with the mother of a 2-year-old female who asks if her daughter's umbilical hernia will require surgery, which of the following would be the nurse's most appropriate response?
    a. "The defect will become smaller and should close by the time your daughter enters school."
    b. "Yes, it is important that you ask your pediatrician to refer you to a surgeon as soon as possible."
    c. "I have no idea. That question is a good one to ask your pediatrician."
    d. "Yes, there is a chance she may need surgery. However, if you tape it shut, it should close more quickly."

13. When planning a discharge teaching program for parents of a child who has undergone surgery to repair an inguinal hernia, the nurse should include information concerning which of the following possible sequelae?
    a. sterility
    b. wound infection
    c. wound rupture
    d. excessive scar formation

ANSWER KEY

1. *Correct response: b*
Disease pathophysiology involves the absence of parasympathetic ganglion cells in one segment of the colon, leading to lack of innervation in that segment.
  a. Chronic constipation is a clinical manifestation.
  c. Abnormality results in the absence of propulsive movements.
  d. Failure to pass meconium stool aids diagnosis.
Knowledge/Physiologic/Assessment

2. *Correct response: c*
Intussusception is characterized by invagination of the bowel into a proximal portion.
  a. Stenosis refers to an abnormal narrowing.
  b. Herniation involves the protrusion of a bowel segment through an abnormal opening in the abdominal wall.
  d. Atresia refers to an abnormal closure.
Comprehension/Physiologic/Assessment

3. *Correct response: c*
Dietary restrictions must be maintained throughout life to prevent recurrence of clinical manifestations.
  a, b, and d. Symptoms will recur if dietary restrictions are not maintained.
Analysis/Health promotion/Planning

4. *Correct response: d*
Holding the infant in a semi-upright position helps prevent aspiration.
  a. Positioning on the abdomen could allow the infant to rub his or her face and disrupt the suture line. The infant should be placed on his or her side with the head slightly elevated after feeding.
  b. The infant should be burped more frequently to prevent regurgitation and aspiration.
  c. The Logan bow must be kept in

place postoperatively to protect the suture line.
Application/Safe care/Implementation

5. *Correct response: d*
These interventions will help facilitate the family's acceptance of the infant.
  a. Family members need to be allowed to express their feelings.
  b. The infant and mother need to be together to promote bonding.
  c. The nurse should focus on the family's feelings concerning their own infant's defect.
Application/Psychosocial/Evaluation

6. *Correct response: c*
An Asepto syringe with a rubber tip provides a safe, effective feeding device for an infant with cleft lip.
  a. Gastric gavage usually is not necessary.
  b. IV fluids usually are necessary only in the immediate postoperative period until the infant can tolerate oral fluids.
  d. Thickening the formula is not necessary.
Application/Safe care/Implementation

7. *Correct response: d*
These are common clinical manifestations of pyloric stenosis.
  a. These are not the clinical manifestations of intussusception.
  b. These are not the clinical manifestations of GER.
  c. These are not the clinical manifestations of a hernia.
Knowledge/Physiologic/Assessment

8. *Correct response: c*
Feeding smaller amounts more frequently helps prevent vomiting.
  a. The infant should be positioned either in an upright position or prone in a body harness.
  b. Formula may be thickened to prevent vomiting.
  d. Nissen fundoplication may be per-

formed when conservative management fails.

Application/Safe care/Implementation

9. Correct response: c

Chicken is gluten-free and is a potential diet choice for a child with celiac disease.

a. Spaghetti contains gluten.
b. Most soups—except for clear broth—contain gluten.
d. Macaroni noodles contain gluten.

Comprehension/Health promotion/Planning

10. Correct response: a

Failure of a newborn to pass meconium is an important diagnostic indicator of Hirschsprung's disease.

b. This manifestation is not associated with celiac disease.
c. This manifestation is not associated with intussusception.
d. This manifestation is not associated with an abdominal wall defect.

Comprehension/Physiologic/Assessment

11. Correct response: c

Intussusception is not believed to have a familial tendency.

a. "Currant jelly" stools, containing blood and mucus, are a common manifestation in intussusception.
b. Acute, episodic abdominal pain often is the first sign of intussusception.
d. In intussusception, a sausage-shaped mass often can be palpated

in the upper right abdominal quadrant.

Analysis/Physiologic/Analysis (Dx)

12. Correct response: a

Umbilical hernia usually closes spontaneously by age 3 or 4 years.

b. Surgery usually is required only if the defect has not resolved by the time the child enters school.
c. To provide effective nursing care, a nurse should be knowledgeable concerning disease causes and treatments and should be able to answer many of his or her client's questions without referring to the physician.
d. The nurse should caution clients that home remedies such as taping the umbilical hernia could be harmful to the skin and actually delay closure.

Application/Safe care/Evaluation

13. Correct response: b

The most likely complication of this surgery is wound infection. Parents should be taught signs and symptoms of infection before discharge.

a. Sterility is not associated with inguinal hernia repair.
c. Rupture of the wound is a rare complication of this surgery.
d. Excessive scar formation is a rare complication of this surgery.

Analysis/Health promotion/Planning

Hematologic Dysfunction

I. Essential concepts: hematologic anatomy and physiology

    A. Hematopoiesis

        1. Hematopoiesis is defined as the formation and development of blood cells.

2. Hematopoietic activity occurs by the second week of embryonic life; blood islands arise from the yolk sac and liver.
3. From the second to fifth month of gestation, the liver is the most active site of hematopoiesis.
4. Bone marrow becomes active around the fourth month; within 2 to 3 weeks after birth, the bone marrow is the main site of hematopoietic activity.

B. **Function of blood cells and cellular elements**
1. Blood consists of liquid plasma and formed elements: erythrocytes, leukocytes, and thrombocytes.
2. Plasma transports formed elements and helps maintain homeostasis.
3. *Erythrocytes* (red blood cells, RBCs) primarily transport oxygen to and carbon dioxide away from body tissues; this activity relies on hemoglobin, an erythrocyte component. Erythrocytes also give blood its red color. Their typical life span is about 120 days.
4. The primary function of *leukocytes* (white blood cells, WBCs) is to protect the body against infection. Two types of leukocytes exist: granulocytes and agranulocytes.
5. *Thrombocytes* (platelets), the smallest blood cells, contain coagulation factors and help regulate hemostasis through a sequence of events known as the coagulation process.

II. Hematologic system overview
A. Assessment
1. Health history questions should focus on bleeding or bruising tendencies, medication use, and family history of bleeding problems.
2. History and physical assessment findings pointing to possible hematologic problems include:
   a. Skin: pallor, flushing, jaundice, purpura, petechiae, ecchymoses, pruritus, cyanosis, brownish discoloration, decreased capillary refill time
   b. Eyes: jaundiced sclera, conjunctival pallor, retinal hemorrhage, blurred vision
   c. Mouth: gingival and mucosal pallor
   d. Lymph nodes: lymphadenopathy, tenderness
   e. Cardiac: tachycardia, murmurs, signs and symptoms of congestive heart failure
   f. Pulmonary: tachypnea, orthopnea, dyspnea
   g. Neurologic: headache, vertigo, irritability, depression, impaired thought processes, lethargy, cold sensitivity
   h. Gastrointestinal: anorexia, hepatomegaly, splenomegaly
   i. Musculoskeletal: weight loss, decreased muscle mass, bone pain, joint swelling and pain

B. **Laboratory studies and diagnostic tests**
1. Complete blood count provides a fairly complete picture of the blood's formed elements; it usually includes the following components (Tables 10–1 and 10–2):
   a. RBC count
   b. WBC count
   c. Differential WBC count (neutrophils and lymphocytes)
   d. Hemoglobin (Hgb)
   e. Hematocrit (Hct)
   f. Mean corpuscular volume
   g. Mean corpuscular Hgb
   h. Mean corpuscular Hgb concentration
   i. Platelet count
2. Bone marrow aspiration aids diagnosis of aplastic anemia, pernicious anemia, agranulocytosis, thrombocytopenia, and leukemia.
3. Reticulocyte count helps differentiate between types of anemias.
4. Coagulation and hemostasis studies aid in differential diagnosis of hemorrhagic disorders.

C. **Psychosocial implications**
1. Children with hematologic dysfunction commonly undergo a multitude of invasive diagnostic tests, procedures, and treatments, which leads to anxiety and stress. Permitting the child to handle the equipment to be used may help decrease fears.
2. These children also often depend on others for care and support, and need the opportunity to perform as many self-care activities as possible to develop a normal sense of self-esteem and independence.

III. Iron-deficiency anemia

A. **Description: anemia caused by inadequate supply of iron for normal RBC formation, resulting in smaller cells, depleted RBC mass, decreased Hgb concentration, and decreased oxygen-carrying capacity of the blood**

B. **Etiology and incidence**
1. Common causes include inadequate dietary iron intake, iron malabsorption, low iron stores at birth, and significant blood loss.
2. Iron deficiency anemia is the most prevalent nutritional disorder in the United States and a major health problem in many developing countries.
3. It occurs most commonly in children between ages 6 months and 3 years; adolescents and premature infants also are at increased risk.

C. **Pathophysiology**
1. Inadequate supply of iron for normal RBC formation results in formation of microcytic cells.

TABLE 10-1.
Normal Peripheral Blood Values

AGE	WBCS (PER MM₃ [µL])	NEUTROPHILS (%)	LYMPHOCYTES (%)	PLATELETS (PER MM₃ [µL])	HEMOGLOBIN (G/DL)	HEMATOCRIT (%)	MCV (FL)
Birth	9,000–30,000	60	30	84,000–478,000	13.5–21	42–65	100–140
1 week	5,000–21,000	40	50	84,000–478,000	13.5–21	42–65	95–135
1 month	5,000–21,000	35	55	150,000–400,000	10–16	30–48	85–125
6 months	5,000–18,000	30	60	150,000–400,000	11–14	33–42	70–84
1 year	5,000–15,000	30	60	150,000–400,000	11–14	33–42	70–84
4 years	5,000–15,000	50	50	150,000–400,000	11–14	33–42	73–86
8 years	4,000–13,000	60	30	150,000–400,000	11.5–14.5	34–44	75–88
12 years	4,000–13,000	60	30	150,000–400,000	11.5–15.5	34–47	76–91
Adult							
Male	4,000–11,000	60	30	150,000–400,000	14–18	42–54	80–100
Female	4,000–11,000	60	30	150,000–400,000	12–16	36–48	80–100

TABLE 10–2.
Normal Cerebrospinal Fluid Values

PARAMETER	NORMAL VALUE	
Protein	Premature neonate:	65–150 mg/dL
	Term neonate:	75–150 mg/dL
	Child:	10–20 mg/dL
	Adolescent:	15–20 mg/dL
	Adult:	20–40 mg/dL
WBC count	Preterm neonate:	0–25/mm$_2$
	Term neonate:	0–20/mm$_2$
	Infant, child, adolescent, adult:	0–5/mm$_2$
Glucose	All ages: 40–85 mg/dL (or 2/3 of blood glucose level)	
Serum glutaminic–oxaloacetic transminase (SGOT)	All ages: 15 IU	
Gram stain	All ages: no organisms	

2. Body stores of iron decrease, as does transferrin, which binds and transports iron.
3. Insufficient body stores of iron lead to depleted RBC mass and eventually to decreased Hgb concentration and reduced oxygen-carrying capacity of blood.
4. The severity of symptoms is directly related to the degree and duration of iron deficiency.

D.   Assessment findings
   1. Common clinical manifestations include:
      a. Pallor
      b. Poor muscle development and growth retardation
      c. Susceptibility to infection
      d. Fatigue
      e. Irritability
      f. Underweight or overweight due to excessive milk ingestion and decreased intake of solid foods (''milk baby'')
   2. Laboratory test results may reveal:
      a. Decreased Hgb, Hct, reticulocyte count, and mean corpuscular volume
      b. Normal or moderately reduced RBC count
      c. Elevated total iron-binding capacity and reduced serum iron concentration

E.   Nursing diagnoses
   1. Activity Intolerance
   2. Fatigue
   3. Altered Health Maintenance
   4. High Risk for Infection
   5. Knowledge Deficit

6. Altered Nutrition: Less than Body Requirements
7. Social Isolation
8. Altered Peripheral Tissue Perfusion

F. Planning and implementation
1. Administer medications or therapy as appropriate, which may include:
    a. Oral iron (ferrous sulfate), 2 to 4 mg/kg
    b. Iron dextran IV or IM (using the Z-track method), in cases of noncompliance or poor absorption of oral iron
    c. Supplemental oxygen in severe tissue hypoxia
    d. Blood transfusion in severe cases
2. Promote an adequate intake of iron-rich foods; discourage milk as the predominant food source.
3. Provide patient and family teaching, covering:
    a. Proper administration of oral iron supplements: giving two divided doses with vitamin C–containing liquid between meals to enhance absorption and minimize side effects, administering it with a dropper to an infant or through a straw in an older child, and brushing teeth after administration to minimize staining of teeth
    b. Potential side effects, including nausea, vomiting, diarrhea, or constipation; dark green or black tarry stools; tooth discoloration
    c. Prevention of accidental ingestion; storing the preparation in a safe place out of childrens' reach
    d. Prevention of infection through good hygiene, proper nutrition, and adequate rest

G. Evaluation
1. Parents verbalize an understanding of iron deficiency anemia, its causes, and its treatment.
2. Parents relate the importance of routine medical check-ups and evaluation of Hgb level every 6 months to detect recurrence.

IV. Sickle cell anemia

A. Description: a chronic, severe, hemolytic disease associated with the presence of hemoglobin S (HgbS)

B. Etiology and incidence
1. Sickle cell anemia results from homozygous inheritance of the HgbS-producing gene.
2. Heterozygous inheritance of this gene results in sickle cell trait, usually an asymptomatic condition.
3. Sickle cell anemia predominantly affects blacks; among American blacks, incidence is about 1 in 600. Sickle cell trait affects about 8% of the black population (Table 10–3).

C. Pathophysiology
1. Abnormal Hgb (HgbS) replaces all or part of normal Hgb; under

TABLE 10-3.
Transmission of Sickle Cell Disease Probability
of Abnormal Hemoglobin in Offspring

GENOTYPE OF PARENTS	NORMAL	TRAIT	DISEASE
1 Parent with trait	50%	50%	0
Both parents with trait	25%	50%	25%
1 Parent with trait; 1 Parent with disease	0	50%	50%
Both parents with disease	0	0	100%

(Brunner, L.S., and Suddarth, D.S. (1986). Lippincott manual of nursing practice. Philadelphia: J.B. Lippincott, p. 1283)

conditions of decreased oxygen tension and lowered pH, RBCs change from round to sickle or crescent shaped.
2. Sickle cells do not slide through vessels as normal cells do, resulting in clumping, thrombosis, arterial obstruction, increased blood viscosity, hemolysis, and eventually tissue ischemia and necrosis.
3. As sickling progresses, acute and chronic changes develop in various organs and structures.

D. Assessment findings
1. Children with sickle cell anemia usually are asymptomatic unless exposed to a precipitating factor.
2. Periods of exacerbation (called *crises*) may be precipitated by dehydration, infection, fever, cold exposure, hypoxia, strenuous exercise, or extreme fatigue. The frequency and severity of crises vary widely.
3. Crises typically are characterized by:
   a. Fever
   b. Severe pain in joints, back, abdomen, or extremities
   c. Weakness
   d. Anorexia or vomiting lasting for several days
4. Laboratory tests may indicate:
   a. Sickled RBCs seen on stained blood smear
   b. HgbS detected on Hgb electrophoresis
   c. Decreased RBC count, elevated WBC and platelet counts, decreased erythrocyte sedimentation rate, increased serum iron level, decreased RBC survival time, and reticulocytosis
5. Antenatal diagnosis is available through genetic counseling and amniocentesis.

E. Nursing diagnoses
1. Activity Intolerance

2. Body Image Disturbance
3. Altered Family Processes
4. High Risk for Fluid Volume Deficit
5. Altered Health Maintenance
6. High Risk for Infection
7. Knowledge Deficit
8. Pain
9. Social Isolation
10. Altered Peripheral Tissue Perfusion

F. Planning and implementation

1. Implement therapeutic measures as appropriate, which may include:
   a. Oral and IV fluids to increase the fluid volume of blood and help prevent sickling and thrombosis
   b. Electrolyte replacement to counter acidosis caused by hypoxia
   c. Oxygen therapy to promote adequate oxygenation
   d. Bedrest and clustering of caregiving activities to minimize energy expenditure
   e. Blood replacement to treat anemia and reduce the viscosity of blood

2. Relieve pain by assessing the child's need for pain medication, administering prescribed analgesics (acetaminophen for mild pain; meperidine and morphine for extreme pain), and monitoring their effectiveness. Position the child for maximum comfort, and apply heat to affected areas.

3. Help ensure adequate hydration:
   a. Encourage oral fluid intake.
   b. Monitor IV fluid infusion.
   c. Maintain strict intake and output records, and track daily weights.
   d. Monitor for signs of dehydration or electrolyte imbalance.

4. Monitor for signs of infection, and administer antibiotics as ordered.

5. Promote tissue oxygenation by helping the child avoid overexertion or emotional stress and by providing passive range-of-motion exercises.

6. Support the child and family by allowing them to ventilate their fears, concerns, and anger.

7. Provide patient and family teaching, covering:
   a. Disease process, including genetic aspects and early recognition of sickling crisis
   b. Home management of mild crisis
   c. Prevention of sickling episodes by avoiding factors known to precipitate crises

      d.   The importance of regular dental check-ups and ophthalmic examinations

      e.   The importance of maintaining as normal a lifestyle as possible

    8.   Refer parents for questions regarding subsequent pregnancies and genetic counseling if desired.

G.   Evaluation

    1.   The child is free from pain and infection.

    2.   Parents verbalize an understanding of the disease process and major management principles.

    3.   Parents feel comfortable verbalizing any guilt feelings they may have regarding transmission of this potentially fatal, chronic illness to their child.

    4.   Parents verbalize knowledge of differentiating sickle cell trait from actual sickle cell disease.

V. Aplastic anemia

A.   Description: A disorder characterized by pancytopenia (anemia, granulocytopenia, and thrombocytopenia) and bone marrow hypoplasia

B.   Etiology and incidence

    1.   Aplastic anemia may be congenital or acquired.

    2.   Congenital types include:

      a.   Fanconi's syndrome, inherited through an autosomal recessive trait and associated with cytopenia and multiple congenital anomalies

      b.   Hypoplastic anemia (Blackfan-Diamond syndrome), characterized by destruction of RBCs and a slight decrease in WBCs and platelets

    3.   Common causes of acquired aplastic anemia include:

      a.   Idiopathic (half of all cases), with no identifiable precipitating cause

      b.   Radiation therapy

      c.   Drugs such as chloramphenicol, methicillin, sulfonamides, thiazides, and chemotherapeutic agents

      d.   Toxic agents such as industrial and household chemicals, including dyes, glue, paint removers, insecticides, petroleum products, and benzenes

      e.   Infections, particularly hepatitis and sepsis

      f.   Immune deficiencies, such as leukemia and lymphomas

    4.   Aplastic anemia may have a familial tendency and can occur at any age.

C.   Pathophysiology

    1.   In aplastic anemia, the decreased functional capacity of hypoplastic bone marrow results in pancytopenia.

    2.   Severe pancytopenia can produce massive bleeding or infection.

      3.   Prognosis is poor, with a mortality rate over 70%; 50% of patients die within 6 to 12 months of diagnosis.

D.   Assessment findings
1. Common clinical manifestations include:
   a. Abnormal bleeding, bruising, and petechiae due to thrombocytopenia
   b. Fever and infection due to neutropenia
   c. Pallor, weakness, irritability, and lethargy due to anemia
2. Laboratory findings may reveal:
   a. Pancytopenia on peripheral blood smear
   b. Conversion of red bone marrow to yellow, fatty bone marrow with almost complete absence of hematopoietic activity, demonstrated on bone marrow aspiration and biopsy

E.   Nursing diagnoses
1. Activity Intolerance
2. Altered Family Processes
3. Altered Health Maintenance
4. High Risk for Infection
5. High Risk for Injury
6. Knowledge Deficit
7. Altered Oral Mucous Membrane

F.   Planning and implementation
1. Provide supportive treatment, including prevention and control of infection, transfusions, and steroid or hormone therapy.
2. Provide information regarding bone marrow transplantation procedure and follow-up care. Explain that early bone marrow transplantation is associated with a 60% to 80% survival rate.
3. Administer medications and blood products as prescribed, which may include:
   a. Antilymphocyte globulin (ALG) or antithymocyte globulin (ATG), the treatment of choice, which suppresses T-cell dependent autoimmune responses without causing bone marrow suppression
   b. Androgenic steroids (such as testosterone) used in combination with corticosteroids to stimulate erythropoiesis
   c. Blood products such as RBCs, WBCs, and platelets, as well as antibiotics, used as supportive therapy
4. Explain that response to drug therapy is gradual and that no apparent changes may occur until up to 6 months of therapy.
5. Assess for abnormal bleeding tendencies (dipstick urine and guaiac stools).
6. Limit the child's activities when platelet counts are decreased.
7. Monitor for signs and symptoms of infection, and help prevent infection through protective isolation and good hygiene.
8. Monitor for complications of steroid therapy such as gastric irritation, infection, edema, weight gain, and hypertension.

9. Monitor for complications of androgen therapy such as abnormal liver function tests, weight gain, acne, increased hair growth, and deepening of voice.
10. Monitor for complications of ALG or ATG therapy, including fever, chills, rash, serum sickness, severe thrombocytopenia, and anaphylaxis.
11. Attempt to identify and eliminate toxic agents from the child's environment.
12. Support the family in coping with procedures and the disorder's uncertain prognosis and potential fatal outcome.
13. Provide patient and family teaching, covering:
    a. Diagnosis and nature of the disorder
    b. Diagnostic, therapeutic, and surgical procedures
    c. Side effects of therapies
    d. Observation for signs of infection and abnormal bleeding

G. **Evaluation**
   1. The child remains infection free.
   2. Bleeding episodes are managed effectively.
   3. The child achieves remission.

VI. Thalassemia

A. **Description: inherited blood disorders characterized by deficient synthesis of specific globulin chains of the hemoglobulin molecule—in the case of beta-thalassemia, the most common type, of beta-chains**

B. **Etiology and incidence**
   1. Thalassemia is an inherited autosomal recessive disease.
   2. It occurs in two major clinical forms: thalassemia major, the homozygous form (also known as Cooley's anemia), and thalassemia minor, the heterozygous form.
   3. Thalassemia occurs predominantly in persons of Mediterranean (especially Italian and Greek) or Asian origins.

C. **Pathophysiology**
   1. In beta-thalassemia, deficient beta-chain synthesis impairs Hgb synthesis.
   2. In response, the body attempts to compensate through continual production of fetal Hgb beyond the neonatal period.
   3. This results in formation of RBCs that are fragile and easily destroyed, leading to—in beta-thalassemia major—severe anemia and chronic hypoxia.
   4. No known cure exists; children with beta-thalassemia major rarely survive to adulthood although those with thalassemia minor may have a normal life span.

D. **Assessment findings**
   1. Thalassemia minor commonly produces only mild to moderate anemia that may be asymptomatic and often goes undetected.

2. Thalassemia major commonly produces the following clinical manifestations, usually first noted around age 6 months, when the protective effect of fetal Hgb diminishes:
   a. Progressive pallor, poor feeding, and protruding abdomen secondary to hepatosplenomegaly
   b. Signs and symptoms of chronic hypoxia such as headache, lethargy, bone pain, anorexia, and exercise intolerance
3. Long-term complications result from hemochromatosis with resultant cellular damage leading to:
   a. Splenomegaly, usually requiring splenectomy
   b. Skeletal complications such as thickened cranial bones, enlarged head, prominent facial bones, mongoloid appearance to eyes, enlarged maxilla, malocclusion of the teeth, and susceptibility to spontaneous fractures
   c. Cardiac complications such as dysrhythmias, pericarditis, congestive heart failure, and fibrosis of cardiac muscle fibers
   d. Gallbladder disease, including gallstones and possible cholecystectomy
   e. Liver enlargement leading to cirrhosis
   f. Skin changes such as jaundice and brown pigmentation due to iron deposits
   g. Growth retardation and endocrine complications such as delayed sexual maturation and diabetes mellitus possibly due to endocrine gland sensitivity to iron
4. Laboratory test results may reveal:
   a. Characteristic changes in RBCs, such as microcytosis, hypochromia, anisocytosis, poikilocytosis, target cells, and basophilic stippling of immature erythrocytes of various stages
   b. Decreased Hgb, Hct, and reticulocyte count
   c. Fetal Hgb (HgbF) with or without a small amount of normal adult Hgb (HgbA)
   d. Marked increase in erythroid precursors in bone marrow
   e. Folic acid deficiency
5. Prenatal diagnosis through amniocentesis and screening for thalassemia trait may be possible.
E. **Nursing diagnoses**
   1. Activity Intolerance
   2. Body Image Disturbance
   3. Altered Family Processes
   4. Altered Health Maintenance
   5. High Risk for Infection
   6. High Risk for Injury
   7. Knowledge Deficit
   8. Altered Nutrition: Less than Body Requirements

     9.   Pain

F. Planning and implementation

    1.   Implement iron chelation therapy with deferoxamine, as ordered, to eliminate excess iron and its side effects from deposition in tissues.

    2.   Provide information regarding potential splenectomy (for a child with severe splenomegaly) and follow-up care. Explain that prophylactic antibiotics and pneumococcal, meningococcal, and vaccines against *Haemophilus influenzae* are given to prevent complications from splenectomy.

    3.   Administer folic acid as ordered.

    4.   Prevent infection through blood hygiene, avoidance of persons with infections, adequate rest, and good nutrition. Observe for signs of infection.

    5.   Help prevent fractures by encouraging the child to avoid activities that might increase the risk of fractures.

    6.   Promote adequate rest by scheduling caregiving activities to allow for optimal rest.

    7.   Encourage optimal nutrition by taking diet history, determining child's food preferences, and providing those foods in a pleasant mealtime atmosphere. (*Note:* Dietary iron should be decreased as much as possible.)

    8.   Administer blood transfusions as needed, and observe for complications of multiple transfusions.

    9.   Monitor for signs of hepatitis and iron overload.

  10.   Assist the child in coping with disease and its management by exploring the child's feelings about his or her illness and changes in appearance and by preparing him or her for all procedures. Plan treatment to minimize its interference with the child's abilities.

  11.   Support the family by encouraging members to express their feelings about management of life-threatening illness, exploring any feelings of guilt regarding the disorder's hereditary nature, and emphasizing the importance of encouraging the child to lead as normal a life as possible.

  12.   Refer the family to support groups, such as the Cooley's Anemia Foundation.

  13.   Refer the family to genetic counseling, if appropriate.

  14.   Provide patient and family teaching, covering:

       a.   The nature of the disease and its management

       b.   Signs and symptoms of infection, iron overload, and other potential complications to watch for and report

       c.   Home chelation therapy

       d.   Activity restrictions, including avoidance of activities that increase the risk of fractures

       e.   Dietary restrictions

G. **Evaluation**
  1. The child engages in as normal a lifestyle as possible, is free from pain and infection, and copes well with body image changes.
  2. Parents verbalize an understanding of their child's illness and treatment measures.

VII. Hemophilia

A. **Description**
  1. Hemophilia is a group of hereditary bleeding disorders characterized by a deficiency in a blood clotting factor.
  2. The two most common forms are classic hemophilia (hemophilia A or factor VIII deficiency) and Christmas disease (hemophilia B or factor IX deficiency). The classic form accounts for about 75% of all cases.
  3. Hemophilia is classified as severe, moderate, or mild depending on the plasma level of the coagulation factor involved.

B. **Etiology and incidence**
  1. Hemophilia is transmitted by females as an X-linked recessive disorder (Table 10–4).
  2. It predominantly affects males, occurring in about 1 of every 8,000 live male births.

C. **Pathophysiology**
  1. In hemophilia A, factor VIII molecule is present but defective in its clotting function.
  2. Hemophilia B involves a defect or deficiency of factor IX.
  3. Clotting factor malfunction causes abnormal bleeding, due to impaired ability to form a fibrin clot.

D. **Assessment findings**
  1. Diagnosis is based on a history of bleeding episodes, family history, and laboratory studies indicating abnormal partial thromboplastin time and abnormal specific assays for factors VIII or IX. Platelet count, prothrombin test, and bleeding times are normal.

TABLE 10–4.
Transmission of Hemophilia Probability of Abnormality in Offspring

	FEMALE			MALE	
GENOTYPE OF PARENTS	NORMAL	CARRIER	HEMOPHILIAC	NORMAL	HEMOPHILIAC
Female carrier/normal male	50%	50%	0	50%	50%
Noncarrier female/hemophiliac male	0	100%	0	100%	0
Female carrier/hemophiliac male	0	50%	50%	50%	50%

(Brunner, L.S., and Suddarth, D.S. (1986). Lippincott manual of nursing practice. Philadelphia: J.B. Lippincott, p. 1,286)

2. Carrier detection and prenatal diagnosis through amniocentesis are possible.
3. Hemophilia is suspected in a newborn with excessive bleeding from the umbilical cord or after circumcision.
4. Common clinical manifestations in children include:
   a. Easy bruising
   b. Prolonged bleeding from wounds
   c. Spontaneous hematuria
   d. Lower gastrointestinal bleeding
   e. Epistaxis
   f. Hemarthrosis (hemorrhages into joints causing pain, swelling, and limited movement)
5. Disease complications may be manifested as:
   a. Bone changes, osteoporosis, and muscle atrophy, resulting in crippling deformities as a consequence of hemarthrosis
   b. Intracranial bleeding
   c. Gastrointestinal tract hemorrhage, leading to intestinal obstruction
   d. Hematomas in the spinal cord, resulting in paralysis
   e. Airway obstruction due to bleeding into the neck, mouth, or thorax
   f. Secondary complications from factor replacement such as hepatitis and immunodeficiency

E. Nursing diagnoses
   1. Activity Intolerance
   2. Altered Family Processes
   3. High Risk for Injury
   4. Knowledge Deficit
   5. Pain
   6. Self-Esteem Disturbance

F. Planning and implementation
   1. Administer medications as prescribed, which may include:
      a. Plasma products
      b. Fresh frozen plasma
      c. Cryoprecipitated factor VIII
      d. Factor VIII concentrate
      e. Factor IX
      f. Corticosteroids, to reduce inflammation in affected joints
      g. Acetaminophen with or without codeine for pain management (*Note:* Neither aspirin nor any aspirin-containing compound should be used.)
   2. Control bleeding by applying pressure and cold to the injury site and elevating and immobilizing the injured area.
   3. Observe for swelling or tenderness in joints.
   4. Monitor for signs of hypovolemia.

5. Monitor for signs of side effects of therapy such as hepatitis or immunodeficiency.
6. Help prevent crippling effects of joint degeneration through support of a physical therapy program, including passive range-of-motion exercises, and orthopedic measures such as casts, traction, and joint aspiration in joint rehabilitation.
7. Present information regarding surgical replacement of joints in the event of total disability.
8. Foster the child's positive self-image by exploring the child's feelings about the disease and encouraging him or her to engage in activities that increase self-esteem.
9. Assist family members in coping with their child's disease by providing information about the disease and its management and by encouraging family members to verbalize their feelings and concerns and any guilt they may have regarding genetic transmission.
10. Refer the family to support groups such as the National Hemophilia Foundation.
11. Refer parents for genetic counseling if desired.
12. Provide patient and family teaching, covering:
    a. Injury prevention, including the need for judicious limit setting that allows the child to lead as normal a life as possible
    b. Use of a soft toothbrush for oral hygiene and the need for regular dental check-ups
    c. The importance of wearing Medic-alert identification
    d. Passive range-of-motion exercises and other physical therapy measures
    e. Signs and symptoms of hemarthrosis and internal bleeding to watch for and report
    f. Drug administration techniques, including the importance of avoiding aspirin and aspirin-containing compounds
    g. Possible side effects of therapy, such as hepatitis and immunodeficiency
    h. Diet information (increased weight can further stress joints)

G. Evaluation
1. The child is free from pain and does not exhibit joint deformities.
2. The child demonstrates age-appropriate level of independence.
3. Parents verbalize knowledge of disease process and treatment.
4. Parents feel free to verbalize any guilt feelings they may have regarding the genetic aspects of disease.

Bibliography

Brunner, L. S., and Suddarth, D. S. (1986). *Lippincott manual of nursing practice* (4th ed.). Philadelphia: J. B. Lippincott.

Mott, S. R., James, S. R., and Spherac, A. M. (1990). *Nursing care of children and families* (2nd ed.). Menlo Park, CA: Addison-Wesley.

Waechter, E. H., Phillips, J., and Holaday, B. (1985). *Nursing care of children*. Philadelphia: J. B. Lippincott.

Whaley, L. F., and Wong, D. L. (1991). *Nursing care of infants and children* (4th ed.). St. Louis: C. V. Mosby.

STUDY QUESTIONS

1. Which of the following statements best describes iron-deficiency anemia?
   a. It is caused by depression of the hematopoietic system.
   b. It is most commonly seen in the first 2 months of life.
   c. Clinical manifestations are related to a reduction in the amount of oxygen available to tissues.
   d. It often results from a decreased intake of milk and the premature addition of solid foods.

2. In children with sickle cell disease, local tissue damage and pathologic tissue changes result from
   a. a general inflammatory response due to an autoimmune reaction complicated by hypoxia
   b. air hunger and resultant respiratory alkalosis due to deoxygenated RBCs
   c. local tissue damage with ischemia and necrosis due to obstructed circulation
   d. hypersensitivity of the central nervous system due to elevated serum bilirubin levels

3. When planning a patient and family education program for sickle cell disease, the nurse should include which of the following measures?
   a. proper handwashing and isolation from known sources of infection
   b. a high-iron, low-fat, high-protein diet
   c. fluid restrictions of 1 qt/day
   d. aerobic exercise to increase oxygen availability to tissues

4. Which of the following is an appropriate nursing measure to alleviate joint pain in a child with hemophilia?
   a. applying a heating pad
   b. providing passive range-of-motion exercises
   c. applying an ice pack
   d. administering salicylates

5. An adolescent patient in an ambulatory care clinic is diagnosed with iron-deficiency anemia. The most likely cause is
   a. lack of vitamin C
   b. abnormal Hgb structure
   c. hemolysis
   d. inadequate dietary intake of iron

6. In follow-up evaluation of nutritional counseling, the nurse would most like to see which of the following added to the diet of an anemic infant?
   a. orange juice
   b. milk
   c. egg yolks
   d. applesauce

7. Which of the following interventions represents safe and effective nursing management of a child with sickle cell disease?
   a. administration of heparin or other anticoagulants to prevent sickling
   b. health teaching to help reduce the incidence of sickling crises, including preventing infection and avoiding low oxygen environments
   c. observation of imposed fluid restrictions with careful monitoring of intake and output
   d. avoiding the use of narcotics, which promote increased oxygen consumption

8. The mother of a child just admitted to the hospital with sickle cell crisis asks the nurse if she can empty his urine in the toilet. What would be the nurse's best response?
   a. "Yes, thank you. I appreciate your help with your child's care."
   b. "No, I need to measure it each time he urinates."
   c. "That's fine. Can you keep a record of the number of times he urinates?"
   d. "We need to keep track of how much he urinates. I can show you how to measure and record the specific amount."

9. Which of the following statements best describes the pathology of aplastic anemia?

a. There is extensive proliferation of immature RBCs.
b. Only blood clotting mechanisms of the body are affected.
c. Depressed formation of RBCs, WBCs, and platelets occurs.
d. RBCs assume an abnormal size and shape.

10. Which of the following statements regarding thalassemia major is correct?
    a. It is an autosomal dominant disorder.
    b. It involves depressed formation of all formed elements of the blood.
    c. It is an acquired hemorrhagic disorder that results from excessive destruction of platelets.
    d. In the United States, it occurs predominantly in persons of Mediterranean or Asian origins.

11. When planning an education program for the parents of a child with thalassemia major, the nurse should include information regarding
    a. proper administration of oral iron supplements
    b. assessment for signs and symptoms of iron overload
    c. increased daily fluid requirements
    d. complications of hormone therapy

12. Which of the following tests is most definitive in diagnosing hemophilia?

a. bleeding time
b. partial thromboplastin time
c. platelet count
d. complete blood count

13. As the nurse evaluates the effectiveness of parent teaching concerning the transmission of hemophilia, which of the following statements by a parent would best indicate an accurate parental perception?
    a. "Ever since our son was diagnosed with hemophilia, I have had a fear that our daughter also has the disease."
    b. "Our son developed hemophilia because I had measles while I was pregnant with him."
    c. "I am a carrier of hemophilia even though I do not have the disease."
    d. "I am so relieved to know that since my husband is not affected by the disease, none of my daughters can be carriers."

14. Effective nursing management of hemarthrosis includes which of the following interventions?
    a. administering plasma products
    b. providing passive range of motion to the affected joint
    c. ensuring reverse isolation because of decreased platelet counts
    d. applying heat to the affected joint

ANSWER KEY

1. *Correct response: c*
Clinical manifestations result from decreased hemoglobin and reduced oxygen-carrying capacity of blood.
- **a.** Hematopoietic depression is not present.
- **b.** The disorder most commonly occurs between ages 6 months and 3 years.
- **d.** It often results from premature addition of milk and decreased intake of solid foods.

Analysis/Physiologic/Analysis (Dx)

2. *Correct response: c*
Characteristic sickle cells tend to clump, which results in poor circulation to tissue and eventual tissue ischemia and necrosis.
- **a.** Damage is not due to an inflammatory response.
- **b.** Air hunger and respiratory alkalosis are not present.
- **d.** Central nervous system effects are due to ischemia.

Comprehension/Physiologic/Analysis (Dx)

3. *Correct response: a*
Prevention of infection is an important measure in prevention of sickle cell crisis.
- **b.** This diet has no significance in prevention of crisis.
- **c.** Proper hydration should be encouraged to help prevent crisis.
- **d.** Strenuous activity and overexertion should be avoided.

Application/Health promotion/Planning

4. *Correct response: c*
Application of cold promotes vasoconstriction.
- **a.** Heat promotes vasodilation.
- **b.** The affected extremity should be immobilized.
- **d.** Salicylates should never be administered to a child with hemophilia because of their depressive effects on platelet function.

Application/Safe care/Implementation

5. *Correct response: d*
Inadequate dietary iron intake is the most common cause of iron deficiency anemia.
- **a.** Vitamin C deficiency is not a factor in iron deficiency anemia.
- **b.** Abnormal hemoglobin structure occurs in sickle cell anemia, not iron deficiency anemia.
- **c.** Hemolysis occurs in various immune hemolytic anemias, not in iron deficiency anemia.

Analysis/Physiologic/Analysis (Dx)

6. *Correct response: c*
Egg yolks are a good source of iron.
- **a.** Orange juice is not a good source of iron.
- **b.** Milk is not a good source of iron.
- **d.** Applesauce is not a good source of iron.

Application/Health promotion/Evaluation

7. *Correct response: b*
Because there is no cure for sickle cell disease, prevention is one of the main aims of therapeutic management.
- **a.** Anticoagulants do not prevent sickling.
- **c.** Fluids are encouraged to produce an increase in the fluid volume of the blood, which can help prevent sickling.
- **d.** Narcotics may be administered for pain control.

Application/Safe care/Implementation

8. *Correct response: d*
Careful intake and output monitoring is important to assess for possible alterations in fluid balance. Including the mother in the establishment of nursing goals is encouraged.
- **a.** Urine must be measured before it is discarded.
- **b.** This does not provide for the mother's participation.
- **c.** The amount of urine also must be determined.

Analysis/Psychosocial/Planning

9. *Correct response: c*
   Aplastic anemia is manifested by decreased production of blood cells in bone marrow.
   a. RBC production is depressed.
   b. Aplastic anemia also involves RBCs and WBCs.
   d. Aplastic anemia does not involve abnormal shape of cells.
Knowledge/Physiologic/Assessment

10. *Correct response: d*
    Increased incidence occurs in these groups.
    a. Thalassemia major is an autosomal recessive disorder.
    b. The disorder involves a deficiency in beta-chain synthesis of the hemoglobin molecule.
    c. The disorder involves formation of fragile RBCs that are easily destroyed.
Knowledge/Physiologic/Assessment

11. *Correct response: b*
    Iron overload is a potential complication of frequent blood transfusions in a child with thalassemia.
    a. Oral iron supplements are contraindicated in thalassemia.
    c. Fluid requirements are not increased in thalassemia.
    d. Hormone therapy is not indicated in thalassemia.
Application/Health promotion/Planning

12. *Correct response: b*

Partial thromboplastin time is abnormal in hemophilia.
   a. Bleeding times are normal in hemophilia.
   c. Platelet count is normal in hemophilia.
   d. Hemophilia does not affect the complete blood count.
Comprehension/Physiologic/Analysis (Dx)

13. *Correct response: c*
    The mother of a male child with hemophilia is a carrier of the abnormal gene on one of her X chromosomes.
    a. Daughters may be carriers but rarely have the disease themselves.
    b. Communicable diseases are not a factor in hemophilia.
    d. With an unaffected male and a mate who is a carrier, there is a 50% chance that a daughter will be a carrier.
Analysis/Health promotion/Evaluation

14. *Correct response: a*
    Plasma products containing the missing clotting factor are administered to treat joint bleeding in hemophilia.
    b. The affected joint should be immobilized.
    c. Platelet counts are normal in hemophilia.
    d. Ice packs are applied to affected joints to promote vasoconstriction.
Application/Safe care/Implementation

Cardiovascular Dysfunction

11

I. Essential concepts: cardiovascular anatomy and physiology

A. Development

1. Fetal heart development begins in the first month of gestation. At about 21 days of gestation, the fetal heart begins beating, and blood begins circulating.
2. Between the second and seventh weeks of gestation, the primitive fetal heart undergoes a series of changes that create the four-chambered heart and its great arteries.
3. During gestation, the lungs essentially are nonfunctional, and fetal blood oxygenation occurs in the placenta.
4. Key structures of fetal circulation (Fig. 11–1) include:
   a. Foramen ovale: opening between the atria that allows blood flow from the right atrium directly to the left atrium
   b. Ductus arteriosus: conduit between the pulmonary artery and the aorta that shunts blood away from pulmonary circulation
5. Important circulatory changes occurring during the transition to extrauterine life (Fig. 11–2) include:
   a. On lung expansion after delivery, inspired oxygen dilates pulmonary vessels, decreasing pulmonary vascular resistance and increasing pulmonary blood flow.
   b. The foramen ovale closes functionally soon after birth due to compression of the atrial septum.
   c. The ductus arteriosus closes functionally by 48 hours after birth.

B. Function

1. The cardiovascular system's basic function is to pump oxygenated blood to tissues and remove metabolic waste products from tissues.
2. Valves within the heart and pressure differences between the four heart chambers (the left and right atria and the left and right ventricles) regulate blood flow through the heart and into systemic circulation.
3. Blood returning to the heart through the venous system is at about 75% oxygenation saturation.
4. As blood passes through the pulmonary capillaries, it loses CO_2 and binds O_2 from the alveolar air and reaches 97% oxygen saturation.

II. Cardiovascular system overview

A. Assessment

1. Health history findings significant in cardiovascular dysfunction include:
   a. Family history of congenital heart disorders
   b. Presence of murmurs and age at which first noted
   c. Feeding problems, including fatigue or diaphoresis during feeding and poor weight gain

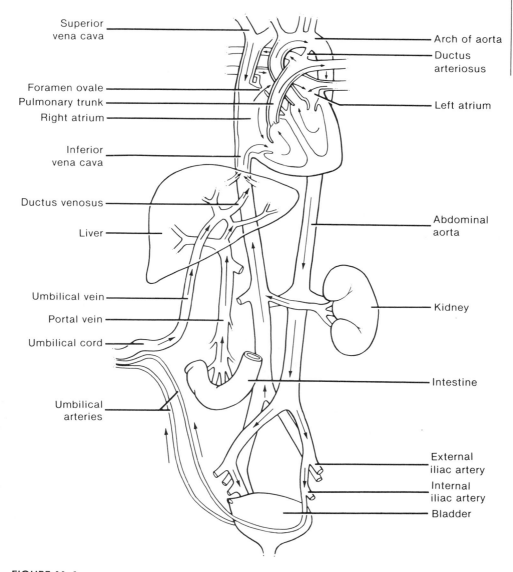

FIGURE 11–1.
Diagram of the fetal circulation shortly before birth; course of blood is indicated by arrows.

        d.   Respiratory difficulties, including tachypnea, dyspnea, shortness of breath, cyanosis, and frequent respiratory infections

        e.   Chronic fatigue or exercise intolerance

    2.   Significant physical assessment findings may include:

        a.   Growth abnormalities

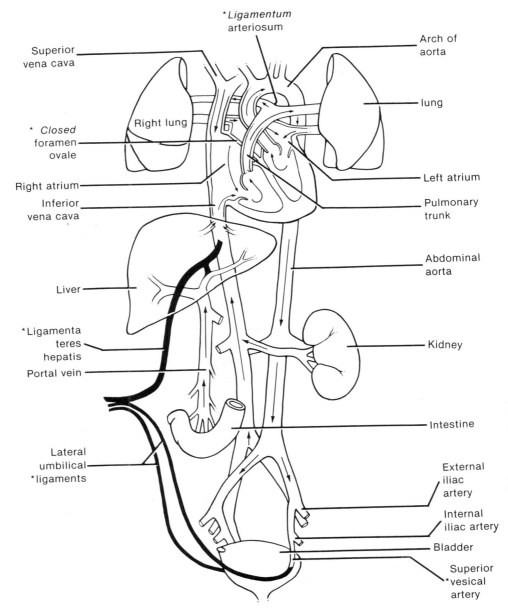

FIGURE 11–2.
Circulation after birth. Note the contrast with Figure 11–1.

      b.   Cyanosis

      c.   Clubbing of fingers and toes

      d.   Periorbital and peripheral edema

      e.   Pulse alterations, including tachycardia or bradycardia, dysrhythmias, diminished peripheral pulses, thready pulse, narrow or wide pulse pressures

      f.   Tachypnea

      g.   Hypotension or unequal blood pressure in arms and legs

      h.   Engorged neck veins

      i.   Murmurs, bruits, thrills (Table 11–1)

      j.   Abdominal distention, hepatomegaly, splenomegaly

B.   **Laboratory studies and diagnostic tests**

    1.   Relevant laboratory results may include:

      a.   Compensatory increase in hematocrit (polycythemia), hemoglobin, and erythrocyte count

      b.   Altered blood gas values

      c.   Abnormalities in hemostasis, such as thrombocytopenia; decreased platelet function; low prothrombin level; decreased or absent clotting factors V, VII, or IX

    2.   Important diagnostic studies include:

      a.   Electrocardiography (ECG), which helps evaluate cardiac musculature, cardiac rate and rhythm, and cardiac impulse conduction (see Table 11–2)

      b.   Chest radiography, which provides information on the size of heart and its chambers and on the prominence and distribution of pulmonary blood flow

TABLE 11–1.
Documenting Cardiac Murmurs

CHARACTERISTIC	DOCUMENTATION
Timing	Occurring in systole or diastole
Location	Where the murmur is best heard: pulmonic, aortic, mitral, or tricuspid areas; described in terms of intercostal space and distance from sternal border or axillary line
Radiation	Other places the murmur can be heard
Loudness	1/6: very faint 2/6: faint but detectable 3/6: readily detectable 4/6: loud 5/6: very loud 6/6: audible before the stethoscope comes in contact with the chest 4–6: associated with a palpable thrill
Quality	Blowing, harsh, musical, or rumbling
Pitch	High-, medium-, or low-pitched
Other	Crescendo, decrescendo, crescendo–decrescendo, or constant; any changes with respiratory cycle and positioning

TABLE 11–2.
Commonly Measured ECG Components

COMPONENT	WHAT IT REPRESENTS	CORRELATION WITH THE CARDIAC CYCLE
P wave	Atrial depolarization	Contraction of the right atrium begins at the peak of the P wave; left atrial contraction follows.
T wave	Ventricular repolarization	Repolarization occurs while the ventricles are still contracting.
P–R interval	Interval between the beginning of the P wave and the beginning of the QRS complex	This is the interval between the onset of atrial depolarization and the onset of ventricular depolarization (i.e., the conduction time between the atria and the ventricles).
Q–T interval	Interval from the beginning of the QRS complex to the end of the T wave	This is the total time of ventricular depolarization and repolarization.
QRS complex	Wave of ventricular depolarizaton	Left ventricular contraction begins at the peak of the R wave; right ventricular contraction, shortly thereafter.

    c.   Echocardiography, which can help assess the thickness of heart walls, the size of cardiac chambers, the motion of valves and septa within the heart, and anatomical relationships of great vessels to various intracardiac structures

    d.   Cardiac catheterization, which provides information on oxygen saturation within heart chambers, pressures within chambers, changes in cardiac output or stroke volume, and anatomic abnormalities (see Section VI for more information on this procedure)

C.   **Psychosocial implications**

    1.   Developmental delays often occur in children with cardiovascular disorders, particularly cyanotic heart defects.

    2.   Allowing the child sufficient time to complete tasks and activities is essential for nurturing a positive self-concept and promoting independence.

    3.   Activity limitations may be essential; however, such restrictions may be difficult to impose in a child with cardiac disease who has no overt symptoms (e.g., as in aortic stenosis).

    4.   With many defects, an older child may be allowed to self-limit activities according to how he or she feels.

    5.   Parents need support and guidance in setting limits, providing discipline, and providing for their child's emotional needs.

III.   **Acyanotic heart defects**

    A.   **Description**

        1.   Congenital heart defects in which no deoxygenated or poorly oxygenated venous blood enters systemic arterial circulation

2. Types of acyanotic defects include:
   a. Left to right shunting through an abnormal opening (e.g., patent ductus arteriosus [PDA], atrial septal defect [ASD], ventricular septal defect [VSD])
   b. Obstructive lesions that restrict ventricular outflow (e.g., aortic valvular stenosis, pulmonic stenosis, coarctation of the aorta)

B. Etiology and incidence
   1. In over 90% of congenital heart defects, the exact etiology is unknown.
   2. Factors associated with increased incidence of congenital heart defects include:
      a. Fetal and maternal infection during the first trimester (especially rubella)
      b. Maternal alcoholism
      c. Maternal use of other drugs with teratogenic effects
      d. Maternal age over 40 years
      e. Maternal dietary deficiencies
      f. Maternal insulin-dependent diabetes
      g. Other congenital defects
   3. Incidence of acyanotic heart defects is as follows:
      a. PDA: occurs in 1 of every 2,000 live births and accounts for 10% of congenital heart defects
      b. ASD: accounts for about 10% of congenital heart defects; occurs almost twice as often in females as in males
      c. VSD: the most common congenital heart disorder, accounting for up to 30% of all congenital heart defects
      d. Pulmonic stenosis: accounts for 5% to 8% of all congenital heart defects
      e. Coarctation of the aorta: accounts for about 7% of all congenital heart defects; twice as common in males as in females

C. Pathophysiology
   1. Patent ductus arteriosus
      a. PDA results from persistence of the fetal ductus arteriosus between the pulmonary artery and aorta (Fig. 11-3).
      b. Oxygenated blood flows from the aorta to the pulmonary artery through the patent ductus arteriosus; eventually, this places a greater volume burden on the left heart.
      c. A large PDA may result in left atrial and left ventricular enlargement, pulmonary edema due to increased pulmonary pressure, and congestive heart failure (CHF); in a small defect, these effects are minimal.
   2. Atrial septal defect.
      a. ASD refers to an abnormal opening in the septum between the left and right atria (Fig. 11-4).

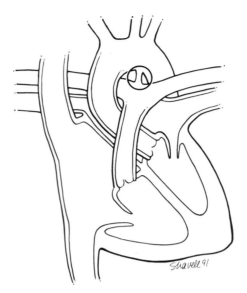

FIGURE 11–3.
Patent ductus arteriosus.

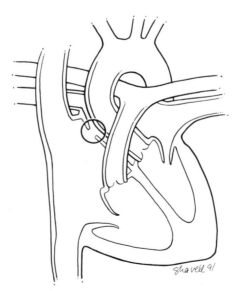

FIGURE 11–4.
Atrial septal defect.

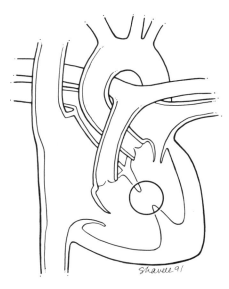

FIGURE 11–5.
Ventricular septal defect.

    b.   This opening may be located at the center of the atrial septum (ostium secundum) or at the base of the atrial septum (ostium primum).

    c.   Oxygenated blood flows through the defect from the left atrium to the right atrium and mixes with systemic venous blood returning to the lungs.

    d.   This increases the total blood flow to the lungs and leads to volume overload of the right ventricle, producing right-sided heart enlargement.

    e.   Increased volume of blood pumped through pulmonary circulation can lead to pulmonary edema and, eventually, CHF.

    f.   Excessive pulmonary resistance and right atrial pressure increase may cause reversal of the left-right shunt, producing cyanosis.

3.   Ventricular septal defect

    a.   VSD involves an abnormal opening in the septum between the right and left ventricles (Fig. 11–5).

    b.   Oxygenated blood flows through this opening from the left ventricle to the right ventricle.

    c.   Thus, an increased amount of blood enters the pulmonary circulation; this may result in increased pulmonary vascular resistance and right-sided heart enlargement.

    d.   Right ventricular and pulmonary arterial pressures increase,

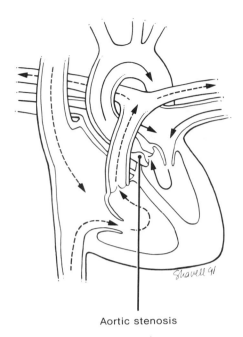

Aortic stenosis

FIGURE 11–6.
Aortic stenosis.

leading eventually to obstructive pulmonary vascular disease.

    e.   High pulmonary resistance and excessive right ventricular pressure increase may cause reversal of the left-right shunt, producing cyanosis.

4.   Aortic valvular stenosis

    a.   This defect primarily involves an obstruction to left ventricular outflow at the valve (Fig. 11–6).

    b.   Left ventricular pressure increases to overcome resistance of the obstructed valve and allow blood flow into the aorta, eventually producing left ventricular hypertrophy.

    c.   Myocardial ischemia may develop as the increased oxygen demands of the hypertrophied left ventricle go unmet.

5.   Pulmonic stenosis

    a.   This defect involves obstruction of blood flow from the right ventricle (Fig. 11–7).

    b.   As a result of right ventricular pressure increase, right ventricular hypertrophy may develop.

    c.   Eventually, right ventricular failure may occur.

6.   Coarctation of the aorta

    a.   This defect involves narrowing of the aorta, most com-

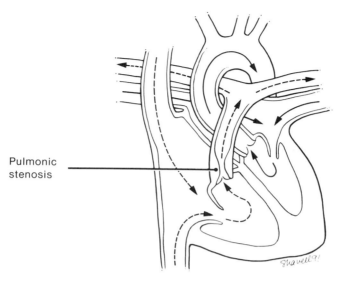

FIGURE 11–7.
Pulmonic stenosis.

monly distal to the origin of the left subclavian artery near the ductus arteriosus (Fig. 11–8).

b. The obstructive process causes hypertension in the aortic branches above the narrowing and diminished pressure in the arteries below the narrowing.

c. Restricted blood flow through the narrowed aorta increases the pressure on the left ventricle and causes dilation of the proximal aorta and left ventricular hypertrophy, which may lead to left ventricular failure.

d. Eventually, collateral vessels develop to bypass the coarctated segment and supply circulation to the lower extremities.

7. Endocardial cushion defects (ECDs)

a. ECDs involve defects in embryonic formation of the endocardium and valve leaflets, resulting in minor to major atrioventricular (AV) canal defects.

b. A *complete AV canal defect* consists of incomplete mitral valve and tricuspid valve formation, an ostium primum ASD, and a high VSD. This allows four-way communication among the left atrium, left ventricle, right atrium, and right ventricle.

c. This defect results in increased pulmonary blood flow and volume overload in the left and right ventricles.

d. The most common congenital heart defects in children with Down's syndrome, ECDs often are asymptomatic un-

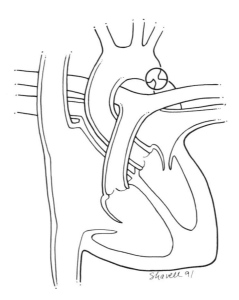

FIGURE 11–8.
Coarctation of the aorta.

til the pulmonary vascular resistance falls in the months after birth and left-to-right shunting occurs.

D. Assessment findings

1. In *PDA*, clinical manifestations and diagnostic findings may include:
   a. A continuous machinerylike murmur heard at the left infraclavicular area in older children
   b. Widened pulse pressure
   c. Slow weight gain and feeding difficulties
   d. Recurrent respiratory infections
   e. Signs and symptoms of CHF
   f. Cardiomegaly
   g. Increased pulmonary vasculature
   h. Possible left ventricular hypertrophy

2. In *ASD*, clinical manifestations and diagnostic findings may include:
   a. Absence of symptoms in a small ASD
   b. Slow weight gain
   c. Easy fatigability
   d. Dyspnea on exertion
   e. Frequent respiratory infections
   f. Signs and symptoms of CHF
   g. Systolic injection murmur heard most prominently at the second left intercostal space
   h. Abnormal S_2 heart sound

      i.   Prominent main pulmonary artery
      j.   Right-sided hypertrophy
      k.   Cardiomegaly
      l.   ECG changes

3. Clinical and diagnostic findings in *VSD* may include:
      a.   Absence of symptoms in a small VSD
      b.   Slow weight gain, failure to thrive, feeding difficulties
      c.   Pallor and diaphoresis
      d.   Frequent respiratory infections
      e.   Tachypnea
      f.   Signs and symptoms of CHF
      g.   Characteristic loud murmur, usually developing a few weeks after birth and best heard at the lower left sternal border
      h.   Biventricular hypertrophy, pulmonary artery enlargement, and left atrial enlargement

4. In *aortic valvular stenosis*, clinical and diagnostic findings typically include:
      a.   Usually absence of symptoms in infants
      b.   In older children, chest pain, dyspnea, and diminished peripheral pulses
      c.   Loud systolic ejection murmur heard best at the second right intercostal space
      d.   ECG changes
      e.   Ascending aorta dilation
      f.   Varying degrees of left ventricular enlargement

5. Clinical manifestations and diagnostic findings in *pulmonic stenosis* commonly include:
      a.   Absence of symptoms in most cases
      b.   In severe cases, decreased exercise tolerance, dyspnea, precordial pain, and generalized cyanosis
      c.   Systolic ejection murmur with thrill
      d.   Right ventricle enlargement
      e.   Main pulmonary artery enlargement
      f.   Right-sided hypertrophy in severe cases

6. In *coarctation of the aorta*, assessment findings may include:
      a.   Usually absence of symptoms in children
      b.   Possibly fatigue, headache, epistaxis, leg cramps, absent or diminished femoral pulses
      c.   Elevated systolic pressure in the arms with decreased pressure in the legs
      d.   Systolic murmur heard along the left sternal border
      e.   Prominent aorta
      f.   Rib notching in older children
      g.   Cardiomegaly
      h.   Increased pulmonary vascularity

            i.   Left ventricular hypertrophy

     7.   Clinical and diagnostic findings in *endocardial cushion defects* commonly include:

         a.   Cyanosis in complete AV canal

         b.   Murmurs characteristic of ASD or VSD

         c.   Signs and symptoms of pulmonary edema and CHF in complete AV canal

         d.   Elevated arterial pressures

         e.   Growth retardation

E.   **Nursing diagnoses** (*Note:* Nursing diagnoses depend on specific manifestations of the defect. Refer also to nursing diagnoses for CHF [section V.E.], cardiac catheterization [section VI.E], and cardiac surgery [section VII.E].)

    1.   Activity Intolerance

    2.   Anxiety

    3.   Altered Family Processes

    4.   Anticipatory Grieving

    5.   Altered Growth and Development

    6.   High Risk for Infection

    7.   High Risk for Injury

    8.   Knowledge Deficit

    9.   Altered Nutrition: Less than Body Requirements

   10.   Self-esteem disturbance

F.   **Planning and implementation**

    1.   Help maintain optimal nutritional status by:

         a.   Promoting a well-balanced diet that's rich in iron and potassium and low in sodium

         b.   Providing small, frequent meals if the child tires easily

         c.   Providing nipples that make it easier for an infant to suck and limiting feedings to 45 minutes or less if the child tires

         d.   Evaluating weight gain regularly

    2.   Help decrease cardiac workload by organizing nursing care to provide for periods of uninterrupted rest, preventing excessive crying in infants, and providing diversional activities that involve only limited energy expenditure for older children.

    3.   Observe for and assist in managing CHF (see section V.F).

    4.   Observe for and assist in managing respiratory distress (marked by manifestations such as tachypnea, tachycardia, retractions, grunting, nasal flaring, cough, and cyanosis) by:

         a.   Administering oxygen therapy as ordered

         b.   Positioning the child to ease breathing

    5.   Observe for and assist in managing hypoxia (marked by manifestations such as tachypnea, cyanosis, bradycardia, tachycardia, restlessness, progressive limpness and syncope) by:

         a.   Placing the child in the knee-chest position

     b.   Administering oxygen, as ordered

     c.   Administering medications, as ordered

     d.   Documenting hypoxic spells

6.   Observe for and assist in managing infective carditis (characterized by fever, pallor, petechiae, anorexia, fatigue) by:

     a.   Ensuring prophylactic administration of antibiotics before dental work, surgery, or laceration repair

     b.   Preventing the child's exposure to ill persons

7.   Monitor for signs and symptoms of thrombosis, such as irritability, restlessness, seizure activity, coma, paralysis, edema, hematuria, oliguria, anuria. To reduce the risk of thrombosis, prevent dehydration, especially during acute illness.

8.   Help prevent infection through careful handwashing, avoiding contact between the child and with infected persons, ensuring that the child's immunizations are up to date, and providing for adequate rest.

9.   Help prevent hypokalemia secondary to diuretic therapy by maintaining a high-potassium diet and administering supplemental potassium, as ordered.

10.   Help prevent anemia by administering iron preparations, as ordered.

11.   Enhance the child's self-concept by encouraging him or her to express feelings about the defect, clarifying any misconceptions he or she expresses concerning the defect and its treatment, and supporting positive coping mechanisms.

12.   Help decrease the child's and family members' anxiety and increase their understanding by providing needed information on medical and surgical treatments for the specific defect.

13.   Provide the following information for *PDA*:

     a.   Surgery may be performed electively by age 1 to 2 years, earlier if CHF develops. Ligation of PDA is not open-heart surgery and does not require cardiopulmonary bypass.

     b.   In premature infants, PDA sometimes can be closed using prostaglandin synthetase inhibitors, such as indomethacin, which stimulate closure of the ductus.

     c.   Some children experience transient unexplained hypertension following repair.

14.   Provide the following information for *ASD*:

     a.   Surgical closure by suture or patch requires cardiopulmonary bypass and usually is performed between age 4 and 6 years.

     b.   Some children develop dysrhythmias despite surgery.

15.   Provide the following information on *VSD*:

     a.   Most VSDs close spontaneously.

     b.   Early surgery, involving closure with a dacron patch and requiring cardiopulmonary bypass, is recommended for children with pulmonary arterial hypertension, CHF, recurrent respiratory infections, and failure to thrive.

    c.   Surgery is complex; pulmonary artery banding may be done as a palliative procedure for infants who are poor surgical candidates.

16.   Provide the following information for *aortic valvular stenosis*:

    a.   If symptomatic, surgical aortic valvulotomy or prosthetic valve replacement is necessary.

    b.   Children with this defect may be restricted from sports and physical exertion.

17.   Provide the following information for *pulmonic stenosis*:

    a.   In moderate to severe cases, surgical valvulotomy is performed.

    b.   Surgery is done immediately in symptomatic newborns and is delayed until excessively high pressure in the right ventricle warrants it in children with mild to moderate stenosis.

18.   Provide the following information for *coarctation of the aorta*:

    a.   Emergency management includes administration of prostaglandin E to dilate the ductus arteriosus and restore lower body blood flow.

    b.   Later intervention involves management of CHF and surgical resection between ages 2 and 4—unless heart failure or severe hypertension presents earlier.

    c.   Postoperatively, most children continue to exhibit some degree of hypertension and ECG changes with exercise.

19.   Provide the following information for *endocardial cushion defects*:

    a.   The goal of treatment is to control pulmonary hypertension and prevent serious pulmonary obstructive disease.

    b.   Optimal treatment is surgical repair involving closure of the septal defect and repair of the mitral and tricuspid valves.

    c.   If the child is a poor surgical risk, pulmonary artery banding may be done to decrease blood flow to the lungs and slow pulmonary changes.

20.   Assist the child's family in coping with diagnosis, treatment, and prognosis by:

    a.   Encouraging family members to ventilate their feelings and concerns

    b.   Encouraging the family to provide as normal a life as possible for the child and to stimulate him or her with age-appropriate activities consistent with his or her activity tolerance

    c.   Initiating a community health nurse referral, as needed

21.   Provide patient and family teaching, covering:

    a.   Nature of the defect, diagnosis, treatment, and potential complications

      b.   Infection prevention and control measures

      c.   Administration, dosage, and side effects of prescribed medications

      d.   The child's nutritional requirements and any special diet information

      e.   The child's need for adequate rest periods and any physical or activity limitations

      f.   The significance of normal developmental tasks and the importance of avoiding overprotecting the child through overstrict activity limitations

G. Evaluation

1. Parents verbalize knowledge of their child's defect, treatments, and potential complications.
2. The child verbalizes an age-appropriate understanding of the disease and its treatment.
3. The child maintains adequate oxygenation, as evidenced by normal color and improved blood gas values.
4. The child remains free from infection.
5. The child's breathing is nonlabored.
6. The child gains or maintains adequate weight.
7. Parents verbalize the date and time of the next scheduled follow-up appointment.

IV. Cyanotic heart defects

A. Description

1. Congenital heart defects in which deoxygenated blood enters systemic arterial circulation
2. Cyanotic heart defects include:
   a. Tetralogy of Fallot
   b. Tricuspid atresia
   c. Transposition of the great vessels
   d. Truncus arteriosus
   e. Total anomalous pulmonary venous communication
   f. Hypoplastic left heart syndrome

B. Etiology and incidence

1. In over 90% of congenital heart defects, the exact etiology is unknown.
2. Factors associated with increased incidence of congenital heart defects include:
   a. Fetal and maternal infection during the first trimester (especially rubella)
   b. Maternal alcoholism
   c. Maternal use of other drugs with teratogenic effects
   d. Maternal age over 40 years
   e. Maternal dietary deficiencies
   f. Maternal insulin-dependent diabetes

g.   Other congenital defects
3.   Approximate relative incidence of cyanotic defects is as follows:
   a.   Tetralogy of Fallot: the most common cyanotic heart defect, accounting for about 10% of all congenital heart defects; affects males and females equally
   b.   Tricuspid atresia: represents about 3% of all congenital heart defects
   c.   Transposition of the great vessels: accounts for about 5% of all congenital heart defects; incidence is about three times greater in males than in females
   d.   Truncus arteriosus: relatively rare, accounting for only about 1% of all congenital heart defects
   e.   Total anomalous pulmonary venous communication: accounts for about 2% of all congenital heart defects
   f.   Hypoplastic left heart syndrome: represents 7% to 9% of all congenital heart defects

C.   Pathophysiology
1.   In all these defects, cyanosis results from right-left shunting of blood through intracardiac communication, mixing of blood in a common heart chamber, or abnormal development of major blood vessels.
2.   Specific pathology and clinical manifestations depend on the severity of the defect and on the amount of pulmonary blood flow involved.
3.   Tetralogy of Fallot
   a.   This defect consists of four abnormalities: a VSD, which shunts unoxygenated blood from the right ventricle through the VSD and into the aorta; overriding of the aorta; pulmonic stenosis, leading to obstruction of blood flow from the right ventricle to pulmonary circulation; and right ventricular hypertrophy due to increased right ventricular pressure.
   b.   Manifestations depend on the size of VSD and the degree of pulmonic stenosis.
4.   Tricuspid atresia
   a.   This disorder involves three major defects: a lack of communication between right atrium and right ventricle due to absence of the tricuspid valve, an ASD, and right ventricular hypoplasia.
   b.   Blood from systemic circulation shunts from the right atrium through an interatrial communication to the left atrium and then to the left ventricle.
   c.   Pulmonary blood flow is generated through a PDA, bronchial circulation, or a VSD.
   d.   Potential complications include cerebrovascular accident,

brain abscess, bacterial endocarditis, and congestive heart failure.

5. Transposition of the great vessels
   a. In this defect, the pulmonary artery originates from the left ventricle, and the aorta originates from the right ventricle.
   b. This defect results in two separate circulations, with the right heart managing systemic circulation and the left heart managing pulmonary circulation.
   c. To sustain life, the patient must have an accompanying defect that enables mixing of oxygenated and unoxygenated blood between the two circulations, such as ASD, VSD, PDA, or patent foramen ovale.
   d. Potential complications of this defect include CHF, infective endocarditis, brain abscess, and cerebrovascular accident due to thrombosis or severe hypoxia.
6. Truncus arteriosus
   a. In this defect, one artery (the truncus), rather than two arteries (the aorta and pulmonary artery), arises from the ventricles and receives blood for pulmonary, systemic, and coronary circulations.
   b. Blood ejected from the left and right ventricles enters this common vessel and flows either to the lungs or to the aorta.
   c. A large intraventricular septal defect is located below the origin of the truncus.
   d. Neonates with this defect often appear normal; but as pulmonary vascular resistance decreases after birth, severe pulmonary edema and CHF commonly develop.
7. Total anomalous pulmonary venous communication
   a. In this defect, also known as total anomalous pulmonary venous return, pulmonary venous blood empties into the right atrium instead of into the left atrium.
   b. This defect can range from simple, with only minor symptoms, to complex, which is immediately life threatening. Variations are described as supracardiac, cardiac, intracardiac, or mixed (or as types A, B, C, or D), depending on how pulmonary venous blood returns to the heart.
   c. The physiologic effects of this defect depend on whether the communication between the common pulmonary venous chamber and the heart or the interatrial septum is unobstructed or obstructed.
   d. If communication is unobstructed, excess blood flow circulates to the right atrium, right ventricle, and pulmonary artery. Also, oxygenated blood returning from the lungs and deoxygenated blood returning from systemic circulation mix, leading to systemic hypoxemia and cyanosis.

       e.   Obstructed communication results in significant pulmonary venous hypertension, which can be fatal if not rapidly relieved.

   8.   Hypoplastic left heart syndrome

       a.   This syndrome involves various left-sided defects, commonly including severe coarctation of the aorta, severe aortic valve stenosis or atresia, and severe mitral valve stenosis or atresia.

       b.   The left ventricle, aortic valve, mitral valve, and ascending aorta are usually small or hypoplastic.

       c.   Survival is possible only while the ductus arteriosus remains patent, which allows systemic blood flow.

       d.   When the ductus arteriosus closes, pulmonary edema and low cardiac output occur, leading to hypoxia, acidosis, and death. Corrective surgery is not feasible.

D.   **Assessment findings**

   1.   Clinical manifestations and diagnostic findings in *tetralogy of Fallot* vary depending on the size of the VSD and the degree of right ventricular outflow obstruction and may include:

       a.   Cyanosis, often observed in the neonate only during crying spells but later in life, as stenosis worsens, occurring even at rest

       b.   Clubbing of fingers and toes

       c.   Squatting (a characteristic posture of older children with this defect that serves to decrease venous return of low oxygen content blood from lower extremities and increase systemic vascular resistance, which increases pulmonary blood flow and eases respiratory effort)

       d.   Slow weight gain

       e.   Dyspnea on exertion

       f.   Hypoxic spells (sometimes called "tet" spells) and transient cerebral ischemia

       g.   A loud systolic murmur heard along the left sternal border, a loud click heard immediately after the S_1 heart sound, a single S_2 sound

       h.   Boot-shaped heart with a small, concave pulmonary segment

       i.   Right ventricular hypertrophy

       j.   Polycythemia and increased hematocrit

   2.   In *tricuspid atresia*, typical assessment findings include:

       a.   Severe cyanosis beginning in the neonatal period

       b.   Respiratory distress

       c.   Clubbing of fingers and toes

       d.   Hypoxic spells

       e.   Failure to thrive

       f.   Possibly, signs and symptoms of congestive heart failure

   g. No murmur or characteristic murmur of associated heart defect, such as VSD or PDA
   h. Normal or mildly increased heart size
   i. Right atrial, left atrial, and left ventricular hypertrophy
   j. Diminutive right ventricular chamber and absence of tricuspid valve
   k. Left axis deviation on ECG

3. *Transposition of the great vessels* produces variable clinical manifestations and diagnostic results, possibly including:
   a. Cyanosis, usually developing shortly after birth
   b. CHF, manifested by tachypnea, cardiomegaly, and hepatomegaly
   c. Easy fatigability
   d. Failure to thrive
   e. Clubbing of fingers and toes
   f. No murmur or murmur characteristic of associated cardiac defect such as PDA or VSD
   g. Single, intense S_2
   h. Normal or moderately enlarged heart
   i. Right ventricular or biventricular hypertrophy
   j. Egg-shaped cardiac silhouette
   k. Right axis deviation on ECG
   l. Polycythemia and thrombocytopenia

4. Assessment findings in *truncus arteriosus* typically include:
   a. Cyanosis, especially on exertion
   b. Signs and symptoms of CHF
   c. Single, loud S_2; systolic ejection click
   d. Loud systolic murmur heart best at the lower left sternal border and radiating throughout the chest
   e. Cardiomegaly
   f. Biventricular and left atrial hypertrophy

5. In *total anomalous pulmonary venous communication*, clinical manifestations and diagnostic findings typically include:
   a. Cyanosis developing soon after birth
   b. Systolic murmur similar to that of ASD in unobstructed communication
   c. No murmurs but an accentuated S_2 in obstructed communication
   d. Right ventricular and right atrial hypertrophy
   e. Pulmonary edema in obstructed communication
   f. Cardiomegaly in unobstructed communication

6. Manifestations of *hypoplastic left heart syndrome* usually are evident by the first 2 weeks after birth and typically include:
   a. Signs and symptoms of pulmonary edema and CHF
   b. Single S_2
   c. Soft systolic ejection murmur

    d.   Cardiomegaly

    e.   Right ventricular and right atrial hypertrophy

E. Nursing diagnoses (See nursing diagnoses for acyanotic defects, section IV.E)

F. Planning and implementation

1.   Nursing interventions for infants and children with cyanotic heart defects are similar to those for patients with acyanotic heart defects (see section III.F), with the exception of patient and family teaching about specific defects and their management.

2.   Help decrease the child's and family members' anxiety and increase their understanding by providing needed information on medical and surgical treatments for the specific defect.

3.   Provide the following information for *tetralogy of Fallot*:

    a.   Intervention is based on symptomatology.

    b.   Early cyanosis requires a palliative procedure to increase blood flow to the lungs, such as the Blalock-Taussig shunt or Waterson shunt.

    c.   Complete surgical repair usually is performed between age 18 and 36 months; the procedure, which requires cardiopulmonary bypass, involves patch closure of the VSD and relief of the pulmonary stenosis.

    d.   Potential complications include heart block, residual VSD or pulmonary stenosis, and pulmonary valve regurgitation.

4.   Provide the following information on *tricuspid atresia*:

    a.   Infants may be given prostaglandin E to keep the ductus arteriosus patent.

    b.   Palliative procedures, such as the Blalock-Taussig shunt, Waterson shunt, or Glenn procedure, may be performed.

    c.   A balloon atrial septostomy may be done to ensure a large interatrial communication.

    d.   Total repair, known as the Fontan procedure, involves open heart surgery to create a communication between the right atrium and the pulmonary artery or the right ventricle via direct anastomosis or conduit; the ASD and VSD are then closed.

    e.   Surgery has proved most successful in children over age 5 years who have relatively normal pulmonary vasculature, adequate left ventricular function, and absence of significant mitral regurgitation.

    f.   Many children experience chronic fluid retention and reduced exercise tolerance.

5.   Provide the following information for *transposition of the great vessels*:

    a.   Prostaglandin E may be administered to maintain a patent ductus arteriosus while further evaluation is done.

    b.   Enlargement of the interatrial communication by balloon septostomy during cardiac catheterization—the Rashkind procedure—is important to maintain adequate mixing of oxygenated and unoxygenated blood.

    c.   The Blalock-Hanlon procedure may be performed to surgically enlarge the foramen ovale.

    d.   Infants with massive pulmonary flow and intractable heart failure require early surgical intervention usually by placing a band around the pulmonary artery and reducing flow to the lungs, which relieves the congestive failure until the child is old enough for definitive repair.

    e.   Surgical procedures for total repair include the Mustard, the Senning, and the arterial switch procedures.

    f.   Potential complications of surgery include superior vena cava or inferior vena cava obstruction, dysrhythmias, tricuspid regurgitation, and pulmonary venous obstruction.

    g.   Without treatment, 90% of infants with this defect die within the first year after birth.

6.   Provide the following information for *truncus arteriosus*:

    a.   CHF is treated medically.

    b.   Palliative surgery involves pulmonary arterial banding.

    c.   Corrective surgery, usually performed before age 2 years, consists of closing the VSD, removing the pulmonary arteries from the truncus arteriosus, and interposing a conduit between the right ventricle and pulmonary artery.

    d.   Possible complications of surgery include residual VSA, truncal valve regurgitation, conduit obstruction, and pulmonary vascular disease.

7.   Provide the following information for *total anomalous pulmonary venous communication*:

    a.   Palliative procedures include the Rashkind balloon septostomy to ensure interatrial communication.

    b.   Surgical repair involves directing the pulmonary venous blood into the left atrium and repairing any associated defects.

    c.   Infants with obstructed communication veins require surgery as soon as possible. Infants with unobstructed communication may be treated for CHF until surgery is performed.

    d.   Potential complications of surgery include pulmonary venous obstruction and dysrhythmias.

8.   Provide the following information on *hypoplastic left heart syndrome*:

    a.   About 95% of infants die by age 1 month unless surgery is performed.

    b.   Palliative procedures have had limited success at extending life. Some cardiac transplantation has been performed.

      c.   Many parents may take their infants home to die; these families may welcome referral to community hospice programs for support.

G. **Evaluation (see evaluation for acyanotic defects, section III.G)**

V. Congestive heart failure

    A. **Description: Severe circulatory congestion due to decreased myocardial contractility resulting in the heart's inability to pump sufficient blood to meet the body's needs**

    B. **Etiology and incidence**

        1.   The primary cause of CHF in the first 3 years of life is congenital heart disease.

        2.   Other causes in children include:

            a.   Other myocardial disorders, such as cardiomyopathies, dysrhythmias, and hypertension

            b.   Pulmonary embolism or chronic lung disease

            c.   Severe hemorrhage or anemia

            d.   Adverse effects of anesthesia or surgery

            e.   Adverse effects of transfusions or infusions

            f.   increased body demands resulting from such conditions as fever, infection, and arteriovenous fistula

            g.   Adverse effects of drugs, such as doxorubicin

            h.   Severe physical or emotional stress

            i.   Excessive sodium intake

        3.   About 80% of CHF cases in children occur before age 1 year.

    C. **Pathophysiology**

        1.   In CHF, the heart is unable to meet the body's oxygenation and nutrition needs, most commonly due to excessive volume or pressure load on the heart or to diminished myocardial function.

        2.   The body attempts to compensate through the following mechanisms:

            a.   Increased heart rate and increased stroke volume, resulting in cardiomegaly

            b.   Release of catecholamines, which increases systemic vascular resistance and leads to decreased renal blood flow

            c.   Decreased glomerular filtration rate and increased tubular reabsorption, leading to diminished urinary output and sodium retention.

        3.   Further myocardial stretching results in progressively ineffective contractions, leading to diminished cardiac output and pulmonary and systemic circulation congestion.

    D. **Assessment findings**

        1.   Signs and symptoms of CHF vary somewhat depending of the child's age and on whether failure occurs on the right or left side of the heart; manifestations of combined right- and left-sided CHF (the usual condition) may include:

    a.   Respiratory distress, marked by tachypnea, dyspnea, orthopnea, retractions, nasal flaring, grunting
    b.   Cough
    c.   Tachycardia, S_3 ventricular gallop
    d.   Pallor, mottling, or cyanosis
    e.   Edema (peripheral and periorbital)
    f.   Feeding difficulties and failure to thrive
    g.   Restlessness and irritability
    h.   Weakness, easy fatigability
    i.   Unexplained weight gain
    j.   Diaphoresis
    k.   Abdominal distention
    l.   Neck vein distention
    m.   Hepatomegaly
2.   Chest radiograph reveals cardiomegaly and pulmonary congestion.
3.   Laboratory study results commonly reveal dilutional hyponatremia, hypochloremia, and hyperkalemia.

E. **Nursing diagnoses**
1.   Activity Intolerance
2.   Anxiety
3.   Ineffective Breathing Pattern
4.   Decreased Cardiac Output
5.   Altered Family Processes
6.   Fluid Volume Excess
7.   High Risk for Injury
8.   High Risk for Infection
9.   Altered Nutrition: Less than Body Requirements

F. **Planning and implementation**
1.   Monitor for signs of respiratory distress. Provide pulmonary hygiene as needed, administer oxygen as ordered, keep the head of the bed elevated, and monitor arterial blood gas values.
2.   Monitor for signs of altered cardiac output, such as signs and symptoms of pulmonary edema; dysrhythmias, including extreme tachycardia or bradycardia; and characteristic ECG and heart sound changes.
3.   Evaluate fluid status by keeping strict intake and output records, monitoring daily weights, assessing for edema and severe diaphoresis, and monitoring electrolyte values and hematocrit level. Maintain fluid restrictions, as ordered.
4.   Help prevent infection through scrupulous handwashing and limiting the child's exposure to persons with infections.
5.   Reduce cardiac demands by keeping the child warm and clustering nursing care activities to allow for periods of uninterrupted rest. Do not allow an infant to feed for more than 45 minutes at

a time, and gavage-feed if the infant becomes fatigued before eating an adequate amount.

6. Help ensure adequate nutrition. As necessary, provide small, frequent meals. Maintain a high-calorie, low-sodium diet, as ordered.

7. Help decrease the child's and parents' anxiety by providing developmentally appropriate explanations, encouraging expression of feelings and concerns, and encouraging parental involvement in the child's care, as appropriate.

8. Administer medications as ordered, which may include:
   a. Digoxin, given to increase cardiac performance.
   b. Diuretics such as furosemide, hydrochlorothiazide, and spironolactone, given to reduce venous and systemic congestion
   c. Iron and folic acid supplements, given to improve nutritional status

9. Monitor for medication side effects, including:
   a. Digitalis toxicity: Extreme bradycardia is a cardinal symptom of toxicity; hold the drug if the child's heart rate falls below the normal range for age, unless the physician specifies a different guideline.
   b. Hypokalemia, due to diuretic therapy: Monitor potassium level closely and administer supplemental potassium, if necessary.

10. As appropriate, refer the family to a community health nurse for follow-up after discharge.

11. Provide patient and family teaching, covering:
    a. Signs and symptoms of CHF to watch for and report
    b. Diet and fluid restrictions
    c. Dosage, administration, and side effects of prescribed medications

G. Evaluation

1. The child exhibits improved cardiac output, as evidenced by clinical condition and laboratory values.

2. The child has normal fluid and electrolyte values and decreased edema.

3. The child exhibits improved oxygenation, as evidenced by normal color and blood gas values within the normal range.

4. The child maintains adequate nutrition for optimal weight gain.

5. Parents verbalize an understanding of signs and symptoms of CHF and possible complications, correct dosage and administration of medications, and necessary follow-up care.

6. The family is referred to a community health nurse for follow-up as appropriate.

VI. Cardiac catheterization

A. Description

1. This invasive diagnostic procedure involves introducing a radiopaque catheter into a peripheral blood vessel and advancing it into the heart.

2. The catheter commonly is introduced through a percutaneous puncture into the femoral vein, then guided into the cardiac chambers with the aid of fluoroscopy.

3. Radiopaque contrast material may be injected through the catheter into the heart to provide more diagnostic information.

B. Purpose: Cardiac catheterization provides information concerning oxygen saturation, pressures within various cardiac chambers, changes in cardiac output or stroke volume, and anatomic abnormalities.

C. Assessment: Preprocedure assessment should include the following components:

1. General health status, including activity level, presence of infection, and history of acute illness

2. Vital signs

3. Complete blood count, clotting studies

4. Urinalysis

D. Nursing diagnoses

1. Preprocedure
   a. Fear
   b. High Risk for Fluid Volume Deficit
   c. Knowledge Deficit
   d. Altered Tissue Perfusion: Cardiopulmonary

2. Postprocedure
   a. Decreased Cardiac Output
   b. Pain
   c. Impaired Skin Integrity
   d. Altered Tissue Perfusion: Cardiopulmonary

E. Planning and implementation: preprocedure

1. Prepare the child and family for the procedure with developmentally appropriate explanations. In general, sensory explanations (e.g., "You will see . . . ", "You will feel . . . ") are most helpful for a child.

2. Help alleviate the child's fears by encouraging him or her to talk about the procedure and express any concerns. As appropriate, initiate therapeutic play to help identify and assuage the child's fears and misconceptions, and allow the child to have a security object, such as a favorite blanket or toy.

3. Support family members by reinforcing and clarifying information provided by the physician.

4. Maintain NPO status for 4 to 6 hours before the procedure; the child may be sedated before catheterization to minimize pain and trauma.

5. Help prevent injury by observing the puncture site for bleeding, swelling, and hematoma formation. If hemorrhage occurs, apply pressure above the site and notify the physician.

F. **Planning and implementation: postprocedure**

1. Maintain the child on bedrest with the affected leg straight, as ordered; usually 4 to 6 hours after venous catheterization and 6 to 8 hours after arterial catheterization. Keep the child quiet, and evaluate extremity color, temperature, pedal pulse, capillary filling time, and sensation frequently.

2. Monitor vital signs, and assess for cardiac dysrhythmias by auscultating the apical pulse to detect irregularities; report any abnormal findings to the physician.

3. Assess hydration status by monitoring intake and output, evaluating urine specific gravity, and observing for signs of dehydration. Encourage oral fluid intake.

4. Assess for pain, and administer analgesics as ordered.

5. Advance the child's diet as tolerated.

6. Explore with parents their feelings regarding the procedure, its results, and their implications.

7. Provide patient and family teaching, covering:
   a. Signs and symptoms: watch for and report any bleeding or swelling at the catheter insertion site.
   b. Home care measures, including bathing: older children may shower; infants and young children should be given sponge baths for the first 3 days.
   c. Catheterization site care: change the bandage over insertion site daily for 3 days, and observe for inflammation or excessive tenderness.

G. **Evaluation**

1. The skin at the catheter insertion site remains intact and noninflamed.

2. The child maintains adequate hydration status.

3. The child exhibits stable vital signs.

4. The child remains quiet and calm.

5. The child or family members verbalize an understanding of and demonstrate proper care of the catheterization site.

6. Parents verbalize dates and times of scheduled appointments for follow-up care.

VII. Cardiac surgery

A. **Description**

1. *Open-heart* surgery involves incising the myocardium to repair intracardiac structures; requires cardiopulmonary bypass.

2. *Closed-heart* surgery involves structures related to the heart but not the heart muscle itself and usually can be done without cardiopulmonary bypass.

B. **Purpose: Cardiac surgery may be performed as an emergency or a planned procedure to correct defects or provide symptomatic relief.**

C. **Assessment: Preoperative assessment should include the following components:**

  1. Health history: cardiac, pulmonary, renal, hepatic, hematologic, and metabolic disorders; medication history, including any allergies or adverse reactions

  2. Baseline assessments of:

    a. Height and weight

    b. Vital signs

    c. Sleep–wake patterns

    d. Elimination patterns

    e. Fluid intake

  3. Laboratory studies:

    a. Complete blood count

    b. Serum electrolyte levels

    c. Clotting studies

    d. Urinalysis

    e. Nose, throat, sputum, and urine cultures

    f. Antibody screen

    g. Renal and hepatic function tests

  4. Radiographic and other diagnostic studies:

    a. Chest radiograph

    b. ECG

    c. Echocardiogram

    d. Cardiac catheterization

D. **Nursing diagnoses: preoperative and postoperative** (*Note:* See also the nursing diagnoses for specific cardiac anomalies that necessitate surgery.)

  1. Activity Intolerance

  2. Anxiety

  3. Ineffective Breathing Patterns

  4. Decreased Cardiac Output

  5. Altered Family Processes

  6. Fear

  7. Fluid Volume Deficit

  8. Altered Growth and Development

  9. Altered Health Maintenance

  10. High Risk for Infection

  11. High Risk for Injury

  12. Pain

  13. Sensory and Perceptual Alterations

  14. Impaired Skin Integrity

E. **Planning and implementation: preoperative**

  1. Reinforce and clarify information provided to the child or family members by the cardiovascular surgeon, as necessary.

2. Help reduce family members' and child's anxiety by:
   a. Providing thorough preoperative preparation, including a visit to the intensive care unit and explanations of what to expect before, during, and after surgery
   b. Providing developmentally appropriate explanations
   c. Allowing and encouraging expression of feelings and concerns regarding surgery
3. Carefully assess vital signs, and notify the surgeon of any signs of infection, which may contraindicate surgery.
4. Prepare skin preoperatively, as ordered.
5. Institute NPO status after midnight on the day of surgery.
6. Administer preoperative medications, as ordered, which may include sedatives and antibiotics.

F. **Planning and implementation: postoperative**
   1. Help maintain optimal respiratory status by monitoring respirations and providing good pulmonary hygiene, as appropriate to the child's status. If the child is intubated, monitor chest tube drainage and patency, monitor blood gases, and observe for early clinical signs of respiratory distress.
   2. Monitor cardiac status; assess:
      a. Heart rate and rhythm
      b. Blood pressure
      c. Central venous pressure (CVP) and other hemodynamic parameters
      d. Heart sounds
      e. Peripheral pulses and perfusion
      f. Blood chemistry values
   3. Help prevent postoperative hypothermia by providing external warmth. Monitor for hyperthermia associated with infection.
   4. Closely monitor input and output, and assess for signs of fluid overload, such as edema. Maintain fluid restrictions, as ordered.
   5. Help maintain skin integrity by inspecting all wound sites at least every 8 hours; changing the child's position frequently; providing good, regular skin care; changing dressings regularly; and monitoring for signs of infection.
   6. Promote comfort by assessing the need for pain medications and administering it as ordered and as needed.
   7. Monitor for complications of surgery, such as hypoxia, acidosis, thromboembolism, electrolyte imbalance, and poor systemic perfusion.
   8. Help prevent problems of sensory overload by keeping the child oriented to time and place, preparing him or her for all procedures, and providing repeated age-appropriate explanations of what is happening. Ensure adequate rest periods and time for uninterrupted sleep. Observe for signs of psychic disturbance and sleep deprivation.

9. During recovery, provide tactile stimulation for infants and distraction activities for older children.
10. Provide emotional support to the child's parents by addressing their concerns and answering questions.
11. Refer the family for community health nurse visits, as appropriate.
12. Provide patient and family teaching, covering:
    a. Activity restrictions
    b. Incision site care
    c. Dosage, administration, and possible side effects of medications
    d. Diet and fluid restrictions
    e. Possible regressive behaviors and psychological distress related to the trauma of surgery and hospitalization
    f. Physiologic complications to watch for and report, such as fever, tachycardia, severe or persistent chest pain, labored breathing or tachypnea, feeding difficulties, and persistent swelling or edema

G. Evaluation
1. The child maintains adequate oxygenation and exhibits nonlabored respiration.
2. The child maintains adequate cardiac output, as evidenced by normal heart rate and blood pressure, adequate urine output, and good peripheral perfusion.
3. The child maintains fluid and electrolyte balance, as evidenced by normal electrolyte values, absence of edema, and clear lungs on auscultation.
4. The child is well oriented and displays no psychologic disturbances.
5. The child is free of life-threatening complications of surgery.
6. The child reports only minimal discomfort.
7. Family members verbalize knowledge of follow-up appointments, home care measures, and proper administration and possible side effects of prescribed medications.
8. The family is referred to a community health nurse, as appropriate.

Bibliography

Brunner, L. S., and Suddarth, D. S. (1991). *Lippincott manual of nursing practice* (5th ed.). Philadelphia: J. B. Lippincott.

Mott, S. R., James, S. R., and Sperhac, A. M. (1990). *Nursing care of children and families* (2nd ed.). Menlo Park, CA: Addison-Wesley.

Waechter, E. H., Phillips, J., and Holaday, B. (1985). *Nursing care of children*. Philadelphia: J. B. Lippincott.

Whaley, L. F., and Wong, D. L. (1991). *Nursing care of infants and children* (4rd ed.). St. Louis: C. V. Mosby.

STUDY QUESTIONS

1. Which of the following congenital heart defects is classified as cyanotic?
   a. pulmonic stenosis
   b. tetralogy of Fallot
   c. aortic stenosis
   d. coarctation of the aorta

2. Jennie, aged 4, is hospitalized for diagnostic evaluation related to her congenital heart disease. Her parents restrict her from going to the playroom because she might "overexert herself." Which of the following statements to the parents by a nurse observing this situation would be most appropriate?
   a. "Jennie needs to realize that playing with peers is too strenuous for a child with a heart defect."
   b. "You must constantly supervise Jennie to make sure she doesn't overexert herself."
   c. "You should allow Jennie to do whatever she wants to prevent crying and emotional stress."
   d. "It's important that you allow Jennie to play and develop as normally as possible."

3. During discharge teaching for the parents of a child who has undergone cardiac surgery, the nurse would assure the parents that which of the following is a common reaction?
   a. regression and behavioral disturbances
   b. a new sense of independence related to experiencing such a traumatic hospitalization
   c. repression
   d. rationalization

4. A nurse involved in preoperative teaching for a preschool child scheduled for cardiac surgery would be sure that her preparation was
   a. detailed in nature so that the child knew everything there was to know about the surgery
   b. geared toward the child's parents since the child is too young to understand anything about the surgery
   c. developmentally appropriate to the child's stage of growth and development
   d. done several days before the actual operation so that the child had the opportunity to think of any questions or concerns

5. A newborn infant is diagnosed as having a patent ductus arteriosus. The knowledgeable pediatric nurse understands that this congenital heart defect involves
   a. narrowing of the aorta
   b. origination of the pulmonary artery from the left ventricle and origination of the aorta from the right ventricle
   c. persistence of the fetal opening between the pulmonary artery and the aorta
   d. obstruction of left ventricular outflow at the level of the aortic valve

6. Pulmonary stenosis involves
   a. return of the pulmonary venous blood to the heart without entering the left atrium
   b. obstruction of blood flow from the right ventricle
   c. obstruction of blood flow from the left ventricle
   d. a single vessel arising from both ventricles

7. Which of the following represents an effective nursing intervention to reduce cardiac demands and decrease cardiac workload?
   a. clustering nursing care to provide for periods of uninterrupted rest
   b. developing and implementing a consistent plan of care
   c. feeding the infant over a longer period of time
   d. allowing the infant to have his or her own way to avoid conflict

8. For a child with congenital heart disease, the nurse should stress the need for prophylactic administration of antibiotics before dental work, surgery, or laceration repair to decrease the risk of

a. infective carditis
b. pneumonia
c. congestive heart failure
d. wound infection

9. Defects associated with tetralogy of Fallot include
   a. severe coarctation of the aorta, severe aortic valve stenosis, and severe mitral valve stenosis
   b. ventricular septal defect, overriding aorta, pulmonic stenosis, and right ventricular hypertrophy
   c. tricuspid valve atresia, atrial septal defect, and hypoplastic right ventricle

d. origin of the aorta from the right ventricle and of the pulmonary artery from the left ventricle

10. A young child with tetralogy of Fallot may assume a characteristic position as a compensatory mechanism to increase pulmonary blood flow. What is this position?
    a. prone
    b. supine
    c. squatting
    d. low Fowler's

ANSWER KEY

1. **Correct response: b**
   Tetralogy of Fallot is classified as cyanotic.
   a, c, and d. These disorders are classified as acyanotic.

   Knowledge/Physiologic/Assessment

2. **Correct response: d**
   The nurse should encourage the family to provide as normal a life as possible for the child and to stimulate the child with age-appropriate activities consistent with the child's activity tolerance. The child usually self-limits activities as necessary.
   a. The child should be encouraged to play with peers and develop normally based on individual activity tolerance.
   b. The parents should be counseled against overprotecting the child.
   c. The parents should be counseled against overindulging the child.

   Application/Psychosocial/Evaluation

3. **Correct response: a**
   Regression and behavioral disturbances are common reactions in children to surgery and hospitalization. Behavior may revert to earlier stages of growth and development. Children may exhibit depression, anger, nightmares, and sleep problems.
   b. Most children regress in behavior and may exhibit overdependence and increased separation anxiety.
   c. Repression is a defense mechanism in which the person puts an unpleasant experience out of their consciousness.
   d. Rationalization is a defense mechanism that consists of the person trying to "rationalize" or make excuses or explanations for unacceptable behavior.

   Application/Psychosocial/Planning

4. **Correct response: c**
   Effective preoperative teaching should be geared toward the individual child's stage of growth and development.

   a. Preschoolers require simple explanations only appropriate to their stage of cognitive development.
   b. A preschool child is cognitively able to understand simple explanations and should be included in preparation.
   d. Preparation done too far ahead of time may be detrimental for the preschool child because it may serve only to magnify his or her fears and fantasies concerning the surgery.

   Analysis/Psychosocial/Implementation

5. **Correct response: c**
   Persistence of the patent ductus arteriosus allows oxygenated blood flow from the aorta to the pulmonary artery.
   a. This describes coarctation of the aorta.
   b. This describes transposition of the great vessels.
   d. This describes aortic valvular stenosis.

   Knowledge/Physiologic/Assessment

6. **Correct response: b**
   Pulmonic stenosis refers to an obstruction of blood flow from the right ventricle.
   a and c. These describe total anomalous pulmonary venous communication.
   d. This describes truncus arteriosus.

   Knowledge/Physiologic/Assessment

7. **Correct response: a**
   Organizing nursing care to provide for uninterrupted periods of sleep reduces cardiac demands.
   b. Developing a consistent plan of care can be important, but it is not related to decreasing workload of the heart.
   c. Feeding time should be restricted to a maximum time of 45 minutes or discontinued sooner if the infant tires.
   d. Excessive crying should be limited in the infant; however, appropriate

limit setting should still be observed.

Analysis/Physiologic/Evaluation

8. Correct response: a

Prophylactic antibiotic administration is geared toward preventing infective carditis (also known as bacterial endocarditis).

b, c, and d. Prophylactic antibiotics are not routinely administered to prevent these conditions.

Application/Health promotion/Planning

9. Correct response: b

These are the defects associated with tetralogy of Fallot.

a. These are the defects associated with tricuspid atresia.

c. These are the defects associated with hypoplastic left heart syndrome.

d. These are the defects associated with transposition of the great vessels.

Knowledge/Physiologic/Assessment

10. Correct response: c

A characteristic squatting position is assumed by a young child with tetralogy of Fallot to increase pulmonary blood flow and help relieve chronic hypoxia.

a, b, and d. These positions will not increase pulmonary blood flow.

Comprehension/Physiologic/Analysis (Dx)

Cancer

I. Essential concepts of cancer in children

A. General characteristics

1. Cancer is a group of disease processes characterized by uncontrolled proliferation of abnormal cells.

2. In adults, cancers most commonly involve epithelial cells (carcinomas), which are largely environmental in origin.

3. Cancers involving connective tissue (sarcomas) occur in both children and adults.

4. Embryonal tumors, which probably originate in intrauterine life, generally are manifested during childhood.

5. Lymphoreticular cancers (leukemias and lymphomas) occur more frequently in children but also occur in adults.

6. Although relatively rare, childhood cancers remain the leading cause of death by disease and the second leading cause of death overall (exceeded only by accidents) in children age 1 to 14 years.

7. Leukemia is the most common form of childhood cancer.
8. In recent years, cancer survival rates have increased so significantly that the term *cure* is now being used cautiously.

B. Classification (by tissue of origin)

1. Blood and related cell cancers include:
   a. Leukemias, originating in hematopoietic cells
   b. Lymphomas, originating in lymphoid tissue: Hodgkin's disease and non-Hodgkin's lymphoma
2. Connective tissue tumors include:
   a. Fibrosarcoma, originating in fibrous tissue
   b. Osteosarcoma, originating in the bone-producing (mesenchymal) cells
   c. Ewing's sarcoma, originating in the midshaft of long bones and flat bones
3. Muscle tissue tumors include rhabdomyosarcoma, originating in striated muscle.
4. Nerve tissue tumors include:
   a. Neuroblastomas, originating from the neural crest during embryonic development from ganglion cells
   b. Glioblastomas, originating from glial cells
   c. Retinoblastomas, originating in the retinal tissue
5. Renal tissue tumors include Wilms' tumor (nephroblastoma), originating in the kidneys.

C. Staging

1. Cancer staging is a system for describing and classifying the extent of malignant neoplasm and its metastases, used to guide therapy and predict prognosis.
2. Various staging criteria and terminology are used, depending on the specific tumor or treatment center; examples include:
   a. The TNM staging classification: T, primary tumor size; N, involvement of regional lymph nodes; M, presence or absence of metastasis
   b. The National Wilms' Tumor Study: a guide to staging Wilms' tumor to guide treatment (total or partial nephrectomy, radiation, chemotherapy or transplantation): groups I and II, completely resectable disease, most curable (90% chance for cure); group III, partially resectable with no evidence of metastasis; group IV, evidence of metastasis; group V, bilateral kidney involvement

II. Overview of cancer in children

A. Assessment

1. Specific clinical findings vary depending on particular body system involvement.
2. Cardinal signs and symptoms of cancer in children include:
   a. Fever, night sweats

> b. Pain
> c. Palpable masses
> d. Purpura, petechiae
> e. Changes in behavior, gait, balance
> f. Unexplained weight loss
> g. Fatigue

B. **Laboratory studies and diagnostic tests**

1. Laboratory studies commonly used to detect, stage, and track cancer include:
   a. Complete blood count
   b. Blood chemistry analyses, especially creatinine
   c. Peripheral blood smears: cell types and level of cell maturity
   d. 24-hour urine for homovanillic acid, vanillylmandelic acid, and catecholamines
   e. Bone marrow aspiration or biopsy for definitive diagnosis of leukemia
   f. Lumbar puncture to analyze cerebrospinal fluid for leukemia cells

2. Radiologic and other imaging studies include:
   a. Intravenous pyelography
   b. Computed tomography
   c. Radiographs

C. **Psychosocial implications**

1. A child and his or her family adjust to the process of living with a life-threatening illness in phases.

2. The first stage, "crisis of discovery," begins with announcement of the diagnoses. In most cases, the child and family initially do not realize the seriousness of the situation.

3. Parents typically respond with shock and disbelief, followed by guilt and self-blame.

4. The child's reaction largely depends on his or her age, the information the child is given, and the physical impact of the disease process on his or her energy level and coping strategies; common responses include:
   a. Under age 3: views death as a reversible event
   b. Age 3 to 6: understands death as something that happens to others; may view cancer as a retribution for his or her "bad" thoughts or actions
   c. Age 6 to 11: begins to view death as a personal event
   d. Preadolescent: vulnerable to intense feelings of guilt in association with death
   e. Early adolescent: intellectually understands the universality and permanence of death; the prospect of "death before fulfillment" is extremely difficult for a youth who is experi-

encing illness during a period when physical beauty and activities are important standards of self-worth and self-esteem

5. After the discovery stage, the child gradually becomes aware of the change in his or her condition and comes to terms with his or her illness and possible impending death; phases of this process include:
   a. Expressions of anger and guilt
   b. Reorganization of relationships with others
   c. Resolution of the loss through active grieving
   d. Reorganization of identity, incorporating the changes that have taken place

6. These phases do not necessarily occur in a linear path but rather can occur in any order and can recur with each disease exacerbation.

7. Because school is the child's "work," a school-age child should engage in school activities to the greatest extent possible throughout the course of illness.

8. Regardless of which family member has cancer, each person in the family is affected by the disease and in turn affects the adjustment of other family members.

III. Leukemia

A. Description

1. Leukemia is a malignant neoplastic disorder of the blood-forming tissues.

2. It can be classified according to its predominant cell type and level of maturity, as follows:
   a. Lympho: involving the lymphoid or lymphatic system
   b. Myelo: of bone marrow origin
   c. Blastic and acute: involving immature cells
   d. Cytic and chronic: involving mature cells

3. Acute leukemias, which represent 98% of cases of childhood leukemia, include:
   a. Acute lymphoblastic leukemia (ALL): accounts for 80% of acute leukemias in children; subclasses include: T lymphocyte, B lymphocyte, pre-B lymphocyte, and null cell (accounting for 75% of cases of ALL; carries the best prognosis of all ALLs)
   b. Acute nonlymphoblastic leukemia (ANLL): accounts for 15% of acute leukemias in children
   c. Acute undifferentiated leukemia (AUL): the least common type of acute leukemia

4. Chronic leukemia accounts for only 2% of childhood leukemias.

B. Etiology and incidence

1. The exact cause of leukemia remains unclear; possible predisposing factors include:

       a.   Genetic influences: Children with Down's syndrome develop leukemia at a rate 15 times higher than the general population.

       b.   Familial predisposition: Siblings of a child with leukemia have a higher risk of developing leukemia themselves.

       c.   Immunologic influences: Immune deficiencies increase the risk of developing many cancers.

       d.   Viral infection: Research suggests the possibility of an oncogenic virus that facilitates the development of cancer (although no direct link has been proved).

       e.   Environmental influences: Evidence suggests that radiation during pregnancy contributes to the development of leukemia in childhood.

  2.   Leukemia accounts for about 31% of all childhood cancers in whites and about 24% in blacks. Peak incidence occurs at age 3 to 4 years.

C. **Pathophysiology**

  1.   Malignant leukemic cells arise from the precursor cells in blood-forming organs.

  2.   These cells accumulate and crowd out normal bone marrow elements, spill into peripheral blood, and eventually can invade all body organs and tissues.

  3.   Replacement of normal hematopoietic elements by leukemic cells results in bone marrow suppression, marked by decreased production of red blood cells (RBCs), normal white blood cells, and platelets.

  4.   Bone marrow suppression results in anemia from decreased RBC production, predisposition to infection due to neutropenia, and bleeding tendencies from decreased platelet production. This puts the patient at increased risk of death from infection or hemorrhage.

  5.   Infiltration of reticuloendothelial organs—the spleen, liver, and lymph glands—causes marked enlargement and, eventually, fibrosis.

  6.   Leukemic infiltration of the central nervous system results in increased intracranial pressure (ICP) and other effects depending on the specific areas of involvement.

  7.   Other possible sites of long-term infiltration include the kidneys, testes, prostate, ovaries, GI tract, and lungs.

  8.   The hypermetabolic leukemic cells eventually deprive all body cells of nutrients necessary for survival. Uncontrolled growth of leukemic cells can actually result in metabolic starvation.

  9.   Leukemia treatment commonly involves a combination of chemotherapy and radiation therapy, provided at four levels:

       a.   Induction of remission: The goal involves reducing the number of leukemic cells. Drugs used commonly include a combination of oral prednisone, intravenous vincristine, and intravenous L-asparaginase.

b. Sanctuary therapy: The goal is to attack leukemic cells in the CNS, which are protected by the blood–brain barrier, or in the testes, which are protected by their peripheral location. Therapy consists of intrathecal chemotherapy—typically a combination of methotrexate, cytosine, arabinoside, and steroids—or irradiation, usually beginning during the first 6 to 8 weeks after diagnosis and lasting for 2 weeks. (*Note:* Irradiation of the testes remains controversial.)

c. Continuation (maintenance) therapy: The goal is to preserve remission and continue to reduce the number of leukemic cells. Therapy begins when CBC values approach normal levels and commonly lasts for $1\frac{1}{2}$ to 3 years.

d. Reinduction therapy: The goal is to reduce the number of leukemic cells in a child who has relapsed; chemotherapy commonly involves prednisone and vincristine, combined with other drugs not used previously in therapy.

10. Bone marrow transplantation may be performed in children facing almost certain death without the procedure. If successful, it destroys the leukemic cells and replenishes bone marrow with healthy cells. Prognosis for long-term survival after transplantation is 25% to 50%.

D. Assessment findings

1. Common clinical manifestations include:

a. Signs and symptoms of anemia: pallor, fatigue, lethargy, cardiac murmurs

b. Poor wound healing, fever, anorexia, lymphadenopathy related to neutropenia

c. Petechiae, ecchymoses, purpura, epistaxis, easy bruising, blood in urine or emesis related to decreased platelet production

d. Bone and joint pain related to leukemic cell invasion into the periosteum

e. Headache, vomiting, papilledema, and other signs and symptoms of increased ICP related to leukemic cell invasion of the CNS

2. Laboratory and diagnostic study results typically reveal:

a. Anemia: normochromic and normocytic, with a low reticulocyte index

b. Thrombocytopenia

c. Neutropenia

d. Blast cells on peripheral blood smear

e. Extensive replacement of normal bone marrow elements

by leukemic cells seen on bone marrow examination, which confirms diagnosis

E. Nursing diagnoses
1. Activity Intolerance
2. Fatigue
3. High Risk for Infection
4. Altered Nutrition: Less than Body Requirements
5. Pain
6. Impaired Skin Integrity

F. Planning and implementation
1. Set realistic patient goals depending on the type of therapy prescribed:
    a. Curative: goal is complete disease eradication
    b. Adjuvant: goal is eradication of disease and subclinical micrometastases with systemic adjunctive modalities
    c. Palliative: goal is not to cure but to provide quality survival with symptom control
2. Prepare the child for diagnostic tests and treatments by:
    a. Assessing the child's level of understanding
    b. Addressing specific fears and misconceptions
    c. Providing information appropriate to the child's age and developmental level
    d. Explaining what he or she will see, smell, hear, and feel rather than merely specifying what will happen
3. Help prevent complications related to bone marrow suppression, such as infection and sepsis, through scrupulous handwashing, limiting the child's exposure to persons with infections (particularly with potentially lethal organisms such as varicella virus), and, if ordered, maintaining reverse isolation. (*Note:* Reverse isolation is a controversial measure.)
4. Prepare the child and family for bone marrow transplantation if this procedure is scheduled.
5. Promote optimum nutrition to maintain and rebuild healthy tissue. Serve small, frequent meals in a pleasant, relaxed environment, and involve the child in food selection, as appropriate.
6. Take measures to prevent hemorrhage, including:
    a. Turning the patient frequently to relieve pressure on bony prominences
    b. Providing meticulous mouth care and good skin care
    c. Measuring temperature via the oral or axillary routes only, avoiding rectal temperature measurement
7. For a child receiving blood transfusions, assess for blood transfusion reaction.
8. Promote adequate rest by providing a calm, quiet environment and by clustering nursing care activities and other procedures to ensure long periods of uninterrupted rest.

9. Take steps to prevent nausea and vomiting resulting from chemo-therapy, such as:
   a. Administering an antiemetic agent 30 minutes to 1 hour before a chemotherapy session
   b. Continuing the antiemetic every 2 to 6 hours for 24 hours after chemotherapy

10. Help prevent constipation resulting from neuropathic side effects of chemotherapy by:
    a. Encouraging a high-fiber diet
    b. Promoting physical activity according to the child's toler-ance
    c. Administering a stool softener

11. Help minimize hemorrhagic cystitis resulting from chemother-apy by:
    a. Encouraging increased fluid intake and frequent voiding
    b. Administering chemotherapy early in the day to allow ade-quate time for significant fluid intake

12. Help prevent renal damage resulting from chemotherapy by:
    a. Administering allopurinol as ordered
    b. Alkalinizing the urine with an acid-ash diet
    c. Providing adequate hydration

13. Help minimize alopecia resulting from chemotherapy by apply-ing a scalp tourniquet before therapy, as ordered. (*Note:* This measure is controversial.)

14. Provide for appropriate play activities based on the child's age, developmental level, and health status.

15. Provide patient and family teaching, covering:
    a. Diagnosis and nature of the disorder
    b. All treatments and other procedures
    c. Side effects of chemotherapy and radiation therapy

G. Evaluation

1. The child or parents verbalize an understanding of the signs and symptoms of infection and the importance of monitoring for these signs and symptoms promptly and notifying the physician if they occur.

2. The child exhibits no evidence of abnormal bleeding.

3. The child engages in usual activities and routines as appropriate for his or her age and developmental level.

4. The child consumes adequate calories balanced among the basic four food groups.

5. The child verbalizes decreased discomfort or absence of pain and appears to rest comfortably.

6. The child or parents verbalize an understanding of treatment pro-tocols and prescribed drugs, including the side effects of medica-tions and treatments to watch for and report.

7.   Family members know the dates and times of scheduled follow-up appointments.

IV.   Wilms' tumor (nephroblastoma)

A.   **Description: a malignant neoplasm of the kidney; the most common intraabdominal tumor and the most curable solid tumor in children**

B.   **Etiology and incidence**

1.   The exact cause is unknown; possible etiologic factors include:

a.   Genetic influence: An autosomal dominant trait seems to account for a rare mode of inheritance. Bilateral Wilms' tumors probably have a genetic influence. About 15% of children diagnosed with Wilms' have other congenital abnormalities such as hypospadias, cryptorchidism, and ambiguous genitalia.

b.   Familial predisposition: Siblings and identical twins of a child with Wilms' tumor have a higher risk of developing the disorder themselves.

2.   Wilms' tumor accounts for 6% of all childhood cancers.

3.   About 75% of cases are diagnosed before age 5.

4.   Incidence is about equal in boys and girls.

C.   **Pathophysiology**

1.   The tumor originates from immature renoblast cells located in the renal parenchyma.

2.   It is well encapsulated in early stages but may later extend into lymph nodes and the renal vein or vena cava and metastasize to the lungs and other sites.

3.   Treatment typically involves surgery to remove the primary tumor, affected lymph nodes, and selected metastases.

4.   Chemotherapy may be effective at all disease stages; commonly used agents include vincristine in combination with either actinomycin D, daunorubicin, or doxorubicin.

5.   Radiation therapy may be performed to eradicate residual tumor cells and selected metastatic foci, such as tumor cells that have seeded the abdomen during surgery area. It usually is not performed in a young child with grade I disease and favorable histology.

D.   **Assessment findings**

1.   Common clinical manifestations of Wilms' tumor include:

a.   Abdominal mass, characteristically firm, nontender, deep, and confined to one side (usually the left)

b.   Abdominal distention, abdominal pain

c.   Pallor, anorexia, and lethargy related to anemia

d.   Hypertension related to excessive renin release from the diseased kidney

e.   Hematuria due to hemorrhage within the kidney

        f.   Weight loss related to anorexia

        g.   Fever related to infection

        h.   Dyspnea and chest pain related to lung metastasis

   2.   Laboratory and diagnostic study results may reveal:

        a.   Anemia, usually secondary to hemorrhage within the tumor

        b.   Evidence of an intrarenal mass on intravenous pyelography

        c.   Evidence of metastases demonstrated by radiographic studies

E.   **Nursing diagnoses**

   1.   Anxiety

   2.   Body Image Disturbance

   3.   Constipation

   4.   Altered Family Processes

   5.   High Risk for Infection

   6.   High Risk for Injury

   7.   Altered Nutrition: Less than Body Requirements

   8.   Altered Oral Mucous Membranes

   9.   Pain

  10.   Powerlessness

  11.   Impaired Skin Integrity

  12.   Spiritual Distress

  13.   Altered Tissue Perfusion

F.   **Planning and implementation**

   1.   Prepare the child for diagnostic tests and treatments by:

        a.   Assessing the child's level of understanding

        b.   Addressing specific fears and misconceptions

        c.   Providing information appropriate to the child's age and developmental level

        d.   Explaining what he or she will see, smell, hear, and feel rather than merely specifying what will happen

   2.   Help prevent rupture of an encapsulated tumor by avoiding abdominal palpation and by promoting careful bathing and handling.

   3.   Monitor bowel sounds and assess for signs and symptoms of intestinal obstruction resulting from abdominal surgery, vincristine-induced adynamic ileus, and radiation-induced edema.

   4.   Help prevent infection by maintaining scrupulous handwashing and limiting the child's exposure to persons with infections. Monitor vital signs for evidence of infection.

   5.   Help prevent postoperative pulmonary complications by providing frequent position changes and encouraging coughing, deep breathing, and ambulation.

   6.   Provide patient and family teaching, covering:

        a.   Diagnosis and nature of the disorder

        b.   Surgery and other treatments

        c.   Side effects of chemotherapy and radiation therapy

G.   Evaluation

1. The child or parents verbalize or demonstrate feelings related to procedures.
2. The child or parents verbalize understanding of treatments and other procedures.
3. The child remains free of signs and symptoms of infection; urine remains clear.
4. The child does not experience any falls or trauma to the abdomen.
5. The child exhibits no evidence of skin breakdown.
6. The child verbalizes concerns regarding hair loss and other body changes, as appropriate.
7. The child or parents verbalize knowledge of the side effects of chemotherapy and radiation therapy.
8. The child or parents verbalize an understanding of the need for precautions to prevent abdominal injury, such as avoiding contact sports and other risky behaviors.
9. The child or parents demonstrate understanding of ways to prevent urinary tract infection (e.g., avoiding bubble baths for girls, providing adequate hydration).
10. The child or parents can specify signs and symptoms of urinary tract infection to watch for and report.
11. Parents have scheduled follow-up appointments for child.

Bibliography

Altman, A., and Schwartz, A. (1983). *Malignant diseases of infancy, childhood, and adolescence.* Philadelphia: W. B. Saunders.

Fochtman, D. (1983). *Nursing care of the child with cancer.* Boston: Little, Brown.

Lanzkowsky, P. (1980). *Pediatric hematology and oncology.* New York: McGraw-Hill.

Mott, S. R., James, S. R., and Sperhac, A. M. (1990). *Nursing care of children and families: A holistic approach* (2nd ed.). Menlo Park, CA: Addison-Wesley.

Sutow, W. W., Fernbach, D. H., and Vretti, T. J. (Eds.) (1984). *Clinical pediatric oncology* (3rd ed.) St. Louis: C. V. Mosby.

Whaley, L. F., and Wong, D. L. (1991). *Nursing care of infants and children* (4th ed.). St. Louis: C. V. Mosby.

STUDY QUESTIONS

1. As a cause of death in children up to age 14, cancer ranks
   a. first
   b. second
   c. third
   d. fourth

2. What is the goal of intrathecal methotrexate therapy in the treating of leukemia?
   a. sanctuary therapy
   b. bone marrow suppression
   c. initial induction of remission
   d. palliative treatment

3. The most common presenting sign of Wilms' tumor is:
   a. hematuria
   b. pain on voiding
   c. nausea and vomiting
   d. abdominal mass

4. When caring for a child awaiting surgery for Wilms' tumor, which of the following nursing interventions would be *most* important?
   a. Handle the child with care, particularly during bathing.
   b. Place the child on low blood count precautions.
   c. Monitor bowel sounds to detect vincristine-induced adynamic ileus.
   d. Place the child in high Fowler's position to facilitate lung expansion.

5. Marsha, aged 5, is hospitalized with a diagnosis of acute lymphocytic leukemia. Admission assessment reveals a pale, listless child with multiple petechiae and fever. Marsha's fever most likely is related to:
   a. anemia
   b. thrombocytopenia
   c. meningeal irritation
   d. neutropenia

6. Marsha is anxious and upset about her upcoming bone marrow aspiration. When preparing Marsha for the procedure, which of the following considerations should the nurse keep in mind?

   a. No small detail of the procedure should be omitted.
   b. With each successive procedure, the child will experience decreasing levels of stress.
   c. Providing details on expected sights, smells, sensations, and sounds helps the child cope.
   d. Marsha needs an explanation of bone marrow function to better understand the reason for the procedure.

7. Side effects of leukemia chemotherapy associated with initial remission include all the following *except*
   a. bone marrow suppression
   b. pneumonitis
   c. alopecia
   d. nausea and vomiting

8. What is the most common form of childhood cancer?
   a. lymphoma
   b. brain tumor
   c. leukemia
   d. osteosarcoma

9. Joseph, aged 3, is scheduled for a laparotomy. Which of the following would be an essential part of the nurse's responsibility preoperatively?
   a. Teach Joseph's parents about the side effects of chemotherapy, especially alopecia.
   b. Assess the parents' understanding of the diagnosis and treatment plan.
   c. Evaluate the parents' understanding of discharge plans.
   d. Assess Joseph for intestinal obstruction related to vincristine-induced adynamic ileus.

10. In the treatment of Wilms' tumor, abdominal radiation therapy is done postoperatively to
    a. irradiate the adjacent adrenal gland
    b. stage the disease
    c. eradicate any tumor cells that may have seeded the abdomen during surgery

d. prepare the body for chemotherapy

11. Which of the following nursing interventions can help prevent or reduce nausea and vomiting during chemotherapy?

 a. Provide a high-fiber diet.

 b. Administer allopurinol 2 hours before a chemotherapy session.

 c. Encourage increased fluid intake.

 d. Administer an antiemetic 30 to 60 minutes before a chemotherapy session.

12. Bobby, aged 4, is about to be discharged after undergoing surgery and follow-up treatments for Wilms' tumor. Which of the following points would be a vital part of the parent teaching program for Bobby's parents?

 a. allowing Bobby to resume normal activities, including contact sports, as soon as his tolerance allows

 b. signs and symptoms of urinary tract infection to watch for and report

 c. the need to make arrangements for a return visit in 6 months

 d. the need to arrange for hospice care since Wilms' tumor is commonly fatal

ANSWER KEY

1. **Correct response: b**
   Cancer is the second leading cause of death in children.
   a. Accidents are the leading cause of death in children of all ages.
   c. Congenital anomalies are the third leading cause of death in children.
   d. Homicide is the fourth leading cause of death in children.
   Knowledge/Health promotion/Assessment

2. **Correct response: a**
   Sanctuary therapy involves administering intrathecal drugs to attack leukemic cells in the CNS.
   b. Bone marrow suppression is a side effect of chemotherapy, not a specific goal of intrathecal therapy, especially with methotrexate.
   c. Initial induction of remission is accomplished by oral prednisone and intravenous chemotherapy.
   d. The goal of palliative treatment is to improve the patient's quality of life rather than to effect a cure.
   Comprehension/Physiologic/Analysis (Dx)

3. **Correct response: d**
   The most common sign of Wilms' tumor is a painless palpable abdominal mass, sometimes marked by an increase in abdominal girth.
   a. Gross hematuria is uncommon; microscopic hematuria may be present.
   b. Pain on voiding is not associated with Wilms' tumor.
   c. Tumor encroachment should not cause abdominal obstruction and resulting nausea and vomiting.
   Comprehension/Physiologic/Assessment

4. **Correct response: a**
   Handling the child carefully is essential to prevent rupture of an encapsulated tumor.
   b. The child usually does not undergo myelosuppression before surgery. In fact, the child may be suffering from polycythemia due to increased production of erythropoietin.
   c. Vincristine is administered postoperatively.
   d. Respiratory difficulty is not a common problem in Wilms' tumor.
   Application/Safe care/Implementation

5. **Correct response: d**
   Neutropenia makes the child vulnerable to infections and resulting fever.
   a. Anemia causes pallor, fatigue, and other effects, but not fever.
   b. Thrombocytopenia causes bruising, petechiae, and other effects, but not fever.
   c. Meningeal irritation, a possible late result of leukemic cell metastasis, is not usually associated with fever.
   Comprehension/Physiologic/Assessment

6. **Correct response: c**
   Children are best prepared and master situations better when they can anticipate sensations rather than just trying to comprehend technical explanations.
   a. A preschool-age child cannot assimilate every detail.
   b. In most cases, the opposite is true.
   d. An explanation of bone marrow function would not be understood by a preschooler and is irrelevant.
   Analysis/Psychosocial/Implementation

7. **Correct response: b**
   Pneumonitis and resulting fibrosis can result from bleomycin therapy.
   a. Bone marrow suppression can result from therapy with vincristine.
   c. Alopecia also can result from vincristine therapy.
   d. Nausea and vomiting commonly result from L-asparaginase therapy.
   Comprehension/Physiologic/Analysis (Dx)

8. **Correct response: c**
   Leukemia accounts for up to 34% of all childhood cancers.
   a. Lymphoma accounts for about 12% of all childhood cancers.

b. Brain tumors account from about 19% of all childhood cancers.

d. Bone cancer accounts for 5%, osteosarcoma being the most common type.

Knowledge/Health promotion/Assessment

9. *Correct response: b*

Assessing the level of parental understanding gives the nurse information that guides further parent teaching.

a. Chemotherapy does not begin until after surgery. Also, the side effect of alopecia does not occur until 2 weeks after initial treatment begins.

c. Staging would not have been done yet; neither would the specific treatment regimen and follow-up plans be identified.

d. Vincristine is started postoperatively not preoperatively.

Application/Health promotion/ Implementation

10. *Correct response: c*

During surgery, rupture of the encapsulated tumor can occur, spreading or seeding tumor cells and thus causing metastases.

a. The adjacent adrenal gland is removed during surgery.

b. Staging occurs during surgery.

d. Radiation therapy does not prepare the body for the assault of chemotherapy.

Comprehension/Physiologic/Planning

11. *Correct response: d*

Antiemetics counteract nausea most effectively when given before administration of an agent that causes nausea. Antiemetics also work best when given on a continuous basis rather than prn.

a. A high-fiber diet does nothing to reduce nausea and vomiting.

b. Allopurinol, an xanthine-oxidase inhibitor, is thought to prevent renal damage due to large releases of uric acid during chemotherapy; it has no antiemetic properties.

c. High fluid intake during periods of nausea only exaggerates the symptom and cause vomiting.

Application/Physiologic/Planning

12. *Correct response: b*

Urinary tract infections can pose a threat to the remaining kidney.

a. Rough play and contact sports should be discouraged because of the residual affect of radiation to the abdomen and because the child needs to protect his or her lone remaining kidney.

c. Six months is too late; all children receive chemotherapy for 6 to 15 months after surgery.

d. Wilms' tumor is the most curable solid tumor of childhood; prognosis is usually favorable.

Application/Safe care/Planning

Endocrine Dysfunction

I. Essential concepts: endocrine system anatomy and physiology
A. Development
1. Most endocrine glands and structures develop during the first trimester of gestation.
2. The thyroid develops in three stages between 7 and 14 weeks of gestation.
3. The parathyroid is recognizable at 5 to 7 weeks of gestation.
4. The pancreas forms from two different cells, which fuse to form a single organ at 7 weeks of gestation; insulin can be detected in beta cells several weeks later.
5. The pituitary originates from fusion of two ectodermal processes. The primordia of anterior and posterior segments can be seen by

week 4 of gestation, and the gland takes its permanent shape and location in the sella turcica between the third and fourth month.

6. The adrenal gland reaches its maximum size by the fourth month of gestation. The medulla arises from the ectoderm via the neural crest; the cortex, from the lateral plate of the embryonic mesoderm. Both corticosterone and aldosterone are secreted in utero.

B. **Function**

1. The endocrine system consists of:
   a. Cells or glands that transmit chemical signals via hormones
   b. Target cells or end organs that receive chemical signals
   c. An environment or medium through which the chemical signals travel: lymph, blood, extracellular fluids
2. This system regulates:
   a. Energy production
   b. Growth
   c. Sexual reproduction
   d. Response to stress
   e. Metabolic processes related to fluid and electrolyte balance
3. Hormonal regulation is based on a negative feedback system.
4. The endocrine system and the autonomic nervous system, collectively known as the neuroendocrine system, work together to maintain homeostasis.
5. The endocrine system transmits its signals primarily via the blood; the autonomic nervous system, via neural impulses.
6. Systemic responses to endocrine system signals are usually slow but long lasting, affecting multiple cells and organs; response to autonomic nervous system signals is usually immediate, short lasting, and localized.
7. Astute and skilled nursing care is especially important for children with endocrine disorders, in whom acute fluid and electrolyte imbalances can develop rapidly—especially in the very young.
8. Most endocrine disorders are chronic in nature and require ongoing care related to health maintenance, education, development, and psychosocial needs.

II. Endocrine system overview

A. Assessment

1. Health history should focus on family history of endocrine disorders, prenatal history, history of chronic childhood disease, and growth and development patterns.
2. Many endocrine disorders present with alterations in weight, height, or sexual development, either alone or in combination.
3. Other common presenting signs and symptoms include:
   a. Neurologic symptoms, such as blurred vision, faintness, nervousness, confusion
   b. Changes in facial features, hair, or skin

       c.   Polydipsia or polyuria

B. **Laboratory studies and diagnostic tests**

    1.   Important blood chemistry studies include thyroid function tests, hormone levels, calcium level, phosphorus level, alkaline phosphatase level, and electrolyte levels.

    2.   Urine studies in endocrine assessment evaluate sodium, calcium, phosphorus, and glucose levels, and specific gravity.

    3.   Radiographic studies are done to evaluate bone age and density, as well as soft tissue calcification.

    4.   Genetic studies may detect enzyme deficiencies (e.g., in congenital adrenogenital hyperplasia).

C. **Psychosocial implications**

    1.   Preparing a child for invasive procedures and tests requires sensitivity to the child's developmental needs.

    2.   Parents and children need the opportunity to express their concerns and fears before and after diagnosis and throughout the course of treatments.

    3.   The nurse should realistically reinforce the parents' and child's expectations of treatment and prospects for improvement.

    4.   A young child may interpret therapy, such as daily or weekly hormone injections, as punishment for wrongdoing; such a child needs clear communication to help him or her distinguish between disease treatment and disciplinary measures.

    5.   Injections may be a source of fearful fantasies; they may enhance a child's body mutilation anxieties.

III. **Hypopituitarism**

  A.   **Description: a condition resulting from diminished or deficient secretion of pituitary hormones, usually growth hormone (GH)**

  B.   **Etiology**

    1.   The most common organic cause is brain tumor, particularly craniopharyngioma.

    2.   Other possible etiologic factors include:

        a.   Primary hypothalamic dysfunction

        b.   Hypoplasia or aplasia of the anterior pituitary

        c.   Idiopathic: genetic or sporadic

        d.   Brain insult (rare)

  C.   **Pathophysiology**

    1.   GH deficiency produces varied effects, including:

        a.   Decreased synthesis of somatomedin (proteins that affect bone and cartilage growth), resulting in decreased linear growth

        b.   Inhibited transport of protein-building amino acids into cells and increased protein catabolism, leading to decreased muscle mass, thin hair, poor skin quality, and delayed growth

       c.   Decreased fat catabolism and increased glucose uptake in muscles, resulting in excessive subcutaneous fat and hypoglycemia

   2.   Associated deficiencies of other hormones, such as adrenocorticotrophic hormone (ACTH), thyroid-stimulating hormone (TSH), leutinizing hormone (LH), and follicle-stimulating hormone (FSH), produce effects related to these hormones' functions.

   3.   Treatment involves GH replacement therapy with a biosynthetic GH created via recombinant DNA (rDNA) technology. Dosage may be as much as 0.06 mg/kg of body weight administered IM or SC three times per week.

D. **Assessment findings**

   1.   Health history may reveal one or more of the following:

       a.   A familial pattern of autosomal recessive inheritance

       b.   Prenatal history of maternal disorders such as malnutrition

       c.   Craniopharyngioma, which can cause deficiency of other pituitary hormones resulting in hypothyroidism, hypoadrenalism, or hypoaldosteronism

       d.   History of normal growth during the first year after birth, with abnormalities not evident until later in life

   2.   Physical assessment findings may include:

       a.   Linear height at or below the 5th percentile on standard growth charts by about age 2 years

       b.   Weight commonly normal or excessive

       c.   Skeletal proportions normal for chronologic age

       d.   Appearance seemingly younger than chronologic age initially (but followed by premature aging later in life)

       e.   Primary tooth eruption not delayed, but permanent tooth eruption delayed; malpositioned teeth due to jaw underdevelopment

       f.   Delayed sexual development, but otherwise normal sexual development if the child is not deficient in gonadotropin

       g.   Normal intelligence

   3.   Progressive growth retardation indicates idiopathic hypopituitarism; sudden slowing in linear growth points to a tumor.

   4.   Diagnostic study results may reveal:

       a.   Bone age younger than chronologic age, depending on the duration of hormone deficiency

       b.   Hypoglycemia

       c.   GH levels below 5 mg/mL after two provocative pharmacologic tests using L-dopa, insulin-arginine, or glucagon, confirming diagnosis

E. **Nursing diagnoses**

   1.   Body Image Disturbance

2. Family Coping: Potential for Growth
3. Altered Growth and Development
4. High Risk for Injury
5. Knowledge Deficit
6. Altered Nutrition: More than Body Requirements
7. Self-Esteem Disturbance
8. Impaired Social Interaction

F. Planning and implementation

1. Help parents promote their child's normal growth and development by teaching them about age-related developmental milestones and encouraging them to notify their physician of any apparent abnormalities.

2. Prepare the child for radiologic and endocrine studies; explain that endocrine studies may require multiple venipunctures or drawing of blood from a heparin lock device.

3. Monitor for early signs and symptoms of hypoglycemia, particularly during provocative tests for GH. If hypoglycemia occurs, elevate the child's blood glucose level rapidly by giving him or her orange juice.

4. Administer GH replacement therapy as ordered; monitor for adverse reactions stemming from antibody production.

5. Assess for acute GH overdose, marked by initial hypoglycemia followed by hyperglycemia, and for long-term GH overdose, characterized by signs and symptoms of acromegaly.

6. Implement meal planning, consulting with a dietitian as necessary, to ensure that the child receives adequate nutrition for growth and development needs.

7. Help promote the child's self-esteem and a positive self-image by encouraging him or her to express feelings and concerns and to focus on personal strengths and assets.

8. Encourage parents to emphasize their child's strengths and abilities, rather than dwell on his or her size, to help him or her develop a more positive self-image.

9. Promote the child's positive social adjustment by encouraging interpersonal relationships with peers and involvement with special peer counseling groups.

10. Promote functional family coping by referring the parents and child to a support group comprised of parents and children with similar disabilities.

11. Provide patient and family teaching, covering:
    a. Diagnosis and nature of the disorder
    b. GH administration, including dosage schedule, administration techniques, what to do if a dose is missed, and adverse reactions.
    c. Realistic expectations for the child's growth, based on age,

personal abilities and strengths, and the effectiveness of GH replacement therapy.

    d. The importance of continual medical supervision, compliance with drug therapy, and follow-up visits.

G. Evaluation

1. The child demonstrates a positive response to GH therapy, manifested by a height increase of 3 to 5 inches during the first year of therapy and less dramatic but measurable increases in subsequent years.

2. Parents verbalize normal growth and developmental milestones for their child.

3. The child and parents verbalize an understanding of signs and symptoms of hypoglycemia and the appropriate actions to take should they occur.

4. The child and parents verbalize an understanding of diet planning, and select appropriate foods.

5. The child interacts appropriately with his or her peer group.

6. The child verbalizes his or her feelings and concerns, as well as personal strengths and assets.

7. Parents verbalize family strengths and identify available community support systems.

8. The child and parents verbalize an understanding that GH deficiency is a chronic problem and that therapeutic care is necessary until young adulthood.

IV. Cushing's syndrome

A. Description: a cluster of clinical abnormalities resulting from excessive levels of adrenocortical hormones, particularly cortisol, and to a lesser extent, related corticosteroids, androgens, and aldosterone

B. Etiology and incidence

1. Causative factors include:

    a. Hyperfunction of the anterior pituitary gland, most commonly due to pituitary adenoma, causing excessive cortisol secretion

    b. An ACTH-producing tumor, adrenal adenoma or adrenal carcinoma, or adrenal hyperplasia

    c. Exogenous cortisol administration to treat other disorders

2. Incidence is 10 times greater in females than in males.

C. Pathophysiology

1. Ineffectiveness of the normal feedback mechanisms that control adrenocortical function results in excessive secretion of cortisol from the adrenal cortex despite adequate levels in circulation.

2. Clinical manifestations are the direct result of hormone excess (glucocorticoids, mineralcorticoids, and sex hormones); the predominant hormone excess—most commonly, glucocorticoids—determines the predominant manifestations.

3. Depending on the underlying cause, treatment may involve surgical removal or irradiation of adrenal or pituitary tumors, or adrenalectomy to resect hyperplastic adrenals.

4. A child undergoing one of these treatments requires lifelong hormone replacement therapy; specific agents depend on the nature of the procedure and on the particular deficiencies.

D. Assessment findings

1. Clinical manifestations commonly include:
   a. Centripedal fat distribution: truncal obesity, fat pads on supraclavicular and neck areas ("buffalo hump")
   b. Rounded or "moon" face, with reddened and oily skin
   c. Muscle wasting, thin extremities, pendulous abdomen
   d. Fragile, thin skin and subcutaneous tissue, acne, excessive bruising, petechiae
   e. Reddish purple abdominal striae
   f. Increased susceptibility to infection, poor wound healing
   g. Elevated blood pressure
   h. Compression fractures of vertebrae, kyphosis, back ache
   i. Retarded linear growth
   j. Irritability, insomnia, euphoria or depression, frank psychoses
   k. Precocious puberty in children
   l. Virilization in adolescent girls, marked by hirsutism, voice deepening, clitoral enlargement, breast atrophy, amenorrhea
   m. Loss of libido, impotence, and gynecomastia in adolescent boys

2. Laboratory and diagnostic study results may reveal:
   a. Excessive plasma cortisol level
   b. Hyperglycemia, glycosuria, latent or overt diabetes
   c. Hypokalemia
   d. Hypocalcemia and alkalosis
   e. Elevated urine levels of 17-hydroxycorticosteroid and 17-ketosteroid
   f. Decreased ACTH production on dexamethasone (cortisone) suppression test, helping establish a more definitive diagnosis
   g. Identification of adrenal tumor on computed tomographic (CT) scan, ultrasonography, or angiography
   h. Location of pituitary tumor on CT scan of the head

E. Nursing diagnoses

1. Activity Intolerance
2. Body Image Disturbance
3. Ineffective Family Coping
4. Ineffective Individual Coping

5. Fluid Volume Excess
6. High Risk for Infection
7. High Risk for Injury
8. Self-Esteem Disturbance
9. High Risk for Impaired Skin Integrity

F. Planning and implementation

1. Prevent infection by practicing good handwashing and limiting the child's exposure to persons with infections.
2. Help maintain skin integrity by providing and promoting good hygiene and skin care.
3. In consultation with a dietitian and in accordance with the physician's orders, implement meal planning to ensure good nutrition. Provide a high-protein, low-sodium diet with potassium supplements.
4. Promote adequate rest to prevent fatigue.
5. Administer medications as ordered, which may include:
   a. Cortical hormone replacement for a child with bilateral adrenalectomy
   b. GH, thyroid extract, antidiuretic hormone, gonadotropin, and steroid replacement for a child who has had a pituitary tumor removed.
6. If Cushing's syndrome results from necessary steroid therapy, reinforce to the child and family that the medication should never be abruptly stopped or a dose missed; either of these actions can precipitate adrenal crises. Explain that cushingoid symptoms caused by steroid therapy may be relieved by administering the steroids on an alternate-day basis and in the early morning.
7. Monitor vital signs for cardiac irregularities and hypertension.
8. Promote the child's positive self-image by encouraging him or her to vent fears and concerns and to identify personal assets and strengths.
9. Provide patient and family teaching, covering:
   a. Diagnosis and nature of the disorder
   b. Purpose of treatments and procedures
   c. Reason for surgery, and its benefits and disadvantages
   d. Dosage schedule, administration techniques, and side effects of all prescribed hormone replacements

G. Evaluation

1. The child exhibits no evidence of infection.
2. The child and family verbalize understanding of meal planning and select appropriate foods.
3. The child engages in activities appropriate to developmental level and condition.
4. The child's skin remains intact with no signs of irritation or breakdown.

5. The child exhibits no evidence of fluid retention.
6. The child verbalizes feelings and concerns.
7. Family members verbalize feelings and concerns regarding the child's special needs and effect on family activities.
8. Family members identify individual family strengths and support systems.
9. The child and family members verbalize an understanding of each prescribed replacement hormone regarding its action, dosage, administration, and possible adverse reactions.
10. The child and family members verbalize an understanding that this syndrome is a chronic illness that requires continual therapeutic management.

V. Diabetes mellitus

A. Description

1. Diabetes mellitus is an autoimmune metabolic disorder characterized by hyperglycemia and abnormal energy metabolism, resulting from absent or deficient insulin secretion or action at the cellular level.
2. Types include:
   a. Insulin-dependent (type I) diabetes mellitus (IDDM)
   b. Non–insulin-dependent (type II) diabetes mellitus (NIDDM)
   c. Maturity-onset diabetes of youth (MODY), a rare form of NIDDM

B. Etiology and incidence

1. The most common endocrine-metabolic disease of childhood, IDDM affects approximately 1 in 500 children and adolescents.
2. Although the precise cause of IDDM is unclear, both genetic and environmental factors play a role, along with autoimmune mechanisms.
3. IDDM apparently develops when a person with a genetic predisposition is exposed to a precipitating factor, such as viral infection.
4. Often asymptomatic, NIDDM is infrequently diagnosed in children and adolescents.
5. NIDDM apparently is inherited as an autosomal dominant trait.

C. Pathophysiology

1. Insulin is needed to support carbohydrate, fat, and protein metabolism, primarily by facilitating entry of these substances into cells.
2. Destruction of 90% or more of the pancreatic beta cells results in a clinically significant drop in insulin secretion.
3. This loss of insulin, the major anabolic hormone, leads to a catabolic state characterized by decreased glucose use and increased glucose production, eventually resulting in *hyperglycemia*.

4. In a state of insulin deficiency, glucagon, epinephrine, GH, and cortisol levels increase, stimulating lipolysis, fatty acid release, and ketone production.

5. Persistent blood glucose concentration above 180 mg/dL (the renal threshold) results in glucosuria, leading to an osmotic diuresis with polyuria and polydipsia.

6. Excessive ketone production can cause *diabetic ketoacidosis* (DKA), an acutely life-threatening condition characterized by marked hyperglycemia, metabolic acidosis, dehydration, and altered level of consciousness ranging from lethargy to coma.

7. The *Somogyi effect*, a unique phenomenon in children late in the course of the disease, involves a temporary decrease in blood glucose level followed by rebound hyperglycemia.

8. Treatment measures in acute care involve restoring homeostasis through IV fluid infusion, continuous regular low-dose insulin, and electrolyte replacement.

9. Goals of long-term care focus on restoring glycemic control through medication, exercise, and diet (Table 13-1).

D. **Assessment findings**

1. Common clinical manifestations of IDDM include:
   a. Polyuria, possibly with nocturia and enuresis
   b. Polydipsia and polyphagia
   c. Significant weight loss
   d. Fatigue
   e. Dry skin
   f. Blurred vision

TABLE 13–1.
Age-Appropriate Diabetes Management Goals

AGE (YEARS)	DIET	INSULIN	TESTING
4–5	Helps pick foods based on likes and dislikes	Helps pick injection sites; pinches up skin; wipes skin	Collects blood or urine; watches parent do testing; colors test results on records
6–7	Can tell if food has no sugar, some sugar, or a lot of sugar	Pushes plunger in after parent gives shot	Performs blood or urine test; records results; might need reminding; will need supervision
8–9	Selects foods based on exchanges	Gives own shots (at least once a day)	Does own blood test
10–13	Knows diet plan	Rotates sites; measures insulin	looks for patterns in test results
14+	Plans meals and snacks	Mixes two insulins in one syringe (if needed)	Suggests insulin changes bases on test patterns

(My child has diabetes: A book of questions and feelings for parents. *Becton Dickinson Consumer Products.* In S.R. Mott, N.F. Fazekas, and S.R. James (1985). Nursing care of children and families: A holistic approach. *Menlo Park, CA: Addison-Wesley)*

      g.   Abdominal pain, nausea, and vomiting

      h.   Hyperventilation, Kussmaul respirations

      i.   Fruity breath odor

  2. Laboratory study and diagnostic test results typically include:

      a.   Random blood glucose level above 200 mg/dL

      b.   Fasting blood glucose level above 120 mg/dL

      c.   Glycosuria

      d.   In DKA: hyperglycemia, ketonemia, acidosis, glycosuria, and ketonuria.

E. **Nursing diagnoses**

  1. Acute care

      a.   Fluid Volume Deficit

      b.   High Risk for Injury

      c.   Impaired Skin Integrity

  2. Long-term care

      a.   Activity Intolerance

      b.   Ineffective Individual Coping

      c.   Altered Family Processes

      d.   Fluid Volume Deficit

      e.   High Risk for Infection

      f.   Knowledge Deficit

      g.   Altered Nutrition: Less than Body Requirements

      h.   Powerlessness

      i.   Impaired Tissue Integrity

F. **Planning and implementation: acute care**

  1. Promote adequate fluid volume by maintaining accurate and careful records of IV fluid infusion, blood glucose level, intake and output, and urine specific gravity.

  2. Monitor cardiac status for signs of hypokalemia.

  3. Administer continuous infusion of low-dose regular insulin, as ordered.

  4. Help prevent hypotension and convulsions by closely monitoring vital signs, cardiac status, and blood glucose levels.

  5. Assess neurologic status by monitoring vital signs and noting any changes in level of consciousness.

  6. Help maintain skin integrity by turning the child frequently and encouraging regular ambulation.

  7. Protect the child from physical injury by keeping side rails up and padding hard surfaces that may cause pressure and injury to soft tissue and extremities.

G. **Planning and implementation: long-term care**

  1. Assess the child's and family's unique learning needs based on age, educational background, capacity to learn, and personal experience.

  2. Assess the child's and family members' emotional and psycholog-

ical state. Initial diagnosis may trigger shock and denial, which will hinder learning; acceptance of the disease is an important first step in learning to cope with long-term management.

3. Create a positive learning environment: comfortable temperature, quiet environment, supplemental materials.

4. Focus patient and family teaching on survival skills, including the disease process, urine and blood glucose testing, insulin therapy, signs and symptoms of hypoglycemia and hyperglycemia, meal planning, exercise, skin care, and special problems.

5. Limit teaching sessions to no more than 15 to 20 minutes. Teach only one new survival skill every 2 to 5 weeks to enable the child and family to assimilate the information completely.

6. Organize and present information from simple to more complex.

7. Evaluate the child's and family members' understanding of information taught by asking for return explanations and demonstrations.

8. Promote a sense of self-esteem in the child by encouraging him or her to express feelings and concerns and to identify personal strengths and positive aspects of his or her situation.

H. **Evaluation**

1. The child maintains adequate fluid balance.

2. The child experiences no cardiac irregularities.

3. The child demonstrates no evidence of injury.

4. The child maintains skin integrity.

5. The child and family members verbalize understanding of disease process, essential skills, and necessary follow-up care.

6. The child or a family member demonstrates proper insulin injection procedure.

7. The child and family members verbalize understanding of exchange diet and proper nutritional planning.

8. The child maintains peer relationships that he or she had before diagnosis.

9. The child becomes involved in special peer support groups.

10. Family members verbalize composite family strengths and incorporate the child's new needs into the family's lifestyle.

11. The child or family members verbalize that diabetes mellitus is a chronic illness that requires ongoing therapeutic management.

Bibliography

Bacon, G. E., Spencer, M. L., and Kelch, R. P. (1982). *A practical approach to pediatric endocrinology*. Chicago: Year Book Medical Publishers.

Bondu, P. K. (1985). Disorders of the adrenal cortex. In R. H. Williams (Ed.), *Textbook of endocrinology* (7th ed.). Philadelphia: W. B. Saunders.

Chambers, J. K. (Ed.) (1987). Common fluid and electrolyte disorders. *Nursing Clinics of North America, 22,* 749-872.

Daughaday, W. H. (1985). The anterior pituitary. In R. H. Williams (Ed.). *Textbook of endocrinology* (7th ed.). Philadelphia: W. B. Saunders.

Guthrie, D., and Guthrie, R. (1983). The disease process of diabetes mellitus. *Nursing Clinics of North America, 18,* 617–630.

Krane, E. J. (1987). Diabetic ketoacidosis: Biochemistry, physiology, treatment, and prevention. *Nursing Clinics of North America, 18.*

Mahoney, C. P. (1987). Evaluating the child with short stature. *Pediatric and Adolescent Endocrinology, 34.*

Mott, S. R., James, S. R., and Sperhac, A. M. (1990). *Nursing care of children and families* (2nd ed.). Menlo Park, CA: Addison-Wesley.

Whaley, L. F., and Wong, D. L. (1991). *Nursing care of infants and children* (4th ed.). St. Louis: C. V. Mosby.

Wilson, D. W., and Rosenfeld, R. G. (1987). Treatment of short stature and delayed adolescence. *Pediatric and Adolescent Endocrinology, 34.*

STUDY QUESTIONS

1. Hypofunction of which hormone causes poor linear growth and insulin sensitivity?
   a. antidiuretic hormone
   b. melanocyte-stimulating hormone
   c. parathyroid hormone
   d. growth hormone

2. Short stature results from
   a. anterior pituitary gland hypofunction
   b. posterior pituitary gland hyperfunction
   c. parathyroid gland hypofunction
   d. thyroid gland hyperfunction

3. Nina, aged 12, is upset that the steroid she is taking for nephrotic syndrome is causing weight gain and a round face. The nurse is afraid Nina may stop taking the drug, precipitating an adrenal crisis. Which of the following suggestions may lessen the cushingoid effects of corticosteroid therapy and help encourage Nina's continued compliance?
   a. Take the corticosteroid on an alternate-day basis.
   b. Take the corticosteroid late in the evening.
   c. Take the corticosteroid only once a week.
   d. Take the corticosteroid with milk.

4. Janet, aged 12 and diagnosed with type I (IDDM) diabetes mellitus, asks the nurse why she cannot take pills like her uncle rather than insulin shots. Which of the following would be the nurse's best reply?
   a. "The pills correct only fat and protein metabolism and not carbohydrate metabolism."
   b. "If you have a Somogyi effect, you can switch to the pill."
   c. "The pills work well only on the adult pancreas."
   d. "The pill adds only to an existing supply of insulin; you do not produce insulin and need replacement."

5. Which of the following phrases best describes hypopituitarism?
   a. normal growth for the first 5 years, followed by progressive linear growth retardation
   b. growth retardation in which height and weight are equally affected
   c. linear growth retardation with skeletal proportions normal for chronologic age
   d. normal growth pattern with precocious puberty

6. David, aged 6, is admitted to the hospital with height measured below the 3rd percentile and weight measured at the 40th percentile. His admitting diagnosis is idiopathic hypopituitarism. One of the nurse's first nursing actions should be to
   a. place David in a room with a 2-year-old boy
   b. arrange for a tutor to instruct David since he appears intellectually precocious
   c. plan for the dietitian to assess David's caloric needs
   d. suggest an orthodontic consultation due to the potential problem of overcrowding of teeth in a small, underdeveloped jaw

7. David's father shares with the nurse David's desire to play organized T-ball, a baseball sport that fosters participation of all team members. However, David's mother expresses her fears that David will get hurt since he is so much shorter than the other boys. In planning anticipatory guidance for David's parents, the nurse should keep in mind that
   a. children with idiopathic hypopituitarism have very fragile and brittle bones and are more prone to injury
   b. activity could aggravate insulin sensitivity, causing hyperglycemia
   c. activity would only aggravate the hip and knee joints already overtasked from David's excessive weight

d. to help promote self-esteem and a positive self-concept, David should be encouraged to participate in normal age-related activities as his condition allows

8. Which of the following endocrine malfunctions commonly results in Cushing's syndrome?
   a. hyperfunction of the anterior pituitary
   b. hypofunction of the anterior pituitary
   c. hyperfunction of the posterior pituitary
   d. hypofunction of the posterior pituitary

9. When caring for a child with Cushing's syndrome, which of the following nursing interventions would be most important?
   a. handling the child carefully to prevent bruising and fractures
   b. monitoring for signs and symptoms of hypoglycemia
   c. observing for signs and symptoms of metabolic acidosis
   d. monitoring vital signs for hypotension and tachycardia

10. Diabetic ketoacidosis results from an excessive accumulation of
    a. glucose from carbohydrate metabolism
    b. ketone bodies from fat metabolism
    c. potassium from cell death
    d. sodium bicarbonate from renal compensation

11. Which of the following is primary nursing action in the care of a child admitted to the intensive care unit with DKA?

    a. Restrict fluids to prevent aggravation of cerebral edema.
    b. Administer intravenous neutral protein Hagedorn (NPH) insulin in high-load doses.
    c. Monitor for hypertension.
    d. Monitor for cardiac irregularities.

12. Which of the following factors represents the best predictor of a successful teaching program for an adolescent with IDDM?
    a. The adolescent's parents accept that their child has diabetes mellitus.
    b. The adolescent accepts the diagnosis of diabetes mellitus.
    c. The adolescent has peers with diabetes mellitus.
    d. Diabetes mellitus survival skills are taught by one nurse.

13. At what age should a child begin self-administering insulin injections, assuming achievement of normal growth and developmental milestones?
    a. 4 to 5 years
    b. 6 to 7 years
    c. 8 to 9 years
    d. 10 to 13 years

14. When preparing a child with IDDM for discharge, the nurse discusses symptoms of hypoglycemia. Which of the following actions should the nurse instruct parents to take when their child displays such symptoms?
    a. Give the child nothing by mouth.
    b. Give the child some type of simple sugar, such as candy.
    c. Give the child some type of complex sugar, such as milk.
    d. Do nothing until they contact a physician.

ANSWER KEY

1. *Correct response: d*
   Growth hormone stimulates protein anabolism, promoting bone and soft tissue growth.
   a. Hypofunction of antidiuretic hormone causes diabetes insipidus, marked by dehydration and hypernatremia.
   b. Hypofunction of melanocyte-stimulating hormone causes diminished or absent skin pigmentation.
   c. Hypofunction of parathyroid hormone causes hypocalcemia, marked by tetany, convulsions, and muscle spasms.
   Comprehension/Physiologic/Assessment

2. *Correct response: a*
   Short stature results from diminished or deficient growth hormone, which is released from the anterior pituitary gland.
   b. Posterior pituitary hyperfunction results in increased secretion of antidiuretic hormone or oxytocin, leading to syndrome of inappropriate ADH secretion (SIADH), marked by fluid retention and hyponatremia.
   c. Parathyroid hypofunction leads to hypocalcemia, marked by tetany, convulsions, muscle spasms.
   d. Thyroid hyperfunction causes increased section of T4, T3, and thyrocalcitonin, resulting in Graves' disease, marked by accelerated linear growth and early epiphyseal closure.
   Knowledge/Physiologic/Analysis (Dx)

3. *Correct response: a*
   An alternate-day schedule allows the anterior pituitary gland to maintain, as much as possible, a normal hypothalamic-pituitary-adrenal control measure.
   b. Administering corticosteroids late in the evening actually increases cortisol levels, producing more pronounced effects.
   c. Once-weekly cortisol therapy usually is not effective.

   d. Taking the drug with milk has no beneficial impact on cushingoid symptoms.
   Application/Health promotion/ Implementation

4. *Correct response: d*
   Oral hypoglycemic agents are indicated only for patients with some functioning beta cells, as in type II (NIDDM) diabetes. Type I (IDDM) diabetics have no functioning beta cells.
   a. Oral hypoglycemics do not correct metabolism.
   b. A child with IDDM cannot substitute a hypoglycemic agent for insulin. The Somogyi effect is only a temporary physiologic reflex that decreases blood glucose level followed by rebound hyperglycemia.
   c. This is an inaccurate statement.
   Application/Health promotion/ Implementation

5. *Correct response: c*
   Although linear growth retardation occurs in hypopituitarism, delayed epiphyseal maturation allows for normal skeletal proportions.
   a. Normal growth may occur for the first year, followed by linear growth retardation thereafter.
   b. Height is affected more profoundly than weight, contributing to obesity.
   d. The child with hypopituitarism commonly experiences delayed sexual maturation.
   Knowledge/Physiologic/Assessment

6. *Correct response: c*
   Because David's weight is excessive for his height, he needs dietary assessment and planning to lose weight.
   a. Placing David in a room with a toddler could contribute to poor self-image.
   b. Arranging for a school teacher to instruct David is an appropriate nurs-

ing action, but the rationale is wrong. Children with hypopituitarism often appear intellectually precocious because of the disparity between height and cognitive ability, when in fact they typically are of normal intelligence.
d. This is not normally a problem in hypopituitarism.

Application/Health promotion/Planning

7. *Correct response: d*
Engaging in peer-group activities can help foster a sense of belonging and a positive self-concept. T-ball is a good choice of sports because physical stature is not an important consideration in the ability to participate, unlike some other sports such as basketball and football.
   a. Hypopituitarism does not affect calcium and phosphorus homeostasis and demineralization of bone.
   b. Physical activity without adequate carbohydrate intake can cause hypoglycemia, not hyperglycemia, although this rarely occurs.
   c. Moderate physical activity increases caloric use and reduces weight without undue strain on weight-bearing joints.

Comprehension/Psychosocial/Planning

8. *Correct response: a*
Cushing's syndrome is caused by excessive circulating cortisol, which can result from hypersecretion of ACTH by the anterior pituitary.
   b. Hypofunction of the anterior pituitary with respect to ACTH causes a low ACTH concentration in the blood, inhibiting adrenal cortex secretion of glucocorticoid and resulting in Addison's disease.
   c. Hyperfunction of the posterior pituitary can lead to SIADH.
   d. Hypofunction of the posterior pituitary causes diabetes insipidus.

Knowledge/Physiologic/Analysis (Dx)

9. *Correct response: a*
Cushing's syndrome causes capillary fragility, resulting in easy bruising and cal-

cium excretion, resulting in osteoporosis.
   b. Cushing's syndrome causes hyperglycemia, not hypoglycemia.
   c. Cushing's syndrome causes increased excretion of potassium and hydrogen ions, resulting in alkalosis.
   d. Cushing's syndrome causes increased water and sodium retention, resulting in hypertension, and hypokalemia, causing a sluggish and irregular heart beat.

Analysis/Physiologic/Implementation

10. *Correct response: b*
Inability to utilize glucose causes lipolysis, fatty acid oxidation, and release of ketones, resulting in metabolic acidosis and coma.
   a. Inability to utilize glucose, not impaired carbohydrate metabolism, is the primary mechanism in diabetes mellitus.
   c. Potassium depletion, not potassium excess, occurs in DKA.
   d. Sodium bicarbonate administration is a treatment for DKA.

Comprehension/Physiologic/Assessment

11. *Correct response: d*
Total body potassium depletion, particularly as fluid volume deficit is corrected, leaves the child vulnerable to cardiac arrest. The nurse should monitor the cardiac cycle for prolonged QT interval, low T wave, and depressed ST segment indicating weakened heart muscle and potential irregular heart beat.
   a. Intravenous fluids should be given to correct dehydration.
   b. Regular insulin is the only insulin that can be given intravenously. NPH is an intermediate-acting insulin; continuous low-dose infusion of a rapid-acting insulin is preferred.
   c. Hypertension is more likely to occur due to dehydration.

Application/Physiologic/Implementation

12. *Correct response: b*
By adolescence, a person begins to assume more responsibility for his or her

own health care practices; thus, his or her involvement in health care teaching can help ensure greater compliance.

a. Although involvement of parents in their adolescent's health care is important, the parents should increasingly transfer responsibility for self-care to the adolescent.

c. Although peer acceptance is important to the adolescent, knowing peers who have diabetes does not necessarily promote the adolescent's acceptance of his or her own disease.

d. Information is best learned when it progresses from simple to complex, builds on previously learned information, includes a variety of audio-visual materials, and is manageable. A well-planned patient education program can be taught by more than one nurse.

Analysis/Health promotion/Planning

13. *Correct response: c*

A child aged 8 to 9 years normally has sufficiently developed hand–eye coordination and motor ability to enable self-injection.

a. A preschool-age child is still clumsy and awkward at skills requiring fine motor coordination for prolonged periods.

b. In a child this age, fine motor coordination is still imprecise and can easily lead to feelings of frustration.

d. Delaying promotion of self-care activities longer than necessary tends to foster dependency.

Comprehension/Self care/Implementation

14. *Correct response: b*

Giving a little sugar temporarily corrects low serum glucose. Simple sugar is converted to glucose more quickly than a complex sugar.

a. A hyperglycemic child needs fluids to prevent dehydration.

c. Complex sugars are absorbed more slowly and do not provide an immediate response.

d. Immediate action is necessary to prevent complications of hypoglycemia.

Analysis/Health promotion/Evaluation

Neurologic Dysfunction

I. Essential concepts: nervous system anatomy and physiology

A. Development

1. The central nervous system (CNS) arises from the neural tube during embryonic development. By the 4th week of gestation, the neural tube has developed; by the 8th to 12th weeks, the cerebrum and cerebellum begin to develop.

2. Two periods of rapid nerve development occur: between the 15th and 20th week of gestation and from the 30th week of gestation through the first year of extrauterine life.

3. In the first year of extrauterine life, the number of brain neurons increases rapidly.
4. Normally comprising about 12% of body weight at birth, the brain doubles its weight by the end of the first year of extrauterine life and triples it by age 5 to 6 years.
5. CNS nerve myelinization, which enables progressive neuromuscular function, follows the cephalocaudal and proximodistal sequence; its rate accelerates rapidly after birth.
6. The peripheral nervous system arises from the neural crest, which originates from the neural tube during embryonic development.

B. Function
1. The neurologic system consists of three main divisions:
   a. CNS
   b. Peripheral nervous system
   c. Autonomic nervous system
2. Major CNS structures include the cerebrum, thalamus, hypothalamus, cerebellum, brain stem, and spinal cord.
3. The *cerebrum* is the center for consciousness, thought, memory, sensory input, and motor activity; consists of two hemispheres (left and right) and four lobes, each with its specific functions:
   a. Frontal lobe: controls voluntary muscle movements and contains motor areas, including the area for speech; center for personality, behavioral, and intellectual functions, for autonomic functions, and for emotional and cardiac responses
   b. Temporal lobe: center for taste, hearing, and smell; in the brain's dominant hemisphere, interprets spoken language
   c. Parietal lobe: coordinates and interprets sensory information from the opposite side of the body
   d. Occipital lobe: interprets visual stimuli
4. The *thalamus* further organizes cerebral function by transmitting impulses to and from the cerebrum. It also is responsible for primitive emotional responses, such as fear, and for distinguishing between pleasant and unpleasant stimuli.
5. Lying beneath the thalamus, the *hypothalamus* is an autonomic center that regulates blood pressure, temperature, libido, appetite, breathing, sleep patterns, and peripheral nerve discharges associated with certain behavior and emotional expression. It also helps control pituitary secretion and stress reaction.
6. The *cerebellum*, or hindbrain, controls smooth muscle movements, coordinates sensory impulses with muscle activity, and maintains muscle tone and equilibrium.
7. The *brain stem*, which includes the mesencephalon, pons, and medulla oblongata, relays nerve impulses between the brain and spinal cord. With the thalamus and hypothalamus, it makes up

the reticular formation, a nerve network that acts as an arousal mechanism.

8. The *spinal cord* forms a two-way conductor pathway between the brain stem and the peripheral nervous system. It also is the reflex center for motor activities that don't involve brain control.

9. Consisting of 31 pairs of spinal nerves and their intricate branches, the *peripheral nervous system* connects the CNS to remote body regions and conducts signals to and from these areas and the spinal cord.

10. The *autonomic nervous system* regulates involuntary body functions, such as digestion, respiration, and cardiovascular function.

II. Nervous system overview

A. Assessment

1. Besides obtaining the usual health history information, the nurse should attempt to determine whether the child's neurologic problem is focal or diffuse, acute or chronic, and stable or progressive.

2. A complete pediatric neurologic examination includes the following components:

   a. General: affect, social interaction, Denver Developmental Screening Test results, emotional state

   b. Head circumference and fontanel assessment (in infants)

   c. Mental status: level of consciousness, orientation, reasoning ability, memory

   d. Sensory status: vision, hearing, taste, smell, touch

   e. Cranial nerve function

   f. Motor function: muscle tone, strength, gait abnormalities, posture

   g. Cerebellar status: balance, coordination

   h. Reflexes: infant reflexes, later reflexes, deep tendon reflexes; superficial reflexes (Table 14–1)

3. In a child with an acute problem, periodic neurologic checks may be done every 4 hours or more often. This assessment, which can be completed in 5 minutes, should include:

   a. Vital signs: temperature, pulse, blood pressure, respirations

   b. Level of consciousness: standing on the Glasgow coma scale (Table 14–2)

   c. Eyes: pupil size, equality, and reaction to light; extraocular movements; corneal reflex; visual disturbances

   d. Motor and sensory function: posture, muscle tone, movement of extremities in response to command or painful stimulus, response to tactile stimuli

   e. Reflexes: gag reflex, Babinski reflex

   f. Head circumference and fontanel inspection (in infants)

TABLE 14–1.
Neonatal Reflexes

REFLEX	NORMAL DURATION
Babinski	Disappears by age 1 year
Crossed extension	Disappears by age 4 to 6 months
Landau	Disappears by age 4 to 6 months
Moro	Diminishes by age 4 months; disappears by age 7 months
Palmar grasp	Diminishes by age 4 months
Perez	Disappears by age 4 to 6 months
Plantar grasp	Diminishes by age 4 months
Prone crawl	Disappears by age 1 to 2 months
Rooting and sucking	Diminishes by age 5 to 6 months; disappears by age 1 year
Startle	Diminishes by age 4 months
Stepping	Disappears by age 1 to 2 months
Swallowing	Persists for life
Tongue extrusion	Disappears by age 4 months
Tonic neck ("fencing")	Diminishes by age 4 months
Trunk incurvation (Galant)	Disappears by age 4 weeks

B. **Laboratory studies and diagnostic tests**
1. Imaging studies include:
   a. Computed tomographic (CT) scan
   b. Magnetic resonance imaging
   c. Skull series
   d. Ultrasonography
   e. Electroencephalography
   f. Isotope brain scan
   g. Electromyography
   h. Myelography
2. Other useful laboratory studies include:
   a. Lumbar puncture to obtain cerebrospinal fluid (CSF) sample for analysis
   b. Subdural and ventricular taps
   c. Blood and urine studies

C. **Psychosocial implications**
1. Many of the specialized tests for neurologic function can be threatening to children; visual pictures of the machinery (e.g., CT scan) and explanations about the need to remain still during scans are helpful to the school-age child.
2. A young child may wish to have a transitional object, such as a favorite blanket or toy, with him or her during diagnostic tests to provide a sense of security.

TABLE 14–2.
Pediatric Coma Scale (Modification of Glasgow Coma Scale)

	SCORE	LESS THAN 1 YEAR	OVER 1 YEAR
Eyes open	4	Spontaneously	Spontaneously
	3	To shout	To verbal command
	2	To pain	To pain
	1	No response	No response
Best motor response	6		Obeys
	5	Localizes pain	Localizes pain
	4	Flexion withdrawal	Flexion withdrawal
	3	Flexion—abnormal (decorticate ridigity)	Flexion—abnormal (decorticate rigidity)
	2	Extension (decerebrate rigidity)	Extension (decerebrate rigidity)
	1	No response	No response

		2–5 YEARS	OVER 5 YEARS
Best verbal response	5	Appropriate words and phrases	Oriented and converses
	4		Disoriented and converses
	3	Inappropriate words	Inappropriate words
	2	Cries or screams	Incomprehensible sounds
	1	Grunts	No response
Total	3–15		

(Whaley, L.F., and Wong, D.L. (1987). Nursing care of infants and children (3rd ed.). St. Louis: C.V. Mosby, p. 1625)

III. Increased intracranial pressure (ICP)

A. Description: excessive pressure within the rigid cranial vault that disrupts neurologic function

B. Etiology

    1. ICP increase can result from any alteration that increases tissue or fluid volume within the cranium, including:

        a. Tumors or other space-occupying lesions

        b. Accumulation of CSF in the ventricular system

        c. Intracranial bleeding

        d. Edema of cerebral tissues

    2. Conditions that can produce increased ICP include:

        a. Craniocerebral trauma

        b. Hydrocephalus

        c. Brain tumor

        d. Meningitis

        e. Encephalitis

        f. Intracerebral hemorrhage

C. Pathophysiology

    1. Normally, ICP remains relatively constant (within its normally fluctuating range) through a system of compensatory alterations among the cranium's contents: brain tissue, meninges, CSF, and blood. Any increase in the volume of one component must be accompanied by a corresponding reduction in one or more of the others.

2. After cranial sutures fuse and fontanels close, only two mechanisms can compensate for increasing intracranial volume: displacement of CSF to the spinal subarachnoid space and increased CSF absorption.

3. An intracranial volume increase that exceeds the ability of these mechanisms to compensate produces signs and symptoms of increased ICP.

4. As ICP rises, it can trigger a cycle of decreasing perfusion, increasing edema, and further increased ICP; if unchecked, this cycle can result in complete loss of cerebral arterial perfusion and brain cell death.

5. Brain stem compression secondary to herniation can cause life-threatening deterioration of vital functions.

6. Treatment of increased ICP focuses on reducing intracranial volume and treating the underlying disorder.

D.   Assessment findings

1. Clinical manifestations of increased ICP in an infant and a young child commonly include:
   a. Irritability and restlessness
   b. Tense, bulging anterior fontanel in child under age 18 months
   c. High-pitched cry
   d. Change in feeding habits
   e. Increased occipital frontal circumference
   f. Crying with cuddling and rocking
   g. "Setting sun" sign
   h. Macewen's ("cracked pot") sign in an infant with unfused cranial sutures

2. In an older child, signs and symptoms may include:
   a. Headache
   b. Anorexia and nausea
   c. Vomiting, often projectile without nausea
   d. Cognitive, personality, and behavioral changes
   e. Diplopia, blurred vision
   f. Seizures

3. Late clinical manifestations of extremely high ICP in any age group include:
   a. Decreased level of consciousness ranging from lethargy and confusion to coma
   b. Decreased motor response to commands
   c. Decreased sensation to painful stimuli

       d.   Alterations in pupil size and reactivity
       e.   Decerebrate or decorticate posturing
       f.   Papilledema
       g.   Cheyne-Stokes respirations

E. Nursing diagnoses
1. Ineffective Airway Clearance
2. Anxiety
3. Altered Family Processes
4. Fear
5. Fluid Volume Deficit
6. Altered Health Maintenance
7. High Risk for Injury
8. Knowledge Deficit
9. Altered Nutrition: Less than Body Requirements
10. Pain
11. Altered Parenting
12. Powerlessness
13. Altered Role Performance
14. Sensory and Perceptual Alterations
15. Impaired Skin Integrity
16. Altered Thought Processes

F. Planning and implementation
1. Assist in reducing intraabdominal and intrathoracic pressure by elevating the head of the bed 15 to 45 degrees.
2. Assess for early changes in ICP by monitoring vital signs, level of consciousness, motor activity, behavior, and pupil size and reactivity.
3. If appropriate, use a transducer to directly monitor ICP.
4. As ordered, assist with treatments and supportive measures such as hyperventilation, mechanical ventilation, and hypothermia.
5. Prevent overhydration or underhydration; monitoring fluid intake and output, and impose fluid restrictions, if ordered.
6. Help the child avoid positions or activities that increase ICP, such as neck vein compression, flexion or extension of the neck, turning the head from side to side, painful or stressful stimuli, and respiratory suctioning or percussion.
7. Promote normal bowel elimination to prevent intraabdominal pressure increase from straining at stool.
8. Help reduce the child's anxiety and fear by providing a quiet, relaxing environment and explaining all procedures before they are performed.
9. Prevent weight loss by providing adequate nutrition in small frequent feedings.
10. Promote normal growth and development without overstimulating child.

11. Prevent skin breakdown by placing the child on a sheepskin or another resilient mattress appliance.
12. As appropriate, prepare the child for surgery to relieve ICP; procedures may include subdural tap, ventriculostomy, epidural evacuation, placement of a ventricular shunt, decompressive craniectomy, or tumor resection.
13. Administer medications as ordered, which may include:
    a. Osmotic diuretics, such as mannitol or urea
    b. Corticosteroids
14. Provide patient and family teaching, covering:
    a. The nature of increased ICP and its underlying cause, if known
    b. All treatments and procedures, including rationales

G. Evaluation
1. The child exhibits decreased ICP and resolution of signs and symptoms subside.
2. The parents verbalize understanding of follow-up care.

IV. Seizures
A. Description
1. A seizure is an excessive, disorderly discharge of electrical impulses by neuronal tissue causing sudden, transient alteration in CNS function.
2. Seizures are classified as follows:
   a. Partial: local focus of abnormal electrical discharge, usually in the cerebral cortex; types include simple partial and complex partial
   b. Generalized: multifocal, arising in the reticular formation and involving both hemispheres of the brain; types include tonic-clonic (grand mal), absence (petit mal), atonic, akinetic, and myoclonic (including infant myoclonic seizures)
   c. Status epilepticus: continuation of grand mal seizures with no recovery period or regaining of consciousness between attacks; a medical emergency

B. Etiology and incidence
1. Most seizures are idiopathic with no known cause.
2. There is some evidence of a genetic factor, in which the seizure threshold is lowered in affected persons; this is seen in children over age 3.
3. Some seizures are acquired in direct relation to an event, such as perinatal injury resulting from trauma, hypoxia, infections, toxins, hypoglycemia, or hypocalcemia.
4. Seizures are more common before age 2 years than at any other period.
5. Up to 5% of all children experience at least one seizure by adolescence; chronic, recurrent seizures, or *epilepsy*, affects 1% to 2% of all children.

C. **Pathophysiology**
1. Seizures result from sudden neuronal discharges of electrical activity resulting from an irritated epileptogenic focus (hyperexcitable cells).
2. The biochemical basis of these discharges is incompletely understood but many appear to be triggered by such factors as cellular dehydration, abnormal blood glucose level, electrolyte imbalance, emotional stress, or endocrine changes.
3. The violent, disorganized burst of electrical energy spreads from the focus to adjacent areas, or may jump to distant areas of the CNS; a seizure results.
4. Specific neurologic effects of a seizure depend on type, focus, intensity, duration, and underlying cause.
5. Primary objectives of treatment include reducing the frequency of seizures, correcting the underlying cause if possible, and promoting as normal a lifestyle as possible.
6. Therapeutic management primarily involves drug therapy and may include diet therapy or surgical intervention.
   a. Drugs: phenobarbital, phenytoin, ethosuximide, primidone, diazepam, carbamazepine
   b. Diet therapy (usually reserved for child with recurrent petit mal, atonic, or myoclonic seizures that are refractive to drug therapy): high-fat, low-protein, low-carbohydrate diet
   c. Surgery: indicated only for well-defined, surgically accessible epileptogenic focus when excision does not interrupt significant life functions; rarely performed

D. **Assessment findings**
1. Clinical manifestations of *simple partial seizures* include:
   a. Twitching of face, hand, or foot; may progress to entire side of body (jacksonian seizure)
   b. Turning of eyes or head away from side of focus (aversive seizure)
   c. Weakness of affected muscle group persisting for hours to days after the seizure
   d. Tingling, numbness, warmth, or other altered sensations in affected body areas
   e. Possible progression to complex partial or generalized seizures
2. *Complex partial seizures* may be marked by:
   a. Prodromal *aura* of anxiety, nausea, and unpleasant taste or smell
   b. Impaired consciousness, confusion, vague stare, mumbling or incomprehensible speech
   c. Repetitive motor activity (automatisms), such as lip-smack-

ing, spitting, chewing, blinking, picking at clothing, kicking, walking in circles

   d. Possible aggressive response to attempts at restraint

   e. Auditory and visual hallucinations

   f. Postseizure confusion and fatigue

   g. Possible progression to generalized seizures

3. Common clinical manifestations of *grand mal seizures* include:

   a. Possible short prodromal aura marked by peculiar sensations, often dizziness, but usually occurs suddenly

   b. Upward rolling of eyes

   c. Loss of consciousness

   d. Characteristic piercing cry as air is forced through tightly closed vocal cords

   e. Generalized and symmetric muscle rigidity lasting 10 to 20 seconds, increased salivation, possible apnea and cyanosis (tonic phase)

   f. After the tonic phase, violent jerking movements as muscles undergo rhythmic relaxation and contraction, possible foaming at the mouth, biting of tongue, and urinary and fecal incontinence (clonic phase); usually lasting about 30 seconds but possibly persisting for up to 30 minutes

   g. Postseizure exhaustion, headache, confusion, inability to recall the episode

4. *Status epilepticus* is marked by grand mal seizures occurring in rapid sequence; the child does not regain consciousness between attacks. Untreated, a succession of uninterrupted seizures can lead to respiratory failure and death.

5. Manifestations of *petit mal seizures* typically include:

   a. Brief (5- to 10-second) loss of consciousness with minimal or no alteration in muscle tone or behavioral changes; may appear to be daydreaming or staring

   b. Possible minor signs such as eye rolling, head nodding, lip smacking, facial twitching, and slight hand movements

   c. Postseizure, normal appearance and sensations but with no awareness of event

6. *Atonic and akinetic seizures* may produce:

   a. Sudden, momentary loss of muscle tone and postural control, causing the child to fall (and often causing serious injury since the child is unable to break the fall by putting out a hand)

   b. Transient loss of consciousness

7. *Myoclonic seizures* are marked by sudden, brief contractures of a muscle or muscle group, occurring singly or repetitively with no alteration in consciousness.

8. *Infant myoclonic seizures* primarily affect infants between age 3 and 6 months and are marked by:

      a. Sudden forceful myoclonic contractions in the trunk, neck, and extremities, either flexion ("salaam" or "jack-knife" seizure) or extension ("spread eagle" seizure); usually lasting no more than 1 minute

      b. Crying or grunting in severe attacks

      c. Grimacing and giggling during and after the seizure

E. **Nursing diagnoses**

  1. Anxiety

  2. Body Image Disturbance

  3. Altered Family Processes

  4. High Risk for Injury

  5. Knowledge Deficit

  6. Altered Parenting

  7. Self-Esteem Disturbance

F. **Planning and implementation**

  1. Protect the child from injury during acute episodes.

  2. During a seizure, carefully observe and document events, including:

      a. Apparent triggering factor, if known or suspected

      b. Behavior before the seizure; aura

      c. Time seizure began and ended

      d. Clinical manifestations of the seizure

      e. Postseizure behavior and symptoms

  3. Help prevent seizures by preventing the child's exposure to factors or situations known to precipitate an attack (e.g., emotional stress, blinking lights).

  4. Minimize the child's anxiety by staying with him or her during seizure activity, providing reassurance and emotional support, explaining all procedures and treatments in terms the child can understand, and allowing him or her as much normal activity as possible.

  5. Promote a positive self-concept in the child by encouraging him or her to express feelings and concerns, assess personal strengths and assets, and set attainable goals.

  6. Provide emotional support to the child's family; encourage them to vent fears and concerns, and assist them in learning to understand and cope with their child's condition and limitations. Refer them to the Epilepsy Foundation of America for further information and support.

  7. Help promote the child's normal growth and development by encouraging activities appropriate to the child's age, developmental level, and physical condition, taking into account any activity limitations imposed by the physician.

  8. Provide patient and family teaching, covering:

      a. The nature of the disorder and possible causes and triggering factors

      b.   Prodromal signs to watch for and steps to take if they occur

      c.   Seizure precaution measures

      d.   Diagnostic tests and procedures, including rationales

      e.   Dosage, administration, and side effects of all prescribed medications

      f.   The importance of never discontinuing drug therapy abruptly (this can precipitate status epilepticus) and of never switching to a different brand of the same medication

      g.   The need for periodic reevaluation of drug therapy effectiveness as well as close monitoring of blood cell counts, electrolytes, liver function, urinalysis, and vital signs

      h.   Other treatment modalities, including diet and surgery as appropriate

      i.   The importance of maintaining as normal a lifestyle as possible and of helping an older child and adolescent achieve independence

      j.   Any activity restrictions imposed by the physician

      k.   The need to share information about the child's special needs with significant others, such as teachers and school nurses

      l.   Follow-up care

G. **Evaluation**

    1.   The child's seizures are well controlled.

    2.   Parents verbalize understanding of the treatment plan (including proper use and possible adverse effects of medications), seizure prevention measures, and the need for continual monitoring.

    3.   The child and parents demonstrate the ability to cope with seizure activity.

    4.   The child exhibits a good self-concept, participates in normal activities to the greatest extent possible, and complies with imposed activity limitations.

V. **Neural tube defects (spina bifida occulta, meningocele, myelomeningocele)**

  A. **Description**

    1.   Neural tube defects are embryologic defects in which midline spinous processes fail to fuse, resulting in varying degrees of protrusion of meninges, CSF, and spinal nerves; may be cystic or noncystic.

    2.   Common neural tube defects include:

      a.   Spina bifida occulta: limitation of the defect to the spinal cord, with no involvement of the spinal cord and meninges

      b.   Meningocele: protrusion of a cystlike sac containing CSF and meninges through an opening in the vertebral arch

      c.   Myelomeningocele (meningomyelocele): CSF, meninges,

and nerve tissue of damaged cord are contained in a protruding cystlike sac covered by a thin membrane

B. Etiology and incidence

1. Hereditary and environmental factors are believed to influence development of neural tube defects.

2. Some speculation exists that virus might contribute to failure of neural tube closure, but this has not yet been confirmed.

3. This defect occurs in about 1 in every 1,000 live births.

C. Pathophysiology

1. The most critical or sensitive period of neural tube closure is at about 4 weeks of gestation. Disruption of normal physiologic processes at this time can result in a neural tube defect.

2. In myelomeningocele, the most serious of the defects discussed in this entry, the degree of neurologic dysfunction is directly related to the defect's location and nerve involvement; neurologic dysfunction occurs at or below the level of the defect.

3. Sensory and motor disturbances are usually parallel.

4. Therapeutic management of myelomeningocele typically involves:

    a. Immediate surgery to reduce the risk of meningitis and further damage to spinal cord and nerve roots

    b. Long-range surgical intervention, which may include tendon release, scoliosis repair, or urinary diversion

    c. Long-term medical therapies directed toward correcting musculoskeletal deformities and achieving bowel and bladder control

D. Assessment findings

1. Clinical manifestations vary with the type and location of the defect, and may include:

    a. Spina bifida occulta: usually asymptomatic; may produce a dimple or hair growth over the malformed vertebra and, as the child grows and develops, such manifestations as foot weakness and bowel and bladder sphincter disturbances

    b. Meningocele: visible herniation of a saclike mass anywhere on the spinal cord; rarely may cause lower extremity weakness and poor sphincter control; hydrocephalus may be an associated finding

    c. Myelomeningocele: a round, raised, possibly bluish protrusion at any point along the spinal cord, but most commonly in the lumbosacral area; fluid leakage may be evident

2. Clinical problems commonly associated with myelomeningocele include:

    a. Arnold-Chiari malformation

    b. Loss of motor control and sensation below the level of the lesion

      c.   Contractures, hip dysplasia, scoliosis, clubfoot

      d.   Urine stasis and susceptibility to urinary tract infections

      e.   Fecal incontinence and constipation

      f.   Susceptibility to skin breakdown in denervated areas

      g.   Tendency toward obesity due to activity limitations

3. Diagnostic tests done to determine the extent of the defect may include spinal radiographs, CT scans, ultrasonography, and myelography.

4. Prenatal detection is now available through amniocentesis and measurement of alpha-fetoprotein level. Testing should be provided to women at risk—those who have the defect themselves or who have given birth to an affected child.

E.   Nursing diagnoses

   1.   Bowel Incontinence

   2.   Constipation

   3.   Altered Family Processes

   4.   High Risk for Infection

   5.   High Risk for Injury

   6.   Impaired Physical Mobility

   7.   Self-Esteem Disturbance

   8.   Sensory and Perceptual Alterations

   9.   Impaired Skin Integrity

   10.   Altered Patterns of Urinary Elimination

F.   Planning and implementation

1. Help prevent infection by applying sterile, moist soaks to the lesion (possibly with an antibacterial agent added) and by not placing a diaper or other covering directly over the lesion, to prevent fecal contamination.

2. Prevent trauma to the sac by placing the infant prone in an isolette or warmer.

3. Position the infant in low Trendelenburg position while prone to reduce the pressure of CSF in the sac.

4. Help prevent hip subluxation by maintaining the legs in abduction with a pad between the knees and the feet in a neutral position with a roll under the ankles.

5. Promote parent–infant relationship by encouraging parent participation with feeding, cuddling, and tactile stimulation.

6. Monitor vital signs, measure occipital frontal circumference daily, assess neurologic checks, assess behavioral changes, and assess anterior fontanel for bulging—all signs of increased ICP.

7. Help prevent skin breakdown by padding bony prominences and placing the child in a side-lying position (postoperatively) if allowed by physician.

8. Encourage parents to express their feelings, fears, and anxieties regarding caring for their chronically ill child.

9. Encourage the parents to contact:

The Spina Bifida Association of America
343 S. Dearborn, #310
Chicago, IL 60604

10. Provide patient and family teaching, covering:
    a. Essentials of infant care with special emphasis on infection prevention, recognizing early signs and symptoms of infection and of increased ICP, bladder and bowel management, and developmental needs
    b. Effects of immobilization and ways to minimize them
    c. The need for lifelong care (in a child with severe defect) requiring maintenance and habilitative care
11. Carefully assess the family's ability to care for the infant, and refer them for further assistance if necessary.

G. Evaluation

1. The child's vital signs, ICP, and neurologic checks reveal findings within acceptable ranges.
2. The child is free of infection, trauma, and skin breakdown.
3. The child displays neutral alignment of legs and hips.
4. Parents demonstrate ability to care for the infant adequately.
5. Parents verbalize understanding of requirements for care, monitoring, and developmental needs of the infant.

VI. Hydrocephalus

A. Description

1. Hydrocephalus refers to an imbalance between the production of CSF and its absorption into the circulation, causing increased CSF accumulation within the intracranial cavity and, in infants, enlargement of the head.
2. Classification is as follows:
   a. Communicating hydrocephalus, involving impaired absorption of CSF in the subarachnoid space; flow is not obstructed
   b. Noncommunicating hydrocephalus, involving obstruction to flow of CSF within ventricles or from ventricles to the subarachnoid space

B. Etiology and incidence

1. Hydrocephalus occurring in first 2 years of life is most often a result of developmental defects such as myelomeningocele.
2. Hydrocephalus occurring in infancy, not caused by developmental defects, is a result of intrauterine infection, anoxia, traumatic birth, or neonatal meningitis.
3. Hydrocephalus occurring in older children is a result of space-occupying lesions, hemorrhage, intracranial infection, or dormant developmental defects.

C. Pathophysiology

1. Regardless of cause, a result of hydrocephalus is impaired absorption of CSF and obstruction to CSF flow.

2. Surgical treatment is the therapy of choice; it involves placing a shunt in a ventricle and threading it into either the peritoneum (VP shunt) or the right atrium (VA shunt).

3. The shunt serves as drain to remove excess CSF. Shunt revisions typically are planned for age 18 to 24 months, again at age 4 to 6 years, and once more when the child has reached about 80% of his or her projected adult height. The primary reason for unscheduled shunt revision is infection of the shunt valve or catheter.

4. Prognosis is related to the underlying cause, rate of hydrocephalus development, duration and degree of increased ICP, and occurrence of postsurgical complications.

D. Assessment findings

1. Common clinical manifestations during infancy include:
   a. Bulging fontanel
   b. Macewen's (cracked pot) sign
   c. Frontal enlargement of skull (bossing)
   d. Setting sun sign
   e. Irritability and lethargy
   f. Persistence of infantile reflexes

2. Clinical manifestations during childhood typically include:
   a. Early morning headache on awakening
   b. Vomiting with or without nausea
   c. Papilledema
   d. Lethargy and irritability
   e. Confusion
   f. Inability to follow commands

3. Diagnostic tests may reveal:
   a. Varying degrees of localized fluid accumulation on cranial transillumination
   b. Evidence of fluid accumulation on CT scan
   c. Widened sutures and fontanels and erosion of intracranial bones seen on skull radiograph

E. Nursing diagnoses

1. Ineffective Airway Clearance
2. Anxiety
3. Altered Family Processes
4. Fear
5. Fluid Volume Deficit
6. Altered Health Maintenance
7. High Risk for Infection
8. High Risk for Injury
9. Altered Nutrition: Less than Body Requirements
10. Pain
11. Altered Role Performance

12. Sensory and Perceptual Alterations
13. Impaired Skin Integrity
14. Altered Thought Processes

F. Planning and implementation (*Note:* See also section III.F for additional interventions related to increased ICP.)
1. Prevent neck injury by supporting the infant's head well when feeding, holding, or moving him or her.
2. Prevent infection by providing meticulous skin care, avoiding contaminating wound dressing, and inspecting wound dressings for CSF leakage.
3. Administer medications as ordered, which may include:
    a. Antibiotics to prevent postoperative infections of shunt or meninges
    b. Acetazolamide to decrease CSF production
    c. An osmotic diuretic such as urea or mannitol to reduce increased ICP
4. Postoperatively, encourage parents to avoid being overprotective of their infant or child.
5. Encourage an older child to resume normal activities, except for contact sports, as soon as is appropriate after surgery.
6. Provide patient and family teaching, covering:
    a. The nature of the condition and its underlying cause, if known
    b. All tests and procedures
    c. The reasons for all therapeutic measures
    d. Signs and symptoms of increased ICP and infection to watch for and report
    e. The fact that hydrocephalus is a lifelong condition necessitating regular evaluation by a physician

G. Evaluation
1. The child is free of infection and neck injury.
2. Parents verbalize understanding of home care and signs and symptoms of increased ICP and infection.
3. Parents verbalize understanding of the need to avoid overprotecting the child and to encourage activity as tolerated.

Bibliography

Blackman, J. A. (1984). *Medical aspects of developmental disabilities in children.* Rockville, MD: Aspen Publications.

Chee, C. M. (1980). Seizure disorders. *Nursing Clinics of North America, 15,* 71–82.

Conway-Rutkowski, B. L. (1982). *Carini and Owen's neurological and neurosurgical nursing* (8th ed.). St. Louis: C. V. Mosby.

Davis, A. T., and Hill, P. M. (1980). Cerebral palsy. *Nursing Clinics of North America, 15,* 35–50.

Downey, J. A., and Low, N. L. (Eds.) (1982). *The child with disabling illness* (2nd ed.). New York: Raven Press.

Menken, J. H. (Ed.) (1985). *Textbook of child neurology* (3rd ed.). Philadelphia: Lea and Febiger.

Mott, S. R., James, S. R., and Sperhac, A. M. (1990). *Nursing care of children and families* (2nd ed.). Menlo Park, CA: Addison-Wesley.

Whaley, L. F., and Wong, D. L. (1991). *Nursing care of infants and children* (4th ed.). St. Louis: C. V. Mosby.

STUDY QUESTIONS

1. As a cause of death in children age 1 to 4 years, congenital malformation ranks
   a. first
   b. second
   c. third
   d. fourth

2. When caring for a child with increased ICP, what is the rationale for elevating the head of the bed 15 to 45 degrees?
   a. to let the child see better without lifting his or her head
   b. to help alleviate headache
   c. to reduce intraabdominal pressure
   d. all the above

3. Mary Shannon, aged 5, is diagnosed with grand mal seizures; therapy includes phenytoin (Dilantin). When formulating a patient and family teaching plan regarding anticonvulsants, which of the following instructions should the nurse stress?
   a. The liquid form of the medication is preferable.
   b. Missing a dose will not disrupt the drug regimen.
   c. Side effects are minimal; drug therapy need not be monitored closely.
   d. Establishing an administration schedule that fits in with the usual family routine can be helpful.

4. In hydrocephalus, which of the following clinical manifestations commonly occurs in infants but not in older children?
   a. irritability
   b. anorexia, refusal to eat
   c. Macewen's (cracked pot) sign
   d. altered level of consciousness

5. Which of the following phrases most accurately describes a myelomeningocele?
   a. complete exposure of the spinal cord and meninges
   b. herniation of the spinal cord and meninges into a sac
   c. sac formation containing meninges and CSF
   d. spinal cord tumor containing nerve roots

6. Leah, a 12-hour-old newborn with a lumbar (L2) myelomeningocele, likely would exhibit all the following clinical manifestations *except*
   a. constipation
   b. foot deformities
   c. paraplegia
   d. decreased sensation in the lower extremities

7. The primary reason to surgically repair a myelomeningocele is to
   a. correct the neurologic deficit
   b. prevent hydrocephalus
   c. prevent epilepsy
   d. decrease the risk of infection

8. Billy, aged 2 years, is recovering from shunt placement surgery done to relieve hydrocephalus. He has a postoperative nursing diagnosis of High Risk for Injury: related to rapid reduction of intracranial pressure. Which of the following would be an appropriate nursing intervention for Billy?
   a. Elevate the head of the bed 15 to 45 degrees.
   b. Place Billy in low Trendelenburg position.
   c. Position Billy flat on the shunt side.
   d. Position Billy flat on the nonshunt side.

9. The most common reason for an unscheduled shunt revision in a child with hydrocephalus is
   a. unexpected growth spurt
   b. infection
   c. seizures
   d. fever

10. What is an epileptogenic focus?
    a. a group of hyperexcitable neuronal cells
    b. a group of atrophied, hypotonic neuronal cells
    c. a clonic movement of tissue
    d. nonchargeable, inhibitory neuronal cells

11. Which of the following is *not* a priority

nursing objective for a child with a seizure disorder?
a. Teach the family about anticonvulsant drug therapy.
b. Assess for signs and symptoms of increased ICP.
c. Ensure safety and protection from injury.
d. Observe and record the seizures.

12. When preparing parents to address their child's unique psychological needs related to epilepsy, the nurse should point out to the parents that the child may experience additional stress related to
a. poor self-image
b. dependency needs
c. feeling different from peers
d. all the above

13. Which of the following is the most useful tool in diagnosing seizure disorder?
a. electroencephalography
b. lumbar puncture
c. brain scan
d. skull radiographs

14. Which of the following therapies has been proved the *least* effective in treating seizure disorders?
a. drug therapy
b. ketogenic diet
c. surgical intervention
d. hypnosis

ANSWER KEY

1. *Correct response: b*
   This information is from the 1986 National Centers for Health Statistics.
   a. Accidents are the number one cause of death in children of all ages.
   c. Cancer is the third-ranking cause of death in children age 1 to 4 years.
   d. Heart disease is the fourth-ranking cause of death in children age 1 to 4 years.
   Knowledge/Health promotion/Assessment

2. *Correct response: d*
   Nursing management focuses on reducing increased ICP by lowering intrathoracic and intraabdominal pressure and by reducing emotional stress.
   Application/Safe care/Implementation

3. *Correct response: d*
   Establishing a regular time that does not disrupt family routines and becomes a part of regular family activities helps promote compliance with the therapeutic regimen.
   a. This preferred form of phenytoin is a tablet.
   b. Skipping a scheduled dose is the most common cause of status epilepticus.
   c. Anticonvulsants carry many serious side effects, including drowsiness, rash, ataxia, and vertigo.
   Comprehension/Health promotion/Planning

4. *Correct response: c*
   Macewen's sign refers to a so-called cracked pot sound heard on cranial percussion in a child with separated cranial sutures.
   a. Irritability and restlessness occur in both infants and older children.
   b. Refusal to eat in an infant is thought to be associated with anorexia, a subjective symptom in older children.
   d. Altered level of consciousness develops in all patients with increased ICP that goes untreated. Infants may have a later onset than older children because the infant cranium

is not as rigid and expands somewhat to accommodate increased ICP.
   Comprehension/Physiologic/Assessment

5. *Correct response: b*
   Myelomeningocele is a herniation of the spinal cord, meninges, and CSF into a sac that protrudes through a defect in the vertebral arch.
   a. Myelomeningocele does not involve complete exposure of the spinal cord and meninges; this is a massive defect incompatible with life.
   c. This is a description of meningocele.
   d. Tumor formation is not associated with myelomeningocele.
   Knowledge/Physiologic/Assessment

6. *Correct response: a*
   Myelomeningocele results in denervation to the bowel and bladder, causing decreased muscle tone and fecal and urinary incontinence.
   b. Foot deformities are usually present, particularly club foot.
   c. Paralysis of the lower extremities commonly occurs.
   d. Sensory nerve involvement decreases sensation below the level of the defect.
   Application/Physiologic/Assessment

7. *Correct response: d*
   Surgical closure decreases the risk of infection stemming from damage to the fragile sac, which can lead to meningitis.
   a. The neurologic deficit cannot be corrected; however, some surgeons believe that early surgery reduces stretching of spinal nerves and prevents further damage.
   b. Surgical repair does not help relieve hydrocephalus—in fact, some researchers believe that repair exaggerates the Arnold-Chiari malformation and decreases the absorptive surface for CSF, leading to more rapid development of hydrocephalus.
   c. Surgical repair of the sac does not

prevent epilepsy, which is an impairment of brain neuronal tissue.
Knowledge/Physiologic/Analysis (Dx)

8. **Correct response: d**
Keeping an infant flat after shunt placement prevents overrapid decompression.
   a. Elevating the head of the bed can help reduce increased ICP. After shunt placement—especially in an infant with a new shunt instead of a shunt revision—this position will cause subdural hematoma as the cerebral cortex pulls away from the dura.
   b. Low Trendelenburg position is used postoperatively after surgery for myelomeningocele to help reduce CSF pressure in the sac.
   c. Positioning the child on the operative site might lead to shunt obstruction.

Application/Safe care/Implementation

9. **Correct response: b**
Infection, obstruction, and disconnection of the tubing are the primary reasons for shunt revision.
   a. Growth spurts usually can be predicted and shunt revisions planned for when the child reaches 80% of his or her projected adult height.
   c. Seizures do not affect CSF flow or cause shunt obstruction.
   d. Although fever is a cardinal sign of infection, the infection may not necessarily be within the shunt system.

Knowledge/Physiologic/Planning

10. **Correct response: a**
An epileptogenic focus is a group of hyperexcitable neuronal cells that are prone to increased electric stimulation and may trigger seizure activity.
   b, c, and d. These are incorrect definitions.

Knowledge/Physiologic/Assessment

11. **Correct response: b**
Signs and symptoms of increased ICP are not associated with seizure activity.
   a. Improper administration of or incomplete compliance with anticonvulsant therapy can lead to status epilepticus.
   c. Safety is always a priority in the care of a child with seizure disorder; seizures may occur at any time.
   d. Careful observation and documentation of seizures provides valuable information to aid prevention and treatment.

Application/Safe care/Planning

12. **Correct response: d**
All these factors can put additional stress on a child trying to understand and manage a chronic illness.
Comprehension/Health promotion/Planning

13. **Correct response: a**
The electroencephalogram detects abnormal electrical activity in the brain. The pattern of the various spikes can help a physician diagnose specific seizure disorders, such as grand mal seizures or petit mal seizures. Absence of electrical activity indicates pathologic conditions such as abscesses or subdural fluid accumulation.
   b. Lumbar puncture confirms problems related to cerebrospinal infection or trauma.
   c. Brain scan confirms space-occupying lesions or brain tissue atrophy.
   d. Skull radiographs can detect fractures and other structural abnormalities.

Knowledge/Physiologic/Assessment

14. **Correct response: d**
Hypnosis, a state analogous to normal sleep that can be artificially induced, does not alter epileptogenic foci.
   a, b, and c. These are all proven therapies in treating seizures.

Knowledge/Health promotion/Planning

Musculoskeletal Dysfunction

I.   Essential concepts: musculoskeletal anatomy and physiology

A.   Development

1.   The musculoskeletal system arises from the embryonic meso-dermal layer, which appears during the second week of gestation.

2. By the eighth week of gestation, all major bones are present in the cartilaginous skeleton.
3. Bone formation occurs via ossification, which begins as early as the eighth week of gestation and continues throughout gestation and childhood.
4. Bone growth occurs in two dimensions: diameter and length. Growth in length occurs at the epiphyseal plate, a vascular area of active cell division. These cells are highly sensitive to the influence of growth hormone, estrogen, and testosterone.
5. Sometime in adolescence, the epiphyseal plate converts to bone, and growth stops.

B. Function
1. Several significant differences in musculoskeletal function between children and adults have important implications for nursing care.
2. The epiphyseal plate in children represents an area of bone weakness that is susceptible to injury through fracture, crushing, or slippage. Damage to the epiphyseal plate can disrupt bone growth.
3. Because a child's bones are still growing, some bony deformities due to injury can be remodeled or straightened over time; conversely, this also can cause some deformities to progress with growth.
4. Because a child's bones are more plastic than an adult's, more force is required to fracture a bone, and specific forces may produce different types of fractures.
5. A child's bones generally heal much faster than an adult's, often greatly reducing the time required for immobilization after injury.

II. Musculoskeletal system overview
A. Assessment
1. In initial assessment of a child's musculoskeletal system, the nurse should obtain a complete health history of problems pertaining to this system, focusing on:
   a. Trauma
   b. Delayed walking or other developmental abnormalities
   c. Pain (dull, boring, or sharp with movement)
   d. Structural abnormalities (e.g., clubfoot, hip dysplasia, Legg-Calvé-Perthes disease, slipped femoral epiphysis, scoliosis, leg length discrepancy, torsional deformities)
   e. Any physical limitations or lifestyle alterations imposed by the problem
   f. Mobility aids used
2. Physical assessment of the musculoskeletal system should include examination for:

      a. Structural abnormalities, including asymmetric limb lengths and spinal deformities
      b. Posture and gait
      c. Range of motion in all joints
      d. Muscle symmetry, mass, tone, strength
      e. Color, temperature, sensation, motion, pain, pulses, capillary filling, and edema in each extremity

B. Laboratory studies and diagnostic tests
  1. Radiologic and other imaging studies to assess bones and joints include:
      a. Radiographs (the most common study to assess injury and healing)
      b. Computed tomographic scan
      c. Bone scan
  2. Other important procedures include:
      a. Arthrography
      b. Arthroscopy
      c. Joint aspiration
      d. Electromyography

C. Psychosocial implications
  1. Treatment for musculoskeletal disorders often involves immobility (casts, traction, body frames), which can be frightening and painful. The impact on the child depends in large part on the child's developmental level.
  2. Play, social interaction, and self-care help the immobilized child gain self-esteem and independence and promote normal growth and development.

III. Immobilization

A. Description: therapeutic or of motion—in extreme cases, confining the child to bed for prolonged periods

B. Etiology and incidence
  1. A child may be immobilized as part of treatment designed to keep body structures at physiologic rest and in proper alignment, or as a result of physical limitations of disease or disability.
  2. Common precursors to immobility include:
      a. Congenital defects
      b. Degenerative neurologic disorders
      c. Integumentary disorders
      d. Musculoskeletal trauma
      e. Imposed bedrest to aid healing and the restorative process
      f. Mechanical restraint as part of therapy

C. Pathophysiology
  1. Over time, muscle disuse leads to atrophy and degeneration of muscle mass and secondarily affects the skeletal, cardiovascular, respiratory, gastrointestinal, urinary, integumentary, and neurosensory systems.

2. Specific physiologic changes result from decreased muscle strength and mass, decreased metabolism, and bone demineralization (Fig. 15–1).
3. Psychologic effects of immobilization commonly include altered body image, altered perception of external environment, sensory deprivation, and impaired mastery of developmental psychosocial tasks.

D. Assessment findings
1. Clinical manifestations of prolonged immobilization may include:
    a. Joint contractures and pain
    b. Muscle atony and weakness
    c. Fatigue
    d. Diminished reflexes
    e. Delayed healing
    f. Orthostatic hypotension
    g. Signs and symptoms of thrombus formation
    h. Shallow respirations
    i. Anorexia
    j. Constipation

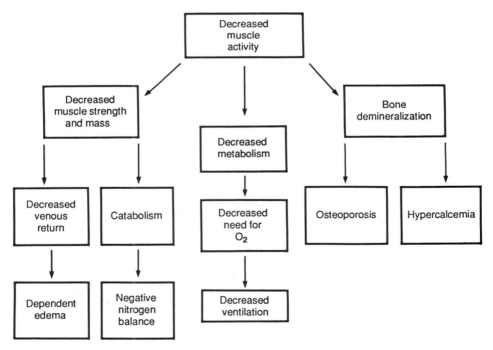

FIGURE 15–1.
Effects of Immobilization. (Whaley, L.F., & Wong, D.L. (1987) Nursing Care of Infants and Children (3rd ed). St. Louis: Mosby. Used with permission.)

       k.   Urinary incontinence
       l.   Signs and symptoms of urinary tract infection
      m.   Skin breakdown and pressure ulcers
      n.   Sensory changes

2. Laboratory study results may reveal:
    a.   Hypercalcemia
    b.   Elevated urinary nitrogen level
    c.   Anemia

E. Nursing diagnoses
1. Activity Intolerance
2. Anxiety
3. Ineffective Breathing Pattern
4. Decreased Cardiac Output
5. Constipation
6. High Risk for Fluid Volume Deficit
7. Altered Growth and Development
8. High Risk for Injury
9. High Risk for Infection
10. Knowledge Deficit
11. Impaired Physical Mobility
12. Altered Nutrition: Less than Body Requirements
13. Altered Role Performance
14. Sensory and Perceptual Alterations
15. Impaired Skin Integrity
16. Sleep Pattern Disturbance
17. Social Isolation
18. Altered Patterns of Urinary Elimination

F. Planning and implementation
1. Protect skin integrity by turning the child frequently and inspecting for early signs of breakdown.
2. Promote adequate hydration by offering the child's favorite fruit juices.
3. Promote good nutrition by offering high-protein, high-caloric foods in small, frequent, and attractively arranged servings.
4. Promote normal bowel elimination by keeping the child well hydrated, including fiber in diet, and providing privacy when toileting.
5. Promote normal urinary elimination by monitoring the frequency and amount of urination and assessing for bladder distention.
6. Promote normal activity, as the child's condition and restrictive devices allow, by providing diversional activities spaced with adequate rest periods.
7. Help prevent respiratory complications by keeping the child well hydrated and changing his or her position frequently to prevent dependent edema.

8. Help maintain adequate cardiac output by changing the child's position frequently and providing active or passive range-of-motion exercises, as appropriate.

9. Protect the child from injury by monitoring physical activities closely; syncope and falling can occur if the child resumes normal activities too quickly.

10. Help prevent urinary tract infections by keeping the child well hydrated; promoting frequent voiding; providing acid–ash foods such as cereal, fish, poultry, cranberry or apple juice, and meats; and limiting calcium intake.

11. Prevent contractures by maintaining proper body alignment, minimizing flexed positions, and providing active and passive range-of-motion exercises.

12. Guard against fractures by moving and positioning the child carefully.

13. Promote self-care by allowing the child to help plan daily routines, select foods, determine the time for bathing, select clothing, and participate in solving toileting problems, as appropriate.

14. Promote the child's orientation to his or her environment by transporting the child out of his or her room as much as possible, providing clocks and calendars (for an older child), and establishing a program of diversional activities.

15. Promote normal growth and development by providing regular social contact, enjoyable diversional activities, and, whenever possible, an age- and sex-appropriate roommate.

16. Promote effective coping by providing play therapy, anticipatory teaching, and explanations of physical restrictions and restraining devices.

17. Administer medications as ordered, which may include:
    a. Antibiotics to treat any infection
    b. Diuretics to remove high levels of calcium
    c. Calcium-mobilizing drugs
    d. Anticoagulants to prevent emboli formation
    e. Stool-softeners to prevent fecal impaction

18. Explain to the child's parents that children may perceive immobilization as a punishment for misdeeds or bad thoughts. Encourage them to help the child cope with immobilization by listening for and correcting any misconceptions the child may express about therapy or physical limitations.

19. Provide patient and family teaching, covering:
    a. The action and purpose of any restraining devices, such as a cast or traction (can demonstrate on a doll for a younger child)
    b. Home care: holding techniques (if appropriate), moving, feeding, bathing, care of restrictive devices, and signs and symptoms of complications (e.g., increased temperature, pain or blood on voiding, difficulty breathing)

G. Evaluation

1. The child maintains skin integrity and exhibits no signs of skin breakdown.
2. The child remains well hydrated with good skin turgor.
3. The child gains weight appropriate for growth.
4. The child maintains normal bowel and urinary elimination patterns.
5. The child engages in age-appropriate diversional activities.
6. The child is free from respiratory complications.
7. The child experiences no physical injury.
8. The child's urine remains clear and free from bacterial infection.
9. The child maintains adequate range of motion in noninjured joints.
10. The child participates in age-appropriate self-care to the best of his or her abilities.
11. The child interacts appropriately with peers and family members.
12. The child expresses fears and concerns related to the cause for immobilization.
13. Family members verbalize understanding of home care measures, signs and symptoms of complications, and follow-up care.

IV. Cerebral palsy

A. Description

1. Cerebral palsy is a group of neuromuscular disorders marked by impaired muscular control resulting from a nonprogressive abnormality in the pyramidal motor system (motor cortex, basal ganglia, cerebellum).
2. Types include:
   a. Spastic (the most common type, accounting for about 65% of all cases)
   b. Dyskinetic (or athetoid)
   c. Ataxic
   d. Mixed type
   e. Rigid type
   f. Tremor type

B. Etiology and incidence

1. The central insult may occur prenatally, perinatally, or postnatally. The many possible causes of cerebral palsy include:
   a. Low birth weight, preterm birth
   b. Prenatal or perinatal anoxia in term infants
   c. Prenatal and postnatal infections, such as cytomegalovirus, rubella, toxoplasma, meningitis
   d. Embryologic malformations
   e. Intracranial hemorrhage
   f. Metabolic disorders, such as hyperbilirubinemia or hypoglycemia
   g. Genetic transmission

2. Cerebral palsy is the most common permanent physical disability of the childhood, occurring in 1.5 to 5 of every 1,000 live births.

C. Pathophysiology

1. Cerebral palsy is distinguished from other neuromuscular disorders by its focus in the brain's motor centers.
2. Specific clinical manifestations reflect the primary area of brain damage—the motor cortex, basal ganglia, or cerebellum.
3. Other associated neurologic impairments result from damage to other areas of the cerebral cortex or brain stem.

D. Assessment findings

1. Common clinical manifestations of cerebral palsy include:
    a. Delayed gross motor development, marked by poor head control and failure to sit, crawl, or stand at normal developmental stages
    b. Abnormal motor performance such as truncal ataxia, early hand preference or dominance, abnormal and asymmetric crawling, and facial grimacing
    c. Increased or decreased muscle tone
    d. Abnormal posturing, with persistent infantile posture beyond age 4 to 5 months
    e. Persistent primitive infantile reflexes
    f. Mild to moderate mental retardation (in about two thirds of children)
    g. Seizure activity (in about one half of children)
    h. Visual problems (strabismus and hemianopia) and hearing loss
    i. Behavioral disorders such as poor attention span, easy distractability, and hyperactivity
2. In addition to general manifestations, specific types of cerebral palsy carry characteristic signs and symptoms, including:
    a. Spastic cerebral palsy: increased muscle tone, muscle weakness, increased stretch reflexes
    b. Dyskinetic cerebral palsy: abnormal involuntary movements, described as slow and writhing, usually of the trunk, neck, facial muscles, tongue, and extremities; abnormal muscular activity absent during sleep, exaggerated during stress and emotional upset
    c. Ataxic cerebral palsy: hypotonia; disintegration of muscular control in hands and arms as the child reaches for objects; wide-based, unsteady gait
    d. Mixed-type cerebral palsy: a combination of spastic and dyskinetic cerebral palsy causing severe disability

E. Nursing diagnoses

1. Activity Intolerance
2. Body Image Disturbance

3. Impaired Verbal Communication
4. Altered Family Processes
5. High Risk for Injury
6. Impaired Physical Mobility
7. Altered Nutrition: Less than Body Requirements
8. Altered Role Performance
9. Self-Esteem Disturbance

F. Planning and implementation

1. Help prevent physical injury by providing the child with a safe environment, appropriate toys, and a protective helmet if necessary.
2. Help prevent physical deformity by ensuring correct use of prescribed braces and other mobilizing devices and by providing appropriate range-of-motion and stretching exercises.
3. Promote mobility by encouraging the child to perform age- and condition-appropriate motor activities.
4. Promote adequate nutrition by providing a high-protein, high-calorie diet.
5. Promote relaxation and general health by providing rest periods scheduled with appropriate recreational activities.
6. Administer medications as ordered, which may include:
    a. Sedatives
    b. Muscle relaxants
    c. Anticonvulsants
    d. Ritalin or dexedrine (for attention deficit disorder)
7. Promote self-care by encouraging the child to participate in activities of daily living, using age- and condition-appropriate utensils and implements.
8. Facilitate communication by talking to the child deliberately and slowly, using pictures to reinforce speech. Encourage early speech therapy to prevent poor or maladaptive communication habits and provide a means of articulate speech; techniques such as computers may help children with severe articulation problems.
9. As necessary, seek referrals for corrective lenses and hearing aids to decrease sensory deprivation related to visual and hearing loss.
10. Help promote a positive self-image in the child by praising his or her accomplishments, setting realistic and attainable goals, encouraging an appealing physical appearance, and encouraging his or her involvement in age- and condition-appropriate peer group activities.
11. Promote optimal family functioning by encouraging family members to express anxieties, frustrations, and concerns and to explore support networks. Provide emotional support and help with problem solving, as necessary, and refer the family to support organizations such as the United Cerebral Palsy Association.
12. Prepare the child and family for each procedure and planned ther-

apy, including, if appropriate, orthopedic surgery to correct abnormal muscle balance and improve function.

13. Teach parents that the child will need considerable help and patience in accomplishment of each new task. Encourage them not to focus solely on their child's inability to accomplish certain physical tasks; urge them to relax, demonstrate patience, and provide positive feedback and compliments on those tasks he or she can perform.

14. Encourage the family to seek appropriate functional and adaptive training and, in an adolescent, vocational training to promote the child's mastery of manual skills and eventual independence. Work with the parents and other health professionals to tailor a program for the child based on his or her individual strengths and limitations.

15. Encourage family members to achieve a balance between caring for the disabled child and other aspects of life to maintain as normal a family life as possible. Point out that every caregiver needs periodic respites from care providing.

G. Evaluation

1. The child experiences no physical injury.

2. The child benefits from physical therapy, and deformities are prevented.

3. The child eats well-balanced diet and maintains appropriate weight for age and size.

4. The child engages in appropriate age and condition activities without fatigue.

5. The child acquires appropriate mobility.

6. The child engages in self-help activities commensurate with individual abilities.

7. The child communicates needs to caregiver.

8. The child expresses feelings and concerns.

9. The child attends school regularly (when appropriate).

10. The child engages in activities with peers when possible.

11. Family members discuss their feelings, concerns, and frustrations.

12. Family members participate in support groups.

13. Family members verbalize an understanding that cerebral palsy is a lifelong disorder.

V. Scoliosis

A. Description

1. Scoliosis refers to an abnormal lateral curvature of the spine associated with rotation of the vertebrae and associated physiologic alterations in the spine, chest, and pelvis.

2. It is classified as:

a. Functional: postural deformity that corrects itself when the child lies down or corrects posture

    b.   Structural: physical changes in spine and supporting struc-
         tures that are not self-correcting

B.   Etiology and incidence

   1.   Functional scoliosis usually results from other musculoskeletal
        deformities, such as unequal leg lengths.
   2.   In 70% to 75% of cases, structural scoliosis is considered idio-
        pathic, with no known cause.
   3.   Evidence increasingly points to a probable genetic autosomal
        dominant trait with incomplete penetrance.
   4.   Other possible causes include:
        a.   Neuromuscular disorders, such as cerebral palsy and mus-
             cular dystrophy
        b.   Trauma
        c.   Spinal cord tumor or infection
   5.   The most common spinal deformity, scoliosis affects 3% to 5%
        of all children. It can appear at any age and in either sex but most
        frequently affects adolescent girls.

C.   Pathophysiology

   1.   Deformity progresses during periods of growth and stabilizes
        when vertebral growth ceases.
   2.   As the spine grows and the lateral curve develops, the vertebrae
        rotate, causing the ribs and spine to rotate toward the convex
        part of the spine. Spinous processes rotate toward the concavity
        of the curve.
   3.   The child attempts to maintain an erect posture, resulting in a
        compensatory curve.
   4.   Vertebrae become wedge shaped, and vertebral disks undergo de-
        generative changes.
   5.   Muscles and ligaments either shorten and thicken or lengthen
        and atrophy, depending on the concavity or convexity of the
        curve. A hump forms from rib rotation backward on the convex
        side of the curve.
   6.   The thoracic cavity becomes asymmetric, leading to severe venti-
        latory compensation. If scoliosis goes uncorrected, respiratory
        function is compromised and vital capacity is reduced; eventually,
        pulmonary hypertension, cor pulmonale, and respiratory acidosis
        may develop.
   7.   Treatment may involve one or more of the following:
        a.   Exercise: can help with postural scoliosis but is rarely of
             value for structural scoliosis
        b.   Bracing: the usual therapy for minor curvatures; the most
             common type is the Milwaukee brace, worn until the spine
             matures or until surgery is performed. The brace is worn
             23 hours a day with 1 hour out of the brace for hygiene
             and skin care; it may eventually be worn only at night after

the spine has matured and the child has been weaned over a period of 1 to 2 years

    c.   Electrical stimulation: involves transmitting electrical impulses to muscles on the convex side of the curve to contract the muscles and straighten the spine

    d.   Skeletal traction: applied preoperatively to achieve greater flexibility and partial correction

    e.   Surgery: the usual treatment of choice for curves greater than 40 degrees; procedures include Harrington rod, Luque segmental instrumentation, Dwyer instrumentation

    f.   Postoperative care: Stryker frame immediately postoperatively to facilitate care and reduce the risk of damaging fusion and indwelling instruments; postoperative casting applied 10 to 14 days after surgery and maintained for 6 months to 1 year

D. **Assessment findings**

    1. Scoliosis rarely produces subjective symptoms until well established; severe deformity may produce backache, fatigue, and dyspnea.

    2. Objective signs may be seen with the child or adolescent undressed and bending forward from the waist. Viewing from behind may reveal the primary curvature and a compensatory curvature and, in severe cases, a rib hump and flank asymmetry.

    3. Because adolescents are often shy about their bodies, the first signs of scoliosis may be uneven hemlines or pant legs.

    4. A scoliometer can measure the extent of deformity.

    5. Diagnosis is based on observation and radiographic examination.

E. **Nursing diagnoses**

    1. General

        a.   Body Image Disturbance

        b.   Ineffective Breathing Patterns

        c.   Altered Family Processes

        d.   High Risk for Injury

        e.   Knowledge Deficit

        f.   Impaired Physical Mobility

        g.   High Risk for Impaired Skin Integrity

        h.   Social Isolation

    2. Postoperative

        a.   Constipation

        b.   Fear

        c.   Impaired Gas Exchange

        d.   High Risk for Injury

        e.   Altered Nutrition: Less than Body Requirements

        f.   Pain

     g.   Altered Role Performance
     h.   Sensory and Perceptual Alterations
     i.   Impaired Skin Integrity
     j.   Altered Tissue Perfusion

F. **Planning and implementation: general care**

1. Help protect the child from injury by assessing for and eliminating or minimizing environmental hazards.
2. Promote adequate respiratory air exchange by keeping the child well hydrated and encouraging periodic deep breathing.
3. Help maintain skin integrity by properly applying braces, and implement corrective action to prevent or treat skin breakdown.
4. Promote mobility by encouraging the child to be up and out of bed and walk two or three times a day.
5. Promote a positive self-concept by assisting the child with personal hygiene and selection of appropriate apparel to wear over the brace, and by encouraging the child to express feelings and concerns.
6. Promote normal growth and development by encouraging socialization with peers and pursuit of age-appropriate activities.
7. Provide family support by referring the parents to social services or a special support group.

G. **Planning and implementation: postoperative care**

1. Help prevent neurologic deficit by monitoring motor, sensory, and neurologic status—particularly in extremities; prompt identification of neurologic deficit and correction can prevent permanent damage.
2. Maintain comfort by administering analgesic and muscle relaxants, as ordered.
3. Detect impending hypoxia by monitoring blood gas values; notify the physician of abnormalities.
4. Assess for hypotension by monitoring intake and output (urine, chest tube, nasogastric tube), monitoring vital signs, and observing skin color for tissue perfusion.
5. Prevent constipation by keeping the child well hydrated, providing privacy, and assessing bowel sounds; keep in mind that immediately postoperatively, the child will have an indwelling (Foley) catheter and some degree of paralytic ileus.
6. Help prevent skin breakdown by turning the child frequently, providing skin care, and gently massaging bony prominences.
7. Help the child maintain a feeling of control by explaining all procedures and listening to the child as he or she vents fears.
8. Promote adequate nutrition by maintaining intravenous therapy until oral fluids are allowed; begin oral intake when allowed in small, frequent, well-liked fluids.
9. Help prevent injury by keeping needed items for care within easy reach, and keep safety restraints on while turning bed.

10. Encourage self-care by arranging hygienic and grooming items and foods and utensils within the child's easy reach; as necessary, administer analgesics before the child performs self-care activities to reduce pain.

11. Promote family functioning by encouraging family members to identify composite strengths, verbalize fears and concerns, and use effective problem-solving strategies.

12. Provide information regarding the defect and therapeutic plan, with particular attention to the long-term nature of treatment and how compliance effects eventual success in straightening the spine.

13. Prepare the child and family for postoperative care with thorough preoperative teaching, including how the Stryker frame works and feels; appearance and sensations of a chest tube, nasogastric tube, and Foley catheter; possible need for respiratory support; discomfort and pain management; logrolling technique for moving in bed.

14. Evaluate the child's acceptance of the prescribed brace and exercises to determine the likelihood of compliance and the need for reinforced teaching. Encourage the positive aspects of wearing a brace, such as improved posture and symptom relief.

H. Evaluation

1. The child is free of neurologic deficit.
2. The child remains free of injury related to compensated balance and brace wearing.
3. The child maintains adequate respirations without complications.
4. The child engages in normal activities that are age and condition appropriate.
5. The child verbalizes feelings and concerns.
6. The child appears well groomed and wears attractive attire.
7. The child engages in social activities with peers.
8. Family members express feelings and concerns.
9. Family members verbalize an understanding that continued follow-up care is necessary until full spinal correction occurs and the child's spine is fully matured.

VI. Congenital hip dysplasia (CHD)

A. Description

1. CHD refers to imperfect hip development affecting the femoral head, acetabulum, or both
2. It is classified as:
   a. Acetabular dysplasia (or preluxation), the mildest form
   b. Subluxation (or incomplete dislocation), the most common form
   c. Dislocation, the most severe form

B. **Etiology and incidence**
1. The cause remains unknown although a genetic factor is suspected; CHD occurs 25 to 30 times more frequently in first-degree relatives of affected persons than in the general population.
2. The defect may be associated with postnatal positioning (i.e., keeping an infant's legs extended and adducted, as commonly occurs in Eskimo and northern Italian populations).
3. Prenatal hormones (principally estrogen) are thought to cause laxity of the maternal pelvis and consequently of the fetal pelvis.
4. Other factors that may affect fetal joint position and contribute to CHD include breech presentation at birth, twinning, and large infant size.
5. The most common congenital defect, CHD occurs in 1 to 2 in 1,000 births.
6. Incidence is about seven times greater in girls than in boys.

C. **Pathophysiology**
1. In *acetabular dysplasia*, the femoral head remains in the acetabulum, but acetabular development is incomplete.
2. *Subluxation* involves incomplete dislocation in which the femoral head remains in contact with the acetabulum but is partially displaced, causing stretching of the ligamentum teres attached to the femoral head.
3. In *dislocation*, the femoral head is displaced superiorly and posteriorly and not in contact with acetabulum, and the ligamentum is elongated and taut.
4. Both hips are affected in 25% to 50% of cases; unilateral CHD most commonly affects the left hip.
5. Other defects, such as spina bifida, may present concurrently.
6. Uncorrected, subluxation or dislocation can lead to abnormal acetabular development and permanent disability.
7. Treatment of CHD commonly depends on the age of the child at diagnosis and on the success of previous treatments, and may involve:
   a. If detected shortly after birth, placing the infant in a dynamic splint (principally the Pavlik harness or Frejka pillow) to center the femoral head into the acetabulum in an attitude of flexion and to deepen the acetabulum by pressure; worn until the hip is clinically and radiographically stable (usually sometime between ages 3 and 6 months)
   b. If adduction is restricted along with hip dysplasia, use of a hip spica cast, changed frequently to accommodate the child's growth, until hip stabilizes
   c. If dislocation is not recognized until the infant starts bearing weight (age 6 to 18 months): gradual reduction of the defect by traction, followed by a plaster cast to immobilize and stabilize the joint

    d.   If traction and casting do not correct the defect: open reduction, followed by spica cast immobilization and later (4 to 6 months) an abduction splint, with the child placed on a Bradford frame

    e.   Generally, the older the child, the more difficult the correction procedures required; between age 2 and 6 years, treatment typically involves open reduction preceded by traction, tenotomy of contracted muscles, and other osteotomy procedures designed to construct an acetabular roof

    f.   Correction of CHD generally is not possible after age 6 years

D.   Assessment findings

    1.   Diagnosis and initiation of treatment before age 22 months yields the greatest chance of successful correction; the primary diagnostic methods are physical examination and ultrasonography.

    2.   In a newborn, acetabular dysplasia or subluxation commonly produces no overt signs or symptoms; dislocation may manifest as unequal leg lengths or a prominent hip.

    3.   Positive Ortolani or Barlow signs indicate congenital dysplasia; these are the most reliable tests during the first 2 months after birth. (*Note:* The Ortolani and Barlow tests should be performed only by experienced personnel; overvigorous testing can lead to persistent hip dislocation.)

    4.   After age 6 to 10 weeks, reliable diagnostic signs include limited leg abduction, positive Gallaezzi sign (shortening of the leg on the affected side), asymmetric thigh and gluteal folds, and broadening of the perineum (seen only in bilateral dysplasia).

    5.   When not detected at birth and corrected promptly, the defect becomes apparent when the child learns to walk. A child with bilateral CHD may have a characteristic "duck waddle," swaying from side to side; unilateral CHD may produce a prominent limp. Other signs may include a visibly prominent greater trochanter and positive Trendelenburg sign.

    6.   Radiographic examination usually does not yield reliable data until age 3 to 6 months, after ossification of the femoral head has occurred.

E.   Nursing diagnosis (*Note:* See also nursing diagnoses related to immobilization, section III.E.)

    1.   Diversional Activity Deficit

    2.   Altered Family Processes

    3.   Fear

    4.   High Risk for Injury

    5.   Pain

    6.   Altered Role Performance

    7.   High Risk for Impaired Skin Integrity

F.   Planning and implementation

    1.   Help prevent complications of immobility by:

      a.   Assessing for and promptly reporting signs of neurovascular changes

      b.   Ensuring correct use of restraining devices

      c.   Performing appropriate range-of-motion exercises

    2.   Maintain cast integrity (when applicable) by promoting complete drying and protecting the cast and cast rim.

    3.   Help prevent circulatory impairment due to cast application by:

      a.   Elevating casted extremities

      b.   Monitoring cardiovascular status (peripheral pulses, blanching)

      c.   Assessing for pain, swelling, coldness, and cyanosis

    4.   Help prevent skin breakdown by:

      a.   Petaling cast edges

      b.   Providing a sheepskin or an alternate pressure mattress

      c.   Frequently inspecting the skin for irritation or pressure areas

      d.   Keeping the skin clean and dry

      e.   Changing the child's position frequently

    5.   Promote growth and development by providing diversional activities that are age and condition appropriate.

    6.   Help the child maintain muscle tone and strength in unaffected areas by encouraging regular range-of-motion exercises and other activities.

    7.   For older children, encourage activities of daily living by assisting with feeding, bathing, dressing, and toileting, as necessary.

    8.   Provide comfort by administering sufficient pain medication and changing the child's position frequently, using pads and pillows for support.

    9.   Support and educate the family by teaching them about the child's defect and treatment plan and helping them modify clothing, supportive devices, and means of transportation.

    10.   Provide patient and family teaching, covering:

      a.   Signs and symptoms of circulatory impairment and infection to monitor for and report

      b.   Cast care and care of the child in cast: correct body mechanics when lifting the child; avoiding use of the cross bar for moving the child; measures to prevent physical and developmental deficits (e.g., age-appropriate toys, a wagon to move the child or take him or her on walks); measures to keep the cast clean and dry (e.g., tucking a disposable diaper beneath the entire perineal opening in the cast); the need to restrain the child when moving him or her

      c.   Feeding tips and techniques for an infant or a small child in a cast: positioning so that the child feels safe; using pillows for support; cuddling the child in their arms; supporting the child in a "football" hold or fashioning a tilt table, depending on the infant's size

d. The need to plan family activities to include the child; a child confined in a cast or brace can be held and transported to areas of activity

e. How to nurture the infant or young child through stroking, holding, and maintaining physical closeness

G. Evaluation

1. Circulation in extremities remains satisfactory.
2. The child exhibits no signs of complications.
3. The child moves his or her extremities when instructed to do so.
4. The child exhibits effective breathing patterns.
5. The child exhibits no signs of infection.
6. Skin remains clean and intact with no signs of irritation.
7. The child engages in activities appropriate to his or her condition and developmental level.
8. The child maintains muscle tone and joint flexibility in his or her unaffected extremities.
9. The child is well hydrated and nourished.
10. The child is well groomed and clean.
11. The child appears comfortable, exhibiting no signs of distress.
12. Family members demonstrate proper brace application and care.
13. Family members demonstrate cast care.
14. Family members verbalize an understanding of the child's defect and the prescribed treatment plan.

Bibliography

Cuddy, C. M. (1986). Caring for the child in a spica cast: A parent's perspective. *Orthopedic Nursing*, 5(3), 17–21.

Farrell, J. (1982). *Illustrated guide to orthopedic nursing* (2nd ed.). Philadelphia: J. B. Lippincott.

Johnson, J., Kirchhoff, K., and Endres, M. (1975). Altering children's behavior during orthopedic cast removal. *Nursing Research*, 24, 404–410.

Mott, S. R., James, S. R., and Sperhac, A. M. (1985). *Nursing care of children and families* (2nd ed.). Menlo Park, CA: Addison-Wesley.

Shesser, L. K. (1986). Practical considerations in caring for a child in a hip spica cast: An evaluation using parental input. *Orthopedic Nursing*, 5(3), 11–15.

Whaley, L. F., and Wong, D. L. (1991). *Nursing care of infants and children* (4th ed.). St. Louis: C. V. Mosby.

Williams, P. F. (1983). *Orthopaedic management in childhood*. St. Louis: C. V. Mosby.

STUDY QUESTIONS

1. The major initial pathophysiologic consequences of immobilization result from all the following factors *except*
   a. decreased muscle strength and mass
   b. bone demineralization
   c. positive nitrogen balance
   d. decreased metabolism

2. Which of the following interventions would best help a child with cerebral palsy achieve the goal of improved self-care ability?
   a. Provide the child with a protective helmet.
   b. Provide age- and condition-appropriate utensils.
   c. Administer medications as ordered.
   d. Provide for adequate rest periods.

3. Sarah, age 14 years, has structural scoliosis, for which she wears a Milwaukee brace. The nurse would determine that Sarah understands the effective use of the brace when Sarah states
   a. "I wonder if I can take the brace off when I go to the opening dance?"
   b. "I'll look forward to taking my bath every day."
   c. "I'm glad I only have to wear this at night!"
   d. "When I get tired I know I can take it off."

4. Positive signs for CHD include positive Ortolani and Barlow tests and
   a. rib hump and flank asymmetry
   b. positive Homan's sign
   c. increased leg abduction
   d. limited leg abduction

5. Which of the following meals represents the best choice for a child who is immobilized and on complete bedrest?
   a. cheeseburger, french fries, and chocolate milk
   b. skim milk, peanut butter and jelly on wholewheat bread, and canned peaches
   c. broiled chicken breast, bran muffins, broccoli, apple, and lemonade
   d. macaroni and cheese, canned spinach, white bread, and orange juice

6. Using dolls or stuffed animals to explain restraining devices is best used as a teaching strategy with which age group?
   a. infants
   b. toddlers
   c. preschoolers
   d. school-age children

7. The most common conservative treatment for cerebral palsy is
   a. traction
   b. orthopedic surgery
   c. recreational therapy
   d. physical therapy

8. Which of the following statements made by a mother of a 4-month-old would indicate to the nurse the possibility that the infant has cerebral palsy?
   a. "My baby has not rolled all the way over yet."
   b. "When I pull the baby to a standing position on my lap, his left hip elevates."
   c. "My baby won't lift his head and look at me; he's so 'floppy.'"
   d. "When I change his diapers, his one leg is so tight and stiff that I have difficulty putting the diaper on."

9. Which of the following statements regarding scoliosis is correct?
   a. Pain is a common presenting symptom.
   b. Disability is confined only to the spine.
   c. A compensatory curve usually results in an effort to maintain an erect posture.
   d. Detection is difficult and requires radiography.

10. Which of the following is the primary mode of therapy for minor curvatures of structural scoliosis?
    a. bracing
    b. traction
    c. instrumentation
    d. exercise

11. Besides assessing neurologic status immediately after a Harrington rod instru-

mentation and spinal fusion, the nurse should be concerned with which of the following factors?

 a. the child's understanding of the procedure
 b. the child's comfort level
 c. the child's physical therapy needs
 d. the child's diet tolerance

12. Which of the following is the most common form of congenital hip dysplasia?
 a. preluxation
 b. subluxation
 c. acetabular dysplasia
 d. dislocation

13. To best assess a mother's understanding of and ability to apply a Pavlik harness or Frejka pillow the nurse would
 a. have the mother verbalize the purpose of the brace
 b. request a home visit by the nurse from a home health agency
 c. have the mother remove and reapply the brace before discharge, allowing time for questions
 d. demonstrate to the mother how to apply the brace

14. Which of the following statements by a mother of a child in a hip spica cast would indicate that the family is having no difficulty including the child in family activities?
 a. "It is so difficult to hold Jeff; I keep him in his bed most of the time."
 b. "We just got a new wagon so that I can move Sarah wherever I am in the house."
 c. "Our new play pen is great! I can leave Mary and not worry that she is getting into anything."
 d. "How do mothers manage a child in a spica cast? All I can do is sit and hold Lisa on the couch."

ANSWER KEY

1. **Correct response: c**
   Negative nitrogen balance (not positive nitrogen balance) is a result of decreased muscle activity and resulting catabolism.
   a, b, and d. All are direct results of decreased muscle activity.
   Knowledge/Physiologic/Assessment

2. **Correct response: b**
   Providing utensils that allow the child some independence and foster self-care.
   a. A protective helmet prevents injury.
   c. Administration of medications is a nursing action that does not relate to self-care.
   d. Adequate rest decreases fatigue but does not foster independence.
   Analysis/Health promotion/Evaluation

3. **Correct response: b**
   The brace should be removed only for 1 hour every 24 hours for hygiene and skin care.
   a. Although physical appearance and social activities with peers are important, the brace should not be removed except for hygiene and skin care.
   c. This statement is true only after radiologic studies indicate the spine has bone maturity and the child has been weaned from the brace over a 1- to 2-year period.
   d. This statement indicates poor understanding of the Milwaukee brace.
   Application/Health promotion/Evaluation

4. **Correct response: a**
   Rib hump and flank asymmetry are positive signs of scoliosis.
   b. Positive Homan sign points to venous thrombosis.
   c. Increased leg abduction occurs in CHD.
   d. Limited leg abduction indicates an adduction contracture.
   Knowledge/Physiologic/Assessment

5. **Correct response: c**
   Children on bedrest need a high-protein, high-calorie, high-fiber, acid–ash diet. This particular meal provides all these and also is low in calcium. (Children develop hypercalcemia when on bedrest due to bone demineralization.)
   a. This meal is fairly high in calcium, high in protein, high in calories, low in fiber, and low in acid-ash.
   b. Skim milk is very high in calcium. Also, this meal has no noticeable fiber.
   d. Macaroni and cheese is high in calcium, moderately high in protein. The spinach adds some fiber to diet, but the fact that it is canned adds additional salt.
   Analysis/Health promotion/Evaluation

6. **Correct response: c**
   A preschooler reasons from what he or she sees and engages in animistic thinking; needs visual, tactile, auditory, and motor images in preparing for an event.
   a. For an infant, communication is conveyed best through soothing, comforting speech.
   b. Explanations for a toddler need to be simple and given immediately before an event.
   d. A school-age child generally engages in more logical thought and reasoning; the most effective strategy may be to use diagrams and models to process more concrete information.
   Application/Psychosocial/Implementation

7. **Correct response: d**
   Physical therapy is directed toward improved control of purposeful acts and improved skeletal alignment.
   a. The goal of traction is to provide immobilization and correct skeletal deformities; cerebral palsy is a neuromuscular disorder of impaired muscular control.
   b. Orthopedic surgery is directed toward decreasing or eliminating spastic muscle imbalances.

c. Recreational therapy provides for social activities and outlets and stimulates the child's interaction with others and builds self-esteem; it is not a treatment modality, and though it provides training programs, the facilities are not always available.

Comprehension/Health promotion/ Implementation

8. **Correct response: c**
   Infant lifts head to 90-degree angle by 4 months; only partial head lag at 2 months; hypotonia or "floppy infant" are early manifestations.
   a. This does not occur until 6 months.
   b. This is a positive Trendelenburg sign seen in infants with congenital hip dysplasia.
   d. Though rigidity and tenseness are possible signs of cerebral palsy, a limitation of one leg adduction indicates congenital hip dysplasia.

Analysis/Physiologic/Evaluation

9. **Correct response: c**
   The child attempts to maintain balance and an erect posture resulting in a compensatory curve.
   a. Pain is rare in children with scoliosis although some children experience chronic discomfort from continually sitting on one buttock.
   b. If the deformity is uncorrected, it will result in respiratory compromise.
   d. Detection is simple and quick by visual examination of the spine as the child bends from the waist; children are exposed unnecessarily to radiographs to detect scoliosis.

Knowledge/Physiologic/Assessment

10. **Correct response: a**
    Bracing is beneficial to halt progression of most curves and correction of minimum curves.
    b. Traction is used preoperatively of a spinal fusion to achieve partial correction and flexibility of the curve.
    c. Instrumentation is an operative procedure reserved for the more difficult-to-correct curves—curves greater than 40 degrees.
    d. Exercise can help postural scoliosis but is of little value with structural scoliosis; however, primary mode of therapy for structure scoliosis is instrumentation to arrest progression of curve.

Knowledge/Physiologic/Planning

11. **Correct response: b**
    Instrumentation and spinal fusion pulling, stretching, manipulation, and insertion of a foreign body into the spinous process causes considerable pain; the child needs vigorous pain management, which involves assessment, administration of medication, and evaluation of response.
    a. Immediately postoperatively, the child is conscious of sensation and surroundings; assessment of understanding of procedure is a preoperative nursing responsibility.
    c. Physical therapy is not an immediate postoperative goal.
    d. The child is not receiving anything by mouth.

Application/Physiologic/Implementation

12. **Correct response: b**
    Subluxation is the most common form of congenital hip dysplasia.
    a. Preluxation is the mildest form of congenital hip dysplasia.
    c. Acetabular dysplasia is another name for preluxation.
    d. Dislocation is complete displacement of the femoral head out of the acetabulum; no percent of incidence quoted.

Knowledge/Physiologic/Assessment

13. **Correct response: c**
    This allows the nurse an opportunity to directly observe the mother's technique and comfort level.
    a. Verbalization allows the nurse to assess understanding but not psychomotor skills.
    b. Requesting a home visit is a further

means of evaluation, but it does not give immediate feedback.

d. Although nurse demonstration is a good teaching technique, it does not permit evaluation of the mother's technique.

Application/Safe care/Implementation

14. *Correct response: b*

This statement indicates that the parents have found a comfortable way to transport the child and involve him or her in their activities.

a. This statement indicates poor coping.

c. Although a play pen is one means of confining a child in a safe area, a child should not be left alone for long periods.

d. This statement indicates that the mother is engaged in minimal activity other than holding the child.

Analysis/Health promotion/Evaluation

Special Problems

I. The child with special needs

A. Overview

1. A child with serious chronic illness or developmental disability often has complex needs that differ from those of unimpaired agemates.

2. A *chronic illness* is any disorder that disrupts daily functioning for more than 3 months or necessitates hospitalization for more than 1 month in any given year.

3. *Developmental disability* refers to a severe physical or mental disability that occurs before age 22 years and usually results in substantial limitation of function.

4. Chronic illness affects an estimated 10% to 15% of all children under age 18 years. Asthma and congenital heart defects account for almost 67% of these chronic illnesses; leukemia, congenital heart defects, and spina bifida carry the highest mortality of all childhood illnesses.

5. Adding speech, learning, sensory, cognitive, and emotional problems, an estimated 40% of children between kindergarten and sixth grade have significant long-term disabilities.

6. In contrast to care of unimpaired children, health care for the child with special needs is related more to developmental age than to chronologic age. Accurate assessment of the child's level of development and adaptation is crucial to planning appropriate interventions.

7. Nursing interventions should be aimed at promoting optimal adjustment of each family member.

B. **Trends in health care**

1. The Education of All Handicapped Children Act of 1975 (Public Law 94-142), probably the most significant recent federal legislation affecting children, provides for the following:

a. Free, appropriate public education for all handicapped children

b. Identification and evaluation of all handicapped children

c. Preparation of an individualized education program for each handicapped child

d. Provision of education in the least restrictive environment possible

e. Procedural safeguards for parental grievances (due process)

f. Protection of the rights of children placed by the state in private schools

g. Inservice training for educators

2. National organizations and local support groups geared to the needs of children with specific disabilities (and their families) provide opportunities for children and parents to improve their understanding of the disability and its management and to develop networks for self-help.

3. In hospitals, parent-care units and rooming-in arrangements provide parents of a disabled child with the opportunity to learn the specialized care measures that their child requires and frees the child from the stress associated with separation from family, allowing the child to mobilize all of his or her emotional resources to cope effectively with the threat posed by the disability.

4. The advent of pediatric home care agencies has enabled shorter hospital stays by providing a variety of continuous or episodic services for disabled children in their home environment.

A. **Description**

1. As defined by the American Association on Mental Retardation

(AAMR), mental retardation is "significantly subaverage intellectual function coexisting with deficits in adaptive behavior and manifested during the developmental period (before age 18)."

2. Mental retardation is classified by the AAMR based on IQ level as follows:
   a. Mild (educable mentally retarded): IQ of 50–55 to about 70
   b. Moderate (trainable mentally retarded): IQ of 35–40 to 50–55
   c. Severe: IQ of 20–25 to 35–40
   d. Profound: IQ below 20–25

B. Etiology and incidence
1. The most common developmental disability, mental retardation affects up to 3% of the population.
2. Causes are classified as idiopathic, acquired, inherited or genetic, and endocrine, as follows:
   a. Idiopathic: all cases of unknown cause (the most common classification)
   b. Acquired: perinatal infections (e.g., maternal infections such as rubella, toxoplasmosis, syphilis, cytomegalovirus); other maternal illnesses; teratogenic effects of prescription or nonprescription drugs used by the mother during pregnancy; maternal abuse of illicit drugs or alcohol; birth injury; prenatal, perinatal, or postnatal hypoxia; kernicterus; trauma in infancy or childhood; lead poisoning; malnutrition; brain tumor; severe psychosocial or psychological deprivation
   c. Inherited or genetic: chromosomal abnormalities, such as Down's syndrome, Turner's syndrome, and Klinefelter's syndrome; autosomal dominant disorders, such as Huntington's chorea, spinocerebellar degeneration, Sturge-Weber disease, tuberous sclerosis, and neurofibromatosis; autosomal recessive disorders, such as galactosemia, glycogen storage disease, phenylketonuria (PKU), Tay-Sachs disease, Neimann-Pick disease, and Hurler's disease
   d. Endocrine: congenital hypothyroidism

C. Pathophysiology: Prognosis depends on cause; early diagnosis and prompt treatment may be particularly important in cases involving an identifiable and possibly correctable cause, such as PKU, malnutrition, or child abuse.

D. Assessment findings
1. Clinical manifestations vary according to the child's age and degree of impairment (Table 16–1); general signs include developmental delays in motor, social, language, or cognitive skills.
2. Diagnostic evaluation typically includes some or all of the following:

TABLE 16–1.
Classification of Mental Retardation

LEVEL (IQ)*	PRESCHOOL (BIRTH TO 5 YEARS) MATURA-TION & DEVELOPMENT	SCHOOL AGE (6–20 YEARS) TRAINING & EDUCATION	ADULT (21 YEARS & OLDER) SOCIAL VO-CATIONAL ADEQUACY
Mild (50–55 to about 70)	Often not noticed as retarded by casual observer but is slower to walk, feed self, and talk than most children; follows same sequence in development as normal children	Can acquire practical skills and useful reading and arithmetic to a third- to sixth-grade level with special education; can be guided toward social conformity; achieves mental age of 8 to 12 years	Can usually achieve social and vocational skills adequate to self-maintenance; may need occasional guidance and support when under unusual social or economic stress; can adjust to marriage but not childbearing
Moderate (35–40 to 50–55)	Noticeable delays in motor development, especially in speech; responds to training in various self-help activities	Can learn simple communication, elementary health and safety habits, an simple manual skills; does not progress in functional reading or arithmetic; achieves mental age of 3 to 7 years	Can perform simple tasks under sheltered condition; participates in simple recreation; travels alone in familiar places; usually incapable of self-maintenance
Severe (20–25 to 35–40)	Marked delay in motor development; little or no communication skills; may respond to training in elementary self-help, for example, self-feeding	Usually walks, barring specific disability; has some understanding of speech and some response; can profit from systematic habit training; achieves mental age of toddler	Can conform to daily routines and repetitive activities; needs continuing direction and supervision in protective environment
Profound (below 20–25)	Gross retardation; minimal capacity for functioning in sensorimotor areas; needs total care	Obvious delays in all areas of development; shows basic emotional responses; may respond to skillful training in use of legs, hands, and jaws; needs close supervision; achieves mental age of young infant	May walk; needs complete custodial care; has primitive speech; usually benefits from regular physical activity

Based on classification from the American Association of Mental Deficiency.
(Whaley, L.F., and Wong, D.L. (1987). Nursing care of infants and children (3rd ed.). St. Louis: C.V. Mosby, p. 987)

a. Neurologic examination, including CT scans, to rule out nervous system pathology
b. Radiologic studies to detect lesions
c. Endocrine studies, including urine screening for abnormal metabolites
d. Developmental screening tests, such as the Denver Developmental Screening Test, to identify apparent developmental delays
e. Intellectual evaluation with standardized tests such as the

Stanford-Binet Intelligence Scale, the Wechster Intelligence Scale for Children, and Gesell Developmental Schedules

f.   Adaptive behavior evaluation using tools such as the AAMD adaptive behavior scale

g.   Chromosomal analysis and genetic screening, in cases of a family history of mental retardation or chromosomal abnormalities

E.   Nursing diagnoses

1.   Impaired Verbal Communication
2.   Altered Family Processes
3.   Altered Growth and Development
4.   Altered Health Maintenance
5.   High Risk for Infection
6.   Altered Role Performance
7.   Self-Care Deficit
8.   High Risk for Impaired Skin Integrity
9.   Impaired Social Interaction
10.   Social Isolation

F.   Planning and implementation

1.   Support the family at time of initial diagnosis by actively listening to their feelings and concerns and assessing their composite strengths.
2.   Perform a task analysis before attempting to teach the child any new task; break down tasks into specific steps with each step building on the last.
3.   Facilitate the child's self-care abilities by encouraging parents to enroll the child in an early stimulation program, establishing a self-feeding program, initiating independent toileting, and establishing an independent grooming program (all developmental-level appropriate).
4.   Promote optimal development by encouraging self-care goals and emphasizing the universal needs of children such as play, social interaction, and parental limit setting.
5.   Promote anticipatory guidance and problem solving by encouraging discussion regarding physical maturation and sexual behaviors.
6.   Assist the family in planning for their child's future needs; refer them to available community agencies.
7.   Provide patient and family teaching, covering:
       a.   Normal developmental milestones and appropriate stimulating activities, including play and socialization activities
       b.   The need for patience with the child's slow attainment of developmental milestones
       c.   Information regarding stimulation, safety, and motivation

      d.   Measures to help prevent skin breakdown: keeping the child's skin clean and well lubricated, applying lip balm during dry weather, and using soap sparingly

      e.   Information regarding normal speech development and how to accentuate nonverbal cues, such as facial expressions and body language, to help cue speech development

      f.   The need for discipline that is simple, consistent, and appropriate to the child's developmental level

      g.   An adolescent's need for simple, practical sexual information, including anatomy, physical development, and conception

      h.   Demonstration as a better way of fostering learning than verbal explanation since the child is better able to deal with concrete objects than abstract concepts

      i.   The benefits of motivating the child to learn through positive reinforcement and shaping and fading principles

      j.   The role of positive self-esteem, built by accomplishing small successes, in motivating the child to accomplish other tasks

G. **Evaluation**

   1.   The child exhibits no evidence of infection or respiratory distress.

   2.   The child's skin remains clean and intact with no evidence of breakdown.

   3.   The child participates in self-care activities appropriate for his or her mental capabilities.

   4.   The child and family are actively involved in early intervention programs and appropriate special education programs.

   5.   Parents verbalize understanding of appropriate discipline and recreational and social activities.

   6.   Family members express feelings and concerns regarding the child's limited mental abilities.

   7.   Family members verbalize realistic goals for care of the child.

   8.   The family demonstrates acceptance of the child into the family structure.

III. Hearing impairment

  A. **Description**

   1.   In this disability, the degree of impairment ranges from mild to profound, including subdivisions or subclasses of deafness (inability to process linguistic information) and hard of hearing (use of a hearing aid enables processing of linguistic information).

   2.   Formal classification of hearing impairment is based on the softest sound that the child can hear unaided, measured in decibels (dB):

      a.   Slight (hard of hearing): 30 dB or softer

      b.   Mild to moderate (hard of hearing): 30 to 55 dB

      c.   Marked (hard of hearing): 55 to 70 dB

    d.   Severe (deaf): 70 to 90 dB

    e.   Extreme (deaf): 90 dB or louder

B.   Etiology and incidence

    1.   Causes of hearing impairment can be grouped into four catego-ries: genetic/familial, intrauterine/prenatal, perinatal, and postna-tal (Table 16–2).

    2.   One of the most common disabilities in the United States, hear-ing impairment affects 11 in 1,000 children ages 6 to 17.

    3.   One third of all hearing-impaired children also have visual or cog-nitive impairments.

C.   Pathophysiology

    1.   Location of the defect determines the nature of interference with transmission of sound along the neural pathway.

    2.   Interference of middle-ear hearing—*conductive* hearing loss—is the most common type of hearing loss. It primarily involves interfer-

TABLE 16–2.
Conditions Associated with Hearing Loss

Familial and Genetic Factors	**Perinatal Factors**
Skeletal defects (Treacher*-Collins and Klippel-Feil syndromes)	Birth weight <1,500 g*
	Prolonged or difficult birth
Retinitis pigmentosa	Hyperbilirubinemia at levels >indications for exchange transfusion*
Cerebral palsy	
Mental retardation	Severe asphyxia
Visual handicaps	Congenital perinatal infection (cytomegalovirus, rubella, herpes, syphilis, toxoplasmosis)
Pigment abnormalities (Waardenburg's syndrome, albinism)	
	Bacterial meningitis*
Anatomic malformations involving the head or neck*	**Postnatal Factors**
Chromosomal abnormalities, such as D & E trisomies	Ear infection (chronic otitis media)
	Acute infection (mumps, rubella, measles, encephalitis, meningitis)
Connective tissue disorders (osteogenesis imperfecta, Hurler's syndrome)	Respiratory conditions hypertrophied adenoids, allergy)
Family history of childhood hearing impairment*	Trauma (burns, frostbite, lacerations, perforations, bone fracture)
Prenatal and Intrauterine Factors	Ototoxic drugs, including topical applications to ear (kanamycin, streptomycin, gentamicin, neomycin, vancomycin, viomycin)
Diabetes mellitus, alcoholism	
Drugs, such as quinine, salicylate, and certain ototoxic antibiotics	Exposure to excessive noise (urban living, loud rock music, model airplanes, snowmobiles, sport shooting, motorcycle and sport racing, heavy machinery)
Maternal anoxia	
Preeclampsia and eclampsia	

* *Indicates need for hearing assessment by 6 months based on recommendations of the American Academy of Pediatrics (1982).*
(Whaley, L.F., and Wong, D.L. (1987). Nursing care of infants and children (3rd ed.). St. Louis: C.V. Mosby)

ence with the loudness of sound; bone conduction remains intact. It can be caused by foreign objects in the middle ear.

3. Damage to inner ear structures or the auditory nerve resulting in distortion of sound and inability to distinguish high-frequency sound—*sensorineural* hearing loss—may be caused by ototoxic drugs, excessive noise exposure, congenital defects, or acquired infections.

4. Interference of sound transmission through the middle ear and along the neural pathway—*mixed conductive–sensorineural* hearing loss commonly results from serous otitis media.

5. Hearing loss that results in receptive–expressive disorder, in which the child has difficulty processing, patterning, and interpreting information, is termed *central-auditory imperception*.

6. Adverse effects of hearing impairment may include:
   a. Delayed language development, which depends in large part on auditory stimulation
   b. Impaired attachment between infant and parents; the parents' voices convey warmth and caring
   c. Impaired learning about the environment; learning is enhanced when the child can associate sounds with various objects
   d. Persistence of immature egocentric behavior for longer than normal without the child's ability to interpret verbal cues regarding sociably acceptable behavior
   e. Impaired locomotion and increased potential for injury; auditory cues enhance locomotion by encouraging rhythmicity, and also alert the child to potential dangers
   f. Impaired cognitive learning, which normally is enhanced by auditory cues such as explanations of directions and verbal feedback
   g. Altered socialization, which normally depends so heavily on verbal communication for interaction; hindering of cooperative play since the child has difficulty interacting and responding in groups

7. Education for the hearing-impaired child should begin as soon as diagnosis is made; the type of educational program depends on the severity of hearing loss and ranges from favorable seating in regular classroom to special education requiring speech, auditory training, and lip reading or signing. Lip reading, signing, and speech therapy are aimed at establishing communicative skills; speech is the most difficult task for the hearing-impaired child, especially since speech is learned by visual and auditory stimulation, imitation, and reinforcement.

8. Hearing aids, which amplify sound, may be useful for children with conductive hearing loss or for those with some types of residual hearing intact.

D.   **Assessment findings**
   1.   Clinical manifestations pointing to hearing impairment may include:
      a.   Failure of an infant to respond to environmental sounds
      b.   Failure of an infant to vocalize by age 6 months
      c.   Abrupt cessation of vocalization in an infant, due to inability to hear verbal feedback from parents
      d.   In an older child with mild hearing impairment, speech distortion or failure to respond to verbal cues
   2.   Diagnostic evaluation may reveal:
      a.   Structural abnormalities or signs of inflammation on visual inspection of the external and internal ear
      b.   Quantitative determination of hearing impairment on audiometric testing
      c.   Impaired acoustic impedance of the tympanic membrane detected on tympanometry
      d.   Abnormal activation of neural pathways in direct response to acoustic stimulation through brainstem auditory-evoked potentials
      e.   Abnormal infant motor response prior to sound via a crib-o-gram (a hearing test that analyzes hearing responses by comparing the infant's response before, during, or after a sound is introduced)
      f.   Abnormal bone or air sound conduction, as evaluated by the Rinne and Weber tests
      g.   Impaired inner ear equilibrium detected on vestibular testing
   3.   Screening for children at risk should be done by age 3 months, no later than 6 months. Such children include those with a history of:
      a.   Low birth weight
      b.   Hyperbilirubinemia
      c.   Severe asphyxia
      d.   Congenital perinatal infection
      e.   Bacterial meningitis
      f.   Family history of childhood hearing impairment
      g.   Anatomic malformation of the head or neck
E.   **Nursing diagnoses**
   1.   Impaired Verbal Communication
   2.   Altered Growth and Development
   3.   Sensory and Perceptual Alterations: Auditory
   4.   Social Isolation
F.   **Planning and implementation**
   1.   Promote communication by encouraging family participation in the child's education.

2. Facilitate lip reading by following specific guidelines to assist the child, such as enface positioning, good lighting on the face, and not moving while speaking.
3. Maximize communication potential by having the child's vision assessed to determine whether any visual problems accompany hearing impairment and thus interfere with learning patterned speech.
4. Maximize residual hearing by investigating reliable hearing devices.
5. Help prevent further hearing loss by encouraging immunizations, teaching parents signs and symptoms of ear infections, and teaching parents to question any prescribed drug that might be ototoxic.
6. Provide opportunities for socialization and play by encouraging the child to participate in age-related and developmentally appropriate activities.
7. Encourage independent development through emphasis on self-care.
8. Assist family members in adjusting to life with a hearing-impaired child; refer them to available community support groups.
9. Promote parent–child attachment by helping parents cue into their child's body language, distress signals, and comfort signs.
10. Provide patient and family teaching, covering:
    a. Goals of rehabilitation: acceptance of the disability and active participation in the child's care and education
    b. The importance of viewing the child primarily as a child and only secondarily as a child with a disability
    c. Information on all local and national organizations that assist persons with hearing impairment
    d. Specific behaviors to enhance parent–child attachment, such as using the enface position when cuddling or talking with an infant
    e. How to operate a hearing aid to reduce ambient noise
    f. Hearing aid care
    g. Strategies for maximizing the child's active participation in peer activities and social events

G. Evaluation
1. The child does not develop additional hearing loss.
2. Family members provide adequate stimulation and communication for the child.
3. Persons communicating with the child practice good technique.
4. The child acquires and uses a hearing aid (when appropriate).
5. The child interacts appropriately with peers.
6. The child attends school regularly.
7. The child practices self-care independently as appropriate.

8. Family members express their concerns and feelings regarding the child's hearing impairment.
9. Family members verbalize the signs and symptoms of ear infection to watch for and report.
10. The family is actively involved in the child's educational program.

IV. Vision impairment

A. Description

1. Vision impairment is defined as a problem with visual acuity that may or may not be correctable with prescriptive lenses.
2. Classification of vision impairment is based on the child's ability to see well enough to engage in common activities, as follows:
   a. School vision: visual acuity between 10/70 and 20/200 (partially sighted); can attend in regular public school system and read normal-size print
   b. Legally blind: visual acuity 20/200 or less (not a medical diagnosis but rather used for legal purposes); unable to accurately see environment without aid of prescription lenses
   c. Travel vision: visual acuity of 20/400, allowing travel in unfamiliar surroundings without aid of another person but with the aid of prescription lenses; can read very large print; however, learning braille is advisable
   d. Light perception: ability to perceive only light and darkness and allow for some mobility with the aid of another person

B. Etiology and incidence

1. Factors associated with vision impairment include familial, prenatal, perinatal, and postnatal, as follows:
   a. Familial: genetically transmitted diseases such as galactosemia, retinoblastoma, Tay-Sachs disease, and albinism
   b. Prenatal: maternal infections such as rubella, toxoplasmosis, herpes simplex, and syphilis
   c. Perinatal: oxygen toxicity, resulting in retrolental fibroplasia; maternal infection resulting in ophthalmia neonatorum
   d. Postnatal: infections, acquired disorders, or trauma (the most common postnatal cause)
2. Incidence of visual impairment, including children with corrective lenses, is estimated at 20 to 35:1,000 children; of this group, 1:1,000 is considered legally blind.

C. Pathophysiology

1. *Refractive errors* primarily involve variations in vision due to imperfect reflection of light rays on the retina: abnormalities of eyeball, cornea, or lens causing nearsightedness (hyperopia) or blurred vision (astigmatism).

2. Reduction of visual stimulation results in amblyopia and potential blindness; blurred vision in affected eye.

3. Structural anomalies of the eye and accessory muscles result in neuromuscular incoordination (strabismus); malalignment of eyes, diplopia, squinting exotropia.

4. *Cataracts* involve opacity of the lens (crystalline lens) and are marked by visible white clouding of lens and reduced visual acuity. Congenital cataracts are the most common cause of blindness in children.

5. Adverse effects of vision impairment may include:

   a. Limited visual–motor perceptions, which can impair learning of spatial relations and other information about the environment

   b. Impaired attachment of young infants to parents, which normally begins with responsiveness and visual alertness and is fostered by reciprocal visual responses

   c. Inhibited sense of object permanence due to a lack of visual cues

   d. Overindulgence in self-stimulation as a substitute for reduced sensorimotor simulation due to vision loss; "blindisms" manifested in ways such as flicking finger in front of eyes, sniffing and smelling, or arm twirling

   e. Delayed autonomy since vision enhances locomotion and exploration of the environment

   f. Delayed locomotion due to loss of depth perception and increased risk of colliding with obstacles

   g. Impaired cognitive learning; normally, children learn the meaning of words by associating sounds and visual images

   h. Altered role identity, hampered by the child's inability to observe and imitate others' behavior

D. **Assessment findings**

1. Clinical manifestations of vision impairment depend on the cause and the child's age at onset and may include:

   a. Excessive tearing, erythema, or discharge; rubbing or blinking of eyes; edema or ptosis

   b. Frequent bumping into or tripping over objects while crawling, walking, or running

   c. Complaints of blurred or double vision, inability to read small print or signs, headache, eye pain, photophobia

   d. Squinting or holding books or other objects close to his or her face

   e. Failure of an infant's eyes to follow an object passed in front of his or her face, or newborn nystagmus persisting for more than 2 weeks after birth

2. Diagnostic evaluation may reveal:

       a.   Impaired visual acuity quantified through age-appropriate visual acuity testing

       b.   Abnormal position, alignment, size, symmetry, color, or motility of external ocular structures detected on inspection

       c.   Abnormal optic nerve function detected on visual field testing

       d.   Abnormal eye movements seen on extraocular muscle assessment

       e.   Strabismus detected through the cover–uncover test

       f.   Asymmetric light reflex on Hirschberg's test

       g.   Absent red reflex, papilledema, retinal hemorrhages, or retinal detachment detected on fundoscopic examination of the fundus (blood vessels, macula, fovea centralis, optic disc).

E. **Nursing diagnoses**
1. Altered Family Processes
2. Altered Growth and Development
3. High Risk for Injury
4. Altered Role Performance
5. Sensory and Perceptual Alterations: Visual
6. Social Isolation

F. **Planning and implementation**
1. Help prevent complications of eye defects by encouraging compliance with corrective therapies.
2. Reinforce information regarding nonoperative or operative management, which may include:
    a.   Prescription glasses
    b.   Contact lenses
    c.   Eye muscle exercises (orthoptics)
    d.   Patching
    e.   Cataract removal
    f.   Goniotomy (for glaucoma)
    g.   Eye muscle surgery
3. Help prevent injury by orienting the child to environment, keeping the environment safe and free of clutter, and arranging room furnishings to allow for maximum mobility.
4. Prevent social isolation by providing opportunities for play and socialization; discourage "blindisms."
5. Promote normal development by providing the child with appropriate visual–motor activities (rattles, swings, crawling).
6. Promote a seriously impaired child's independence by encouraging the parents to enroll him or her in a special education program and to structure the home environment to foster familiarity and a sense of security.

7. Assist the family in accepting their child's disability by listening to family concerns, emphasizing family strengths, and assisting with problem solving and anticipatory guidance.

8. Promote parent–child attachment by instructing parents in specific ways to respond to their child, including how to recognize the child's cues and needs for warmth and comfort.

9. Provide patient and family teaching, covering:
   a. The importance of ensuring environmental safety to allow the child maximum mobility
   b. The need to comply with recommended therapies to prevent further complications, such as eye patching to preserve vision
   c. If prescription glasses are recommended, the need for safety glass lenses
   d. The importance of enrolling a seriously impaired child in an educational program that fosters independent self-help skills
   e. The need for appropriate developmental activities, including social interaction and recreation and various sensory–motor experiences to improve fine motor coordination
   f. The importance of stressing the child's abilities rather than his or her disabilities
   g. Community agencies that assist persons with vision impairment

G. Evaluation
1. The child remains free of physical injury.
2. The child and family comply with corrective therapies.
3. "Blindisms" are minimized or eliminated.
4. The child engages in appropriate actions for developmental level.
5. The child demonstrates an attitude of safety and security within his or her environment.
6. The child and parents express their feelings and concerns related to vision impairment.
7. Parents interact with the child appropriately and participate in activities with the child.
8. The parents and child engage in behavior demonstrating positive regard for each other.

V. Parents of a child with special needs
A. Essential concepts
1. Parenting a child who must master the same developmental achievements as all children, in accordance with individual potentials and limitations, leaves the family unit vulnerable to psychologic and physical problems.
2. Response of family members to the child's disability is influenced by many factors, including perception of the situation, previous coping skills, and support systems.

3. Depending on such variables, a stressful situation may or may not become a crisis for the family.
4. Parents of a disabled child need information, guidance, and support to help them:
   a. Understand and manage their child's illness or problem
   b. Assist their child in understanding and coping with the disability
   c. Meet the needs of the child
   d. Meet the needs of all other family members

B. Parental coping strategies

1. Once parents accept the reality of their child's disability, the task of making adjustments in family life begins. The emerging coping patterns may be adaptive or maladaptive.
2. Adaptive patterns may include:
   a. Assigning special meaning to the disability that provides hope and places the hardship in the context of a meaningful future (e.g., "God selected us to care for this child for His purposes")
   b. Focusing on the child's positive attributes rather than on the negative aspects of the disability
   c. Sharing hardships with others outside the family, such as friends, church members, and formal support groups
   d. Adapting daily family life to the child's special needs without major disruptions in family functioning
   e. Becoming involved in support groups to help parents of other children with similar disabilities
3. Maladaptive strategies can include:
   a. Overprotecting the child and not providing proper discipline and limit setting
   b. Rejecting or becoming emotionally detached from the child or other family members
   c. Directing anger or blame toward the child, spouse, or self

C. Assessing the family

1. Successful parenting of a disabled child hinges on numerous factors, including the parents' reaction to the disability, perception of the disability, parenting style, coping behaviors, composite family strengths, available support systems, concurrent stressors, and the child's developmental level.
2. Common reactions to chronic illness or disability include:
   a. Shock and denial: initial intense emotions, usually adaptive to cushion or soften grief reaction to any type of loss; healthy enabling reaction until it becomes protracted or maladaptive with no or limited recognition of diagnosis; denial allows individual to maintain sense of hope
   b. Adjustment: beginning acknowledgement that disability

or disorder exists; initially manifested by intense feelings of guilt, self-accusation, anger, bitterness; with the most common result being "benevolent overreaction," consequence of unresolved guilt. It is cycle of guilt, overpermissiveness and anger

    c.   Reintegration and acceptance: realistic expectation of child's abilities and reintegration of child into family life; acceptance is interspersed with "chronic sorrow" (periods of intensified sorrow or sadness of loss), especially at times child would have normally been achieving particular developmental milestone

    d.   Freezing-out phase: behavior not experienced by many; not always maladjustive; decision based on need to permanently place child in residential setting, usually institutionalization

3.   The parents' perception of their child's disability involves the meaning or significance that they attach to the situation. This is influenced by such factors as previous knowledge, religious or cultural influence, imagined cause, child's gender and birth order, child's previous health status, and child's prognosis.

4.   Common parenting styles include:

    a.   Authoritarian: parental control of child's behavior by series of rigid, inflexible rules that dictate standards of conduct

    b.   Permissive: laissez-faire style of control over the child's actions with few or no rules determining standards of conduct

    c.   Authoritative: parental direction and guidance of the child's behavior by discussion of reasons for rules with standards of conduct regulated by exchange of ideas between parent and child but with the parent retaining ultimate control

5.   Coping behaviors include actions aimed at reducing tension by crisis and disruption; reflect reactions to previous crisis:

    a.   Approach behaviors: behaviors used to move a person toward adjustment and resolution (e.g., asking for information, seeking support, anticipating future, expressing feelings, planning realistic goals for the future)

    b.   Avoidance behaviors: behaviors, usually maladaptive, aimed at protecting a person by moving him or her away from adjustment and resolution (e.g., failing to recognize the seriousness of the child's condition, refusing to agree to treatment, avoiding staff members or the child, using magical thinking)

6.   The family's composite strengths encompass individual family members' strengths, coping behaviors, and reactions to the child's disability; these can help achieve or impede the goal of optimal development for the family or individual members.

7. Available support systems include:
    a. Marital relationship: prime source of potential support; best predictor of coping behavior; single parent family structure or poorly adjusted family unit contribute to already stressful circumstance of disabled child leaving family unit vulnerable to psychological trauma
    b. Alternate support systems: those available outside marital relationship
    c. Economic support system: financial sources are available for health and rehabilitative care
    d. Emotional support system: system that sustains individual family members during periods of vulnerability
    e. Communication support system: verbal and nonverbal symbols that convey meaning to event; open communication system is one in which verbal and nonverbal cues are congruent with intended message
8. Concurrent stress within the family involves any other difficulties with which family is attempting to deal (e.g., financial, marital, social isolation).
9. The child's development level: Chronically ill children have the same needs and concerns as their well counterparts; however, age of onset influences reaction to diagnosis and psychological adjustment. Early age of onset predisposes child to additional psychosocial problems since critical development stages are interrupted; these stages include:
    a. Infancy: sensorimotor experiences are critical, as well as establishment of sense of trust and attachment to significant other
    b. Toddlerhood: mastery of locomotion and language skills; separation anxiety is at its height; illness interferes with critical foundation of sense of autonomy
    c. Preschool: social development, sexual identity, and body image are developing; interruption in development can interfere with development of sense of initiative and influence development of sense of guilt
    d. School-age: striving for sense of achievement and accomplishment while overcoming sense of doubt; relationships with peers is taking on more importance.
    e. Adolescence: self-esteem, self-image, striving for independence and identity are hallmarks; illness interferes with sense of mastery and control, and adolescent attempts to incorporate disability into self-image; illness or disability is greatest threat during middle adolescence (age 14 to 16 years) when energy is devoted to meet normal development demands

D. Nursing diagnoses
1. Ineffective Family Coping

2. Altered Family Processes
3. Altered Growth and Development
4. Parental Role Conflict
5. Altered Parenting
6. Self-Esteem Disturbance

E. Planning and implementation

1. Promote parental functioning by offering support at times of diagnosis, providing follow-up information, and coordinating services with health care agencies.
2. Promote parental understanding by giving clear and simple explanation of illness or disability and opportunity to ask questions; always remain an active and empathetic listener.
3. Promote the child's development by focusing on his or her strengths and assets and by sharing his or her expected developmental achievements.
4. Promote parenting skills by sharing universal developmental milestones, discipline guidelines, and methods of effective communication.
5. Prevent ineffective coping and dysfunctional parenting by guiding parents to support groups of parents who have children with similar special needs.
6. Promote optimal family functioning by including all significant others and siblings in understanding child's condition; allow family members to vent feelings and concerns; guide family members to identify composite strengths.

F. Evaluation

1. Parents verbalize appropriate use of resources.
2. Parents cope adaptively to stress.
3. Parents demonstrate positive parent–child interaction and use effective discipline without anger, violence, or belligerence.
4. Parents express realistic perception of the child's abilities and disabilities.
5. Parents express realistic expectations of the child's skills and behaviors.
6. Parents express feelings and concerns regarding the child's future.
7. The child's behavior is developmentally appropriate.
8. Parents verbalize support and affirmation of the child's abilities.
9. Parents verbalize understanding that chronic illness or disability will require continuing therapeutic management.

Bibliography

Bess, F. H. (1977). *Childhood deafness: Causation, assessment and management.* New York: Grune & Stratton.

Haynes, U. (1983). *Holistic health care for children with developmental disabilities.* Baltimore: University Park Press.

Hymovich, D. P. (1976). Parents of sick children: Their needs and tasks. *Pediatric Nursing, 2,* 9–13.

Keinberg, S. B. (1982). *Educating the chronically ill child.* Rockwood, MD: Aspen Publications.

Mott, S. R., James, S. R., and Sperhac, A. M. (1985). *Nursing care of children and families* (2nd ed.). Menlo Park, CA: Addison-Wesley.

Olshansky, S. (1962). Chronic sorrow. *Social Casework, 43,* 190–193.

Rapin, I. (1982). Learning disabilities and associated conditions in children with hearing impairment. In K. F. Swainan and F. S. Wright (Eds.). *The practice of pediatric neurology* (2nd ed.) St. Louis: C. V. Mosby.

Riddle, I. (1973). Caring for children and their families. In E. Anderson (Ed.). *Current concepts in clinical nursing,* Vol. 4. St. Louis: C. V. Mosby.

Solnit, A. J., and Stark, M. H. (1962). Mourning the birth of a defective child. *Psychoanalytic Study of the Child, 16,* 523–237.

Waisbren, S. E. (1980). Parents' reactions after the birth of a developmentally disabled child. *American Journal of Mental Deficiency, 84,* 345–351.

Wassenberg, C. (1981). Common visual disorders in children. *Nursing Clinics of North America, 16,* 479–485.

Whaley, L. F., and Wong, D. L. (1991). *Nursing care of infants and children* (4th ed.). St. Louis: C. V. Mosby.

Wikler, L., Wasow, M., and Hattfield, E. (1981). Chronic sorrow revisited. *American Journal of Orthopsychiatry, 51,* 96–70.

Young, R. K. (1977). Chronic sorrow: Parents' response to the birth of a child with a defect. *American Journal of Maternal–Child Nursing, 2,* 38–42.

Zamerowski, S. T. (1982). Helping families cope with a handicapped child. *Topics in Clinical Nursing, 4,* 41–56.

STUDY QUESTIONS

1. Which of the following is the term applied to a severe physical or mental disability that occurs before age 22 years and likely will result in substantial limitation of function?
   a. developmental
   b. handicap
   c. chronic illness
   d. disability

2. Which parenting style allows for discussion between parent and child but with parent retaining ultimate control?
   a. authoritarian
   b. permissive
   c. authoritative
   d. laissez-faire

3. David Childers, aged 4 years, has leukemia. During the initial discussions with Mrs. Childers regarding David's treatment plan, Mrs. Childers states, "No, no this can't be true; there's nothing wrong with David." Mrs. Childer's denial
   a. gives her a sense of hope
   b. is maladaptive
   c. is an example of "chronic sorrow"
   d. is typical and should be ignored

4. Mr. Jacob's 18-year-old daughter, who has been diagnosed as educably mentally retarded, has expressed a physical attraction to a young man in her vocational training class. Mr. Jacob asks the nurse for guidance with this matter. Which of the following would be the nurse's best response?
   a. "Mr. Jacob, you should think about having your daughter sterilized soon."
   b. "Mr. Jacob, your daughter needs simple and practical sexual information."
   c. "Mr. Jacob, it is best to ignore this. If you bring up the idea of sex, it will just make her curious."
   d. "Mr. Jacob, don't worry, absolutely nothing will come of this infatuation. Your daughter is unable to respond sexually."

5. David, aged 4 years, is admitted to a pediatric hospital for readjustment of anticonvulsant medication. David has myelomeningocele and is unable to walk. David's mother states, "There are times I find myself breaking down and crying. David is never going to walk like other children." From this comment, the nurse could assess that David's mother is
   a. experiencing benevolent overreaction
   b. experiencing chronic sorrow
   c. filled with anger and consequently maladjusted
   d. experiencing shock and denial

6. According to Riddle, the support system that sustains individuals during periods of vulnerability is the
   a. economic support system
   b. emotional support system
   c. communication support system
   d. system of seeking and using help

7. Mrs. Woodlawn's 8-month-old daughter is blind. During a health history interview, Mrs. Woodlawn comments to the nurse that the child's loss of sight was caused by the copper bracelet she wears around her wrist. This statement represents an example of
   a. adjustment and resolution
   b. approach behavior
   c. avoidance behavior
   d. seeking and using help

8. All the following are principles of normalization *except*
   a. protection
   b. preparation
   c. participation
   d. sharing

9. The American Association of Mental Deficiency's definition of mental retardation stresses
   a. no responsiveness to contact
   b. deficits in adaptive behavior along with intellectual impairment
   c. cognitive impairment occurring after age 22 years

d. IQ level must be below 50

10. After amniocentesis, Mr. and Mrs. Davis find out that their unborn child— their first—has Down's syndrome. Extremely upset, they ask the nurse what they should do about terminating the pregnancy. Which of the following would be the nurse's best response?
    a. "It's wrong to take the life of another human being."
    b. "I would terminate the pregnancy if it were me."
    c. "I know several children with Down's syndrome, and they are a delight to their families. I think you should complete the pregnancy."
    d. "Tell me how you feel about the pregnancy."

11. Steven, aged 9 years, wants to learn to tie his shoes. What would be the nurse's best first step in teaching this skill to Steven?
    a. Explain the steps involved in tying shoes.
    b. Do a task analysis by breaking the task down into simple steps.
    c. Assess Steven's motivation to learn.
    d. Cluster or pair the information that Steven needs to learn.

12. Which of the following descriptions of sensorineural hearing loss is correct?
    a. most common type of hearing loss in which the primary interference with transmission of sound is the loudness; interference of middle-ear hearing
    b. damage to inner ear or auditory nerve causing distortion of sound

and loss of discrimination of high frequencies
    c. difficulty processing, patterning, and interpreting the given information
    d. interference of sound transmission through the middle ear and along the auditory nerve

13. Mrs. Thompson has given birth to a little boy, Jason. On examination, Jason's startle reflex is only to quick physical movements and not to loud sounds. After a battery of tests, Jason is diagnosed with a possible hearing loss. As the nurse prepares Mrs. Thompson and Jason for discharge, which of the following statements would call for immediate attention so as not to adversely effect development?
    a. Babbling and cooing will disappear if not reinforced.
    b. Parent–infant attachment is enhanced by auditory cues; therefore, Mrs. Thompson will need to walk with Jason more.
    c. Locomotion is enhanced by auditory cues; therefore, Mrs. Thompson will need to learn to walk with Jason more.
    d. Academic learning will be slowed.

14. Of the following behaviors seen in the visually impaired child, which one should the nurse work toward diminishing or eliminating?
    a. orienting
    b. clumsiness
    c. blindisms
    d. hitching

ANSWER KEY

1. **Correct response: a**
   Developmental disabilities either are severe physical or mental disabilities that limit function, may continue indefinitely, and occur before the age of 22 years.
   b. A handicap is not necessarily a disability but rather an environmental barrier that makes it difficult for an individual to fully participate.
   c. Chronic illness is any disorder that disrupts daily functioning for more than 3 months or causes hospitalization for more than a month, each in a given year.
   d. Disability refers to loss of function.
   Knowledge/Health promotion/Assessment

2. **Correct response: c**
   Authoritative style directs and guides the child's behavior by discussion of reason for rules, and yet the parent retains ultimate control.
   a. Authoritarian style orders and controls by a series of rigid, inflexible rules.
   b. Permissive style operates with no or few rules that determine conduct.
   d. Laissez-faire style operates with no or few rules that determine conduct.
   Knowledge/Psychosocial/Assessment

3. **Correct response: a**
   Denial is adaptive during initial periods of intense emotions and is an enabling reaction that allows the individual a sense of hope.
   b. Denial is maladaptive only when it limits true recognition of a diagnosis and disallows needed treatment.
   c. Chronic sorrow is intense sadness or sorrow that occurs at each developmental period when the child is unable to achieve a universal task.
   d. No emotion should ever be ignored or discounted in the care of another, especially when that emotion may hinder or help.
   Analysis/Health promotion/Evaluation

4. **Correct response: b**
   Dealing with the subject of the sexuality of their mentally retarded child is difficult for parents, yet half of mildly retarded persons have experienced sexual intercourse during adolescence. Mentally retarded adolescents need simple, practical, and understandable information regarding their anatomy, physical development, and conception.
   a. Sterilization will not provide any immediate answers for the child. It is an issue that must be discussed between parent and child and is an issue of competency, morality, human rights, and ethics.
   c. Ignoring the issue will not lessen the physical response and the possibility that the child will act on the physical signals for sexual fulfillment.
   d. This simply is not true.
   Application/Health promotion/Implementation

5. **Correct response: b**
   Chronic sorrow is periods of intensified sorrow or sadness of loss, particularly during periods when developmental milestones should be normally occurring.
   a. Benevolent overreaction is exhibited by a cycle of overpermissiveness followed by anger and overwhelming guilt.
   c. David's mother's feelings are very normal, and she grieves the loss of function that her child will not achieve.
   d. David's mother is past the initial stage of shock and denial.
   Comprehension/Psychosocial/Assessment

6. **Correct response: b**
   A strong emotional support system supports family members during periods of vulnerability because of the need for feeling safe and having a dependable system to assure support when needed.

a. Important for financial maintenance of family unit.

c. Open and congruent expression of meaning is accomplished through verbal and nonverbal symbols.

d. Implies understanding and a willingness to take responsibility.

Knowledge/Health promotion/Assessment

7. *Correct response: c*
Avoidance behaviors are used to protect the individual; magical thinking is a type of avoidance behavior.

a. Adjustment and resolution implies acceptance of the disability, magical thinking is protection against disintegration, in the mist of a loss.

b. Approach behaviors are coping behaviors used to move the individual toward adjustment and resolution.

d. Seeking and using help implies understanding of the condition and a willingness to receive additional information; magical thinking avoids accurate and precise understanding.

Analysis/Health promotion/Evaluation

8. *Correct response: a*
Protection implies shielding the child or alleviating him or her from discomfort; although children must be given only what they can psychologically handle for their developmental age, protection fosters dependence rather than independence, and consequently normalization does not happen.

b. Preparation is one principle of normalization that allows for planning and anticipation of events to come. It prepares the child for some control of the situation.

c. Participation includes the child in decision making and fosters independence.

d. Sharing allows for full participation of care with significant family members, allowing for the normal event of ''give and take'' within a family, all part of normalization.

Knowledge/Health promotion/Assessment

9. *Correct response: b*

The definition states that in addition to subaverage intellectual functioning that the child must exhibit deficits in adaptive behavior.

a. An early behavioral sign suggestive of cognitive impairment but not part of the definition

c. The definition states that cognitive compromise or impairment must occur before age 18 to 22 (depending on different authors defining developmental period).

d. IQ 70 or below is considered significantly subaverage intellectual functioning

Knowledge/Psychosocial/Assessment

10. *Correct response: d*
Counseling should be nonjudgmental and nondirective, and gives the parents opportunities to explore all available options. The parents are the ones who must deal with their decision, thus it should be guided by how they feel about their actions, not the nurse's opinion.

a, b, and c. These statements express the nurse's opinion and thus are not appropriate responses.

Application/Health promotion/ Implementation

11. *Correct response: b*
A task analysis is always done first to break down the task to be learned into very simple steps.

a. Demonstration is preferable to abstract concepts needed with verbal explanation.

c. Motivation is always important in teaching a task, to reinforce learning, but task analysis is necessary first to determine what is to be taught.

d. Clustering and pairing the information to be learned helps, particularly since the cognitively impaired child usually has a deficit in short-term memory, but task analysis precedes determining the method of instruction.

12. **Correct response: b**

    Auditory nerve and inner ear structures are the structures of sensorineural hearing.
    a. conductive hearing
    c. receptive–expressive disorder
    d. mixed conductive-sensorineural

    Knowledge/Physiologic/Assessment

13. **Correct response: b**

    Parent–infant attachment is important for healthy emotional development, and parents of special needs children must be sensitive to other ways to enhance their children's development (i.e., eye contact, cuddling, holding).
    a. Babbling and cooing do not occur until around 4 months of age.
    c. Locomotion does not occur until about 10 months of age.
    d. Academic learning will be slowed

but is not an immediate concern in the newborn period.

Analysis/Psychosocial/Evaluation

14. **Correct response: c**

    Blindisms are self-stimulating behaviors that serve as a substitute for diminished sensorimotor stimulation; blindisms hinder stimulation; blindisms hinder social integration.
    a. Orienting behaviors are those in which the individual assesses the physical environment and attempts to maneuver about with minimum interference.
    b. Clumsiness is part of locomotion particularly since people normally rely on visual cues to smoothly guide direction.
    d. Hitching is a substitute for crawling in which children use their legs to propel themselves forward while in a sitting position; allows them to feel objects with their hands instead of their head.

Knowledge/Safe care/Planning

COMPREHENSIVE TEST—QUESTIONS

1. When talking with Mrs. Cohen, the nurse also reviews the proper method of measuring temperature. Which of the following routes is most appropriate for a 2-month-old infant?
   a. oral
   b. rectal
   c. skin
   d. axillary

2. Further evaluation of Ms. Jones's hemoglobin and nutritional intake leads to the determination that her diet is deficient in iron. Based on this determination, the nurse would recommend all the following measures *except*
   a. providing supplemental bottle-feedings with an iron-fortified formula two times each day
   b. gradually weaning the infant from breast-feeding over the next 2 weeks
   c. administering supplemental iron drops to the infant
   d. adding iron-fortified cereal to the infant's daily feeding schedule

3. On family assessment, the nurse notes that Ms. Jones's 2-year-old son, George, is listless and appears pale. Analysis reveals that George's hemoglobin level is 8 g/dL. Further assessment reveals that George dislikes solid food except pudding, bananas, rice, and milk shakes; he drinks six 8-oz bottles of 2% milk each day. In collaboration with a dietitian and Ms. Jones, the nurse devises a care plan to improve George's nutritional status to be phased in over the next 3 weeks. Which of the following would *not* be appropriate for this plan?
   a. Change the "white" solid foods to peanut butter on whole wheat bread, grapes, salami, and boiled egg slices.

   b. Provide instructions for administering liquid iron supplements.
   c. Decrease milk intake to 6 oz six times per day.
   d. Provide a written food plan for George involving six small meals per day.

4. What is the primary purpose of providing anticipatory guidance to parents?
   a. to provide professional input from the health care team for more optimal parenting styles
   b. to aid in problem solving
   c. to provide supportive counseling in groups
   d. to prepare them for the child's next stage of development

5. During an interview with parents, the nurse might take a "universal approach" to provide additional information. Such an approach might begin with
   a. "Many parents find that . . ."
   b. "All the parents I know . . ."
   c. "I wonder why you don't consider . . ."
   d. "Have you thought about . . ."

6. When assessing a child's social development, the best approach would be to focus on the child's
   a. toys
   b. interaction with the parents or caregiver
   c. drawings
   d. choice of books

7. A "typical" toddler stands
   a. with a characteristic pot belly
   b. tall and slender
   c. with a rounded back
   d. with assistance only

8. Aaron Kaiser, aged 30 months, demonstrates increasing skill in climbing on furniture and stairs. When talking with the nurse, Mrs. Kaiser—who is 6 months pregnant with her second child—expresses the desire to move

Answer sheet provided on page 343.

Aaron from a crib to a bed. Guidelines for this change include all the following *except*

a. talking to Aaron about his becoming "big" and needing a different bed
b. letting him move his "belongings" from the crib to the bed
c. making sure that the bedtime ritual stays the same
d. moving him to the bed while Mrs. Kaiser is at the hospital having the new baby

9. Toddlers' basic emotional needs must be met to ensure development of a healthy personality. Between ages 1 and 3 years, a child needs

a. unlimited freedom to do what he or she wants to gain the independence desired
b. rigid rules set by parents to protect him or her from harm
c. reasonable limits that are loosened as he or she shows readiness
d. recognition that the toddler can determine his or her own limits for behavior

10. During a discussion on injury prevention with a toddler's parents, the nurse should explain that toddlers are especially prone to accidental injury because

a. They are curious about the environment.
b. They have the ability to run and climb with ease.
c. They have an increased need for peer approval and thus engage in dangerous acts.
d. They have a drive for increased strenuous activity.

11. Lakiesha Smith, aged 28 months, is admitted to the hospital with a serum lead level of 66 μg/dL, signs of neurologic impairment, and lead lines on her teeth. Lakiesha's mother states that she habitually eats paint chips off the window frame in her room. Based on these data, which of the following nursing diagnoses would be most appropriate?

a. Powerlessness related to interpersonal interaction
b. High Risk for Injury, trauma related to neglect
c. High Risk for Injury, poisoning related to pica
d. Altered Family Processes related to sudden hospitalization

12. Mrs. Smith is concerned with the medical diagnosis of lead poisoning for Lakiesha. Her questions indicate concern and the need for more information. Which of the following instructions would be of most help to Mrs. Smith in preventing further lead ingestion?

a. Place Lakiesha in foster care until all sources of lead are removed from the home.
b. Because Lakiesha must have greater than normal oral needs, provide her with safe objects for chewing.
c. Decrease environmental stimulation to decrease Lakiesha's interest in ingesting nonfood substances.
d. Remove all lead paint from the environment to eliminate the source of exposure.

13. Lakiesha does not have encephalopathy and can receive prescribed chelating agents by IV rather than by injection. The most helpful information that the nurse can provide to a toddler like Lakiesha to prepare her for the IV infusion is

a. how long the procedure will take
b. where her parents will be during the procedure
c. which room she will be in
d. what the equipment will look like

14. A 4-year-old child must have the capacity for self-awareness to

a. develop gender identity
b. eliminate fear of the dark
c. maintain self-control
d. focus on more than one dimension of an object

15. A preschool-age child's moral development is
  a. limited by labels of good and bad
  b. marked by consistent conformation to rules
  c. in a reward and punishment mode
  d. based on a sense of right and wrong

16. When preparing a preschool-age child for the following procedures, which of the following statements by the nurse would be *inappropriate*?
  a. Surgery: "The doctor is going to help you so you can run and play and won't get as tired as you do now."
  b. Temperature measurement: "I'm going to put this thermometer in your mouth to measure how warm you are."
  c. Cardiac catheterization: "The doctor will make a cut in your leg so a small tube can be inserted to your heart."
  d. Leg radiograph: "I'll go with you to the special room so a picture can be taken of your leg."

17. Communicable diseases are common to preschool children who have not been immunized because of their increased contact with other children of the same age. Which of the following communicable diseases does *not* have a vaccine developed for widespread use?
  a. rubeola (measles)
  b. varicella (chickenpox)
  c. *Haemophilus influenzae* type B
  d. parotitis (mumps)

18. Billy Bates, aged 3 years, is hospitalized for a severe infection. Based on knowledge of normal growth and development, the nurse would expect that the skill Billy has most recently acquired is
  a. alternating his feet while walking upstairs
  b. throwing a large ball 4 to 5 feet
  c. eating with a spoon without spilling the contents
  d. speaking in three- to four-word sentences

19. The nurse needs to administer a liquid medicine per os to 3-year-old Jenny. Which of the following approaches would best help ensure success?
  a. "It's time to take your medicine, Jenny—do you want to use a straw or drink it from this cup?"
  b. "Here is your medicine, Jenny. Why don't you drink it for me now?"
  c. "It's time to drink your medicine because the doctor says it will make you feel better."
  d. "See how well Susie took her medicine? Now take yours."

20. The school nurse at an elementary school is an important role model and teacher of health. All the following areas are important for fourth- and fifth-grade children *except*
  a. stress reduction techniques
  b. hazards of drugs, alcohol, and cigarettes
  c. sex education
  d. defensive driving techniques

21. Sixth- and seventh-grade children may comprehend why they become ill, but they do not understand their role in illness prevention. A teaching plan for 11- and 12-year-old children needs to stress all the following *except*
  a. understanding that outside forces determine illness prevention
  b. eating a balanced diet from the basic four food groups
  c. dressing in appropriate layers for the temperature
  d. ensuring proper handwashing practices

22. The nurse should encourage school-age children to become active participants in learning about health care by
  a. asking questions
  b. cooperating with the health care professional in the design of the health care plan
  c. clarifying their responsibilities for self-care
  d. all the above

23. Susie, aged 9 years, is hospitalized at 4

AM for lower right quadrant pain; appendicitis is confirmed with diagnostic tests. An appendectomy is scheduled for this morning. Susie's major nursing diagnosis is High Risk for Infection related to presence of infective organisms. Preoperative nursing interventions should focus on all the following *except*

a. placing Susie in a low Fowler's position
b. applying a warm pack to the abdomen
c. keeping Susie NPO
d. gently palpating Susie's abdomen to detect swelling

24. Surgery has gone well, and Susie is in the postoperative phase of recovery. Nursing diagnoses that will guide care from this point likely would include all the following *except*
   a. Pain related to surgical incision
   b. High Risk for Fluid Volume Deficit related to NPO status
   c. High Risk for Infection related to surgical incision
   d. Altered Family Processes related to separation anxiety

25. As Susie is recovering and feeling better, nursing assessment determines that she has had a growth-promoting experience versus a stressful–regressive experience. This could be attributed to all the following factors *except*
   a. assignment to a primary nurse
   b. presence of family and siblings
   c. gifts provided from staff
   d. self-mastery in coping with a surgical experience

26. Nearly half of the accidents in the adolescent age group are caused by
   a. poisoning
   b. motor vehicles
   c. burns
   d. guns

27. Besides adolescents, children in which of the following age groups experience the most rapid growth?
   a. infancy

   b. toddler stage
   c. preschool age
   d. school age

28. Which of the following statements regarding adolescent sexual maturation is correct?
   a. Boys begin developing at different ages but develop at about the same rate.
   b. Boys finish maturing before girls.
   c. The rate of development differs greatly from individual to individual.
   d. Boys usually mature faster than girls.

29. On average, the adolescent growth spurt begins
   a. earlier for boys than for girls
   b. earlier for girls than for boys
   c. at approximately the same time for both sexes
   d. between the seventh and eigthth years

30. Which of the following factors does *not* have an effect on the onset of menstruation?
   a. climate
   b. urban vs. rural life
   c. genetics
   d. nutrition

31. Tom, aged 16, has been admitted to the adolescent unit to recover from a suicide attempt—not his first. Tom's parents are beside themselves with grief. When helping clients such as Tom's parents cope with a crisis, what is the most important message the nurse can convey?
   a. They can deal with it; everyone has to cope with crises.
   b. They are competent people, and counselors are available to help them work through this crisis.
   c. The nurse can solve the problem if they give him or her enough information.
   d. There must be a community agency that can help them.

32. Nursing interventions for adolescent

suicide attempts include which of the following?

a. Ignoring threats of suicide since they are usually merely bids for attention
b. Recognizing the prodromal signs and symptoms
c. Emphasizing to the patient that a suicide attempt is an immature way of dealing with stress
d. Recognizing that a suicide attempt is an impulsive act resulting from a temporary crisis

33. During his 3 weeks of hospitalization, Tom has had a positive change in feelings about himself. His mood swings are stabilized, and he is more positive in his interactions and in his comments about himself. In collaborating with the health care team to design a discharge plan for Tom and his parents, the nurse would want to include all the following *except*

a. follow-up counseling on a weekly basis
b. communication that his parents and the health care professionals care about him
c. identification of a sensible schedule of activities that Tom is interested in pursuing
d. heavy doses of mood elevators to fight any depression he may experience

34. Which of the following is a sign of dehydration in an infant?

a. urine specific gravity of 1.035
b. bulging anterior fontanel
c. elevated blood pressure
d. increased lacrimation

35. Which of the following factors predisposes a child to urinary tract infection?

a. short urethral structure
b. circumcision
c. frequent emptying of the bladder
d. increased fluid intake

36. When talking with the parents of a child with vesicoureteral reflux who was admitted for surgical reimplanta-

tion of the ureters, the nurse should explain that surgery is necessary to

a. increase urine output
b. prevent renal damage
c. lower BUN level
d. enable toilet training

37. Andrew Jones, aged 3, is admitted to the pediatric unit with ascites and decreased urinary output. The physician diagnoses nephrotic syndrome. What is the cause of edema in nephrotic syndrome?

a. increased colloidal osmotic pressure
b. suppression of ADH
c. hypervolemia
d. increased permeability in the glomeruli to protein

38. Skin care is important for Andrew because of his severe edema. Which of the following nursing interventions related to skin care would be most appropriate?

a. Maintain strict bedrest to prevent trauma to the skin.
b. Apply tight-fitting diapers to prevent leakage of urine onto the skin.
c. Keep Andrew flat in bed to minimize fluid shifts.
d. Change Andrew's position frequently.

39. When assessing a child with acute glomerulonephritis, the nurse would expect to see which of the following signs?

a. frothy, yellow urine
b. decreased blood pressure
c. peripheral edema
d. tremors in the extremities

40. In a nursing care plan for a school-aged child with acute glomerulonephritis, which of the following interventions would be most appropriate to meet the child's need for diversional activities while still allowing him or her to rest?

a. Do not allow the child to perform any self-care.

b. Encourage the child's mother to spend all of her time with him or her.

c. Determine what type of quiet activities the child likes.

d. Keep the child in a room alone.

41. Which of the following statements concerning acute otitis media is correct?

a. *Staphylococcus aureus* is the most common causative organism.

b. Amoxicillin or ampicillin are the drugs of choice.

c. Otitis media usually results in a permanent hearing loss.

d. Breast-fed infants have a higher incidence than formula-fed infants.

42. In planning a teaching session with parents of an infant who has just been treated for acute otitis media, the nurse should include which of the following instructions?

a. Discontinue the use of antibiotics once the child is afebrile.

b. Continue to administer prophylactic low-dose antibiotics indefinitely.

c. Have the child blow his of her nose well and often.

d. Do not give the child a bottle once he or she is in bed.

43. Bobby Baer, aged 2 years, is admitted to the hospital with a diagnosis of croup. He is tachypneic with stridor and circumoral cyanosis. Which of the following would *not* be an appropriate nursing intervention for Bobby?

a. Assess vital signs and respiratory status closely.

b. Force oral fluids to prevent dehydration.

c. Place Bobby in a high-humidity mist tent or place cool mist vaporizer at the bedside.

d. Administer oxygen therapy.

44. As part of the nursing care plan for Bobby, the nurse plans to concentrate her nursing interventions to allow him long periods of undisturbed rest in the cool mist tent. This nursing goal is

a. appropriate because the cool mist maintains good hydration

b. appropriate because this action promotes decreased oxygen demands

c. inappropriate because frequent assessment by auscultation is required

d. inappropriate because Bobby should be awakened and assessed often for stridor

45. Mrs. Martin brings her 4-year-old son to the emergency department in the middle of the night. He is irritable, febrile, stridorous, and drooling, and complains of a sore throat. The nurse in the emergency room does not examine the child's throat but rather notifies the physician immediately. What is the best rationale for the nurse's action?

a. The child's stridor may become worse if the throat is examined.

b. Examination of the throat may cause complete airway obstruction.

c. The child is irritable, and it is best not to upset him more by examining his throat.

d. Examination of the throat may initiate a respiratory tract infection.

46. Three major organisms cause bacterial pneumonia in children. Which of the following organisms is *not* in this group?

a. staphylococcus

b. *Haemophilus influenzae* type B

c. streptococcus

d. pneumococcus

47. When assessing the respiratory status of a child admitted to the hospital with an acute asthma attack, the nurse would most likely find

a. periods of apnea

b. expiratory wheezing

c. inspiratory stridor

d. absent breath sounds

48. A nurse is asked by the mother of a patient with cystic fibrosis why the physician told her to be especially cautious during hot weather. An appropriate response by the nurse would be

a. "Your child has no sweat glands, and hot weather may be hazardous."

b. "Your child has little skin pigment to prevent sunburn."

c. "Your child has a poorly functioning temperature control center, and hot weather may be hazardous."

d. "Your child may experience an unusually high salt loss through perspiration in hot weather."

49. All the following interventions would be appropriate in postoperative care of an infant with a cleft lip repair *except*

a. cleaning the suture line after each feeding

b. using elbow restraints at all times

c. maintaining the child in a side-lying or prone position

d. providing slow feedings with frequent burping

50. Of the following interventions for postoperative care of an infant with a cleft lip repair, which one would be of *highest* priority?

a. maintaining a patent airway

b. keeping the infant from crying

c. administering medications to reduce oral secretions

d. administering IV fluids

51. One danger of pyloric stenosis is the altered electrolyte balance due to excessive vomiting. Which of the following imbalances would most likely result from excessive vomiting?

a. metabolic alkalosis

b. metabolic acidosis

c. decreased hematocrit and hemoglobin levels

d. hypernatremia

52. All the following symptoms would be characteristic of the child with celiac disease *except*

a. steatorrhea

b. general malnutrition

c. periorbital edema

d. abdominal distention

53. In celiac disease, the main nursing consideration is assisting the parents and child to adhere to the diet. In planning nursing strategies to achieve this goal, the nurse might include all the following approaches *except*

a. stressing that diet compliance need be only a temporary measure

b. encouraging the child and parents to express feelings about the diet, illness, and lifestyle changes

c. stressing the positive benefits of adhering to the diet

d. focusing on ways to make the diet as normal as possible

54. Which of the following statements made by the nurse to the parents of a child with intussusception demonstrates an accurate understanding of the pathology of this condition?

a. "This condition involves hypertrophy and hyperplasia of the muscular layer around the pylorus."

b. "This condition involves relaxation or incompetence of the lower esophageal sphincter."

c. "This condition involves absence of autonomic parasympathetic ganglion cells in one segment of the colon."

d. "This condition involves a telescoping of the bowel into the portion immediately next to it."

55. Samuel Jones, aged 4 months, has been diagnosed with an inguinal hernia. It is visible only when he cries, and he apparently is not experiencing any related discomfort. His parents ask the nurse when their child's hernia will be repaired. Which of the following replies best indicates that the nurse has an accurate understanding of the medical management of inguinal hernia?

a. "An inguinal hernia will usually close by age 3 to 4 years and will require surgery only if it doesn't close by age 6 or so."

b. "Inguinal hernias are repaired as a prompt, elective surgical procedure. The surgeon will probably schedule surgery for sometime in the next few weeks."

c. "An inguinal hernia is treated as a surgical emergency. The surgeon will be scheduling your child for surgery later today."

d. "Surgical repair of an inguinal hernia will be done if there is no spontaneous resolution by about age 1 year. The doctor will wait until then to see if the hernia is reduced on its own."

56. A nurse would expect a child with iron deficiency anemia to display all the following signs and symptoms *except*
   a. pallor
   b. increased resistance to infection
   c. fatigue
   d. growth retardation

57. In planning nutritional counseling for an adolescent with iron deficiency anemia, the best approach for the nurse would be to
   a. plan a dietary regimen for the client and emphasize the importance of compliance
   b. let the client choose foods that he or she prefers and that contain iron and assist the client in planning menus that contain those foods
   c. recommend to the client that he or she see a nutritionist and proceed to make an appointment for the client
   d. inform the client's parents of his or her diagnosis and discuss a plan for care with them

58. When administering oral iron supplements to a patient, the nurse should
   a. give the medication between meals with orange juice
   b. give the medication with milk to prevent gastric irritation
   c. give the pill at bedtime since rest promotes absorption
   d. give the pill after meals

59. Which of the following represents the most accurate and supportive response to parental concerns for a child with sickle cell anemia experiencing frequent recurrence of crises?
   a. "As your child grows older, he likely will have fewer episodes of crisis."
   b. "Crisis is a part of sickle cell disease. You can do nothing to prevent them."
   c. "Don't worry about anything. We are taking good care of your child, and it's senseless to worry."
   d. "I know you're concerned for your child, but crises don't really have any long-term adverse effects."

60. Intermittent painful swelling of the hands and feet, known as hand–foot syndrome, commonly occurs in infants with
   a. thalassemia major
   b. hemophilia
   c. sickle cell disease
   d. iron-deficiency anemia

61. Through understanding the pathology of thalassemia major, the nurse understands that deferoxamine is administered to reduce the side effects of
   a. chronic lead ingestion
   b. ammonia accumulation
   c. excessive iron deposits in tissues
   d. splenomegaly

62. Parent education centered around reducing the risk of injury for a toddler with hemophilia should include all the following instructions *except*
   a. pad the side rails of the crib
   b. dress the child in clothes with padding over the elbows and knees
   c. limit exploratory behavior
   d. inspect toys frequently for hazards

63. A left-to-right shunt can be created by all the following congenital heart defects *except*
   a. patent ductus arteriosus
   b. atrial septal defect
   c. ventricular septal defect

d. tetralogy of Fallot

64. The mother of a toddler with a cyanotic congenital heart defect states "My husband says I really need to keep him quiet or it'll damage his heart more." Which of the following would be the most appropriate response by the nurse?

a. "Your son was born with his defect, and there's nothing you can do that will damage his heart more than it already is."

b. "Your husband means well, but obviously he does not know much about children with cardiac defects."

c. "Your husband is right. It is important for you to limit you son's activities to prevent cyanosis."

d. "It's important to let your child play and develop as normally as possible based on his own activity tolerance."

65. In planning nursing care for a child undergoing cardiac catheterization, it is important for the nurse to be aware of possible complications following the procedure. Common complications include all the following *except*

a. hemorrhage

b. cardiac dysrhythmias

c. overhydration

d. infection

66. Which of the following statements about ventricular septal defect (VSD) is *incorrect*?

a. A VSD is an abnormal opening in the septum between the right and left ventricles.

b. Most VSDs close spontaneously.

c. This type of defect is inoperable.

d. A VSD can be surgically repaired.

67. An infants born with transposition of the great vessels cannot sustain life unless

a. an accompanying defect exists, such as an ASD, VSD, PDA, or patent foramen ovale

b. intubation and assisted ventilation is begun immediately after birth

c. total corrective surgery is done in the first week of life

d. high concentrations of oxygen are administered

68. In planning discharge teaching with the family of a child with a congenital heart defect, the nurse would stress all the following *except*

a. avoiding contact with people

b. administering medications properly and monitoring for side effects

c. meeting with a community health nurse for home care assistance

d. scheduling follow-up appointments with the cardiologist

69. A nurse who administers medications to children should be aware of the action of the medication. Digoxin, a medication commonly given to children with congestive heart failure, acts to

a. increase the heart rate

b. increase the force of cardiac contractions

c. stabilize electrolytes in the myocardium

d. decrease the PR interval on the ECG

70. Appropriate nursing interventions for digoxin administration include all the following *except*

a. Assess apical pulse before administration.

b. Administer the medication, and notify the physician if the heart rate is below normal.

c. Observe for signs of toxicity.

d. Double-check the dosage with another nurse before administering the medication.

71. Kevin is not placed in reverse isolation, but the nurse will employ all other measures to restrict the spread of pathogenic organisms to Kevin, including

a. administering immunizations to prevent common childhood illnesses

b. giving Kevin several baths a day

c. administering platelet transfusions
d. placing Kevin in a private room and screening all visitors for recent exposure to illnesses

72. Kevin's physician needs to determine if leukemic cells have entered the central nervous system. Which procedure would provide this information?
    a. venipuncture
    b. bone marrow biopsy
    c. lumbar puncture
    d. peripheral blood smear

73. As a preschooler, Kevin's response to hospitalization and subsequent mastery is most influenced by which of the following?
    a. the need for sustained rituals
    b. fear of separation
    c. fear of body mutilation
    d. awareness of the finality of death

74. Postsurgically, Kelly is diagnosed with stage II tumor and will need radiation and chemotherapy. Nursing care aimed at reducing skin breakdown due to radiotherapy includes all the following *except*
    a. avoiding sun exposure
    b. providing daily baths, using soap sparingly
    c. applying skin lubrication to counteract dry skin
    d. referring to skin changes as a "burn"

75. Postoperatively, the nurse should assess Kelly for intestinal obstruction, performing all the following *except*
    a. auscultating bowel sounds
    b. monitoring bowel movements
    c. assessing for abdominal distention or vomiting
    d. monitoring serum creatinine level

76. As a toddler, Kelly's response to hospitalization and subsequent mastery is influenced by which of the following?
    a. separation anxiety
    b. magical thinking
    c. causality
    d. identity crisis

77. Michael, aged 7, is admitted to a pediatric unit for evaluation of short stature. The nurse using good observation and interviewing skills can gather information that may help establish a diagnosis of hypopituitarism. Which of the following statements by the mother would indicate the likelihood of progressive idiopathic hypopituitarism?
    a. "Michael grew as well as my other children until 18 months ago, when he just stopped getting taller."
    b. "Michael has always been a child who has worn out his clothes before he outgrew them."
    c. "Michael has been complaining of a headache and trouble seeing for several months."
    d. "Maybe Michael will have another growth spurt as he did for the first couple of years."

78. While undergoing an endocrine test to provoke growth hormone blood levels, Michael becomes irritable, refusing to respond to the nurse's questions and crying that he wants to go back to his room. The nurse should suspect which of the following problems?
    a. hypoglycemia
    b. a behavior disorder
    c. separation anxiety
    d. hospitalism

79. Michael is scheduled to receive GH therapy three times a week. Michael's mother is so hopeful that Michael will achieve a normal height that she asks the nurse if increasing GH injections to six times a week would double Michael's chances for increased growth. Which response by the nurse would be most appropriate?
    a. "An acute overdose of growth hormone would lead to an initial hyperglycemia followed by a severe hypoglycemia."
    b. "Long-term overdosage could result in signs and symptoms of acromegaly—enlargement of facial features."

c. "Since there are few adverse side effects, doubling the dosage couldn't do any harm."

d. "Doubling the dosage would shock the body and cause a reversal in skeletal growth, resulting in dwarfism."

80. Matthew, aged 14, is admitted to the pediatric unit with mood swings, truncal obesity, acne, hypertension, and ecchymotic areas. He is to undergo several endocrine studies and radiologic examination to determine if he has Cushing's syndrome. The nurse caring for Matthew should keep in mind that a major threat to a hospitalized adolescent is

a. fear of body mutilation

b. separation from home and family

c. poor self-image and fear of losing peer acceptance

d. getting behind in school work

81. In teaching Matthew about Cushing's syndrome, the nurse would want to stress which of the following?

a. the signs and symptoms of adrenal insufficiency

b. the need to avoid other persons to guard against infection

c. the importance of vigorous exercise to rebuild muscle tissue in the extremities

d. the need for diet modifications to limit calories and fats

82. Julia, aged 8, is admitted to a pediatric hospital with deep, rapid Kussmaul respirations and a flushed, dry face. Her mother states the she has been sick the last several days with "flu" symptoms. When evaluating Julia's laboratory study results, the nurse would expect to find which the following?

a. blood pH of 7.40

b. blood glucose of 100 mg/dL

c. bicarbonate level of 21 mEq/L

d. urine test results of 4+ for sugar and acetone

83. When administering the type of insulin Julia should be receiving while in ketoacidosis, the nurse would anticipate its *peak* action to be within

a. 30 to 60 minutes

b. 2 to 3 hours

c. 4 to 6 hours

d. 8 to 10 hours

84. In planning care for Julia, the nurse should keep in mind which of the following developmental considerations?

a. Peer acceptance and influence is decreasing in importance.

b. Formal operational thought provides Julia with abstract cognition.

c. Julia will enjoy participation in her care.

d. Julia is developing a sense of identity, her current developmental task.

85. Sarah Jane, a newborn, is admitted to the pediatric hospital with the diagnosis of myelomeningocele. In the initial assessment, the nurse would need to understand which of the following?

a. Sensory and motor disturbances are usually not parallel and thus motor dysfunction and sensation are not correlated.

b. Urine and feces in the diaper indicate intact innervation to the bladder and the anal sphincter.

c. Joint contractures and hip dislocation occur due to complete denervation of extensors and flexors.

d. The nature and degree of neurologic dysfunction is directly related to the defect's location and nerve involvement.

86. Sarah Jane's mother is upset and thinks that a fall she experienced at 16 weeks gestation is the cause of the defect. The most appropriate response by the nurse would be

a. "The cause of the defect is a virus that the mother passes on to her unborn child, not a result of a fall."

b. "We don't know what the cause is, but we do know that the defect results at around 4 weeks of gestation when mothers usually don't know that they are pregnant."

   c. "Your baby has a genetic defect. Did someone in your family have this too?"

   d. "Anything could have caused this at any time, so don't blame yourself."

87. Sarah Jane undergoes surgery to have the myelomeningocele sac repaired. An important nursing intervention when caring for Sarah Jane postoperatively would be to

   a. Facilitate drying and toughening of the sac by applying heat treatment via a heat lamp.

   b. Measure the occipitofrontal circumference daily to detect early signs of hydrocephalus.

   c. Prevent hip dislocation by applying a triple diaper.

   d. Place the infant up in a pumpkin seat to relieve strain on the back muscles.

88. Postoperative assessment of Sarah Jane reveals bulging anterior fontanel, irritability, and crying when the nurse attempts to cuddle and hold her. These are signs and symptoms of all the following *except*

   a. hydrocephalus

   b. meningitis

   c. dehydration

   d. Arnold-Chiari syndrome

89. Before Sarah Jane's discharge, the nurse should teach her parents that

   a. Sarah Jane's immobility will not hamper her struggle for independence.

   b. Immobility may leave Sarah Jane with little means to reduce stress.

   c. Sarah Jane's physical restraints will have little impact on language development.

   d. Although immobility may contribute to sensory deprivation, behavioral changes should be minimal.

90. Jason, aged 6 years, is admitted to a pediatric hospital for diagnosis and treatment of a seizure disorder. On admission assessment, the nurse would want to obtain all the following information *except*

   a. age of onset

   b. sensations prior to onset of seizures

   c. birth weight, height, and head circumference

   d. any factors that might have precipitated the seizure

91. Emergency treatment for Jason during a seizure would include which of the following measures?

   a. Ease him to the floor if he is sitting in a wheelchair or standing at the beginning of the attack.

   b. Insert a padded tongue blade into the mouth to unclamp his jaw.

   c. Attempt to restrain him to avoid additional injury.

   d. Get help from other personnel even if it requires leaving him alone for a moment.

92. Jason is diagnosed with grand mal seizures; dilantin and phenobarbital are prescribed. When teaching Jason and his parents about dilantin therapy, the nurse should include which of the following?

   a. the importance of good, daily oral hygiene

   b. the need for monthly platelet counts to assess for bleeding

   c. the need for daily blood pressure assessment

   d. the possibility of alopecia developing about 2 weeks after therapy begins

93. When planning for Jason's discharge, the nurse should stress the importance of normal healthy play activities with limitations based on

   a. the type of seizure disorder

   b. the frequency of seizures

   c. the severity of seizures

   d. any coexisting learning disability

94. On returning for a clinic visit, Jason seems quiet and withdrawn. The nurse would want to follow up on which of the following statements made by Jason?

a. "School is going okay. My grades are about the same."

b. "My best friend's mom let me come over the other night. Billy has seizures too!"

c. "Mom and Dad let me go fishing with Uncle Bill. He knows what to do if I get sick."

d. "The teacher wouldn't let me go out to recess. She's afraid I'll have an attack and hit my head."

95. Lisa, aged 4 months, is admitted to the pediatric unit with persistent primitive infantile reflexes, early hand dominance, and increased muscle tone. Lisa does not lift her head or grasp objects; her left side seems more affected than her right side. She is diagnosed with hemiparesis spastic cerebral palsy. Which of the following statements by Lisa's mother would indicate to the nurse that Lisa's parents have misinterpreted information that the physician has given them regarding Lisa?

a. "We're going to have to put Lisa in an institution since she is severely mentally retarded."

b. "The doctor said they can't cure Lisa but they might be able to help her walk."

c. "The doctor is going to do some hearing tests; Lisa might be deaf."

d. "Lisa eventually may experience seizures, but that won't happen for a while."

96. Anticipating future mobilizing devices, the nurse should mention all the following to Lisa's parents *except*

a. braces

b. wheeled scooter board

c. walker

d. stroller

97. Lisa's parents are preparing for their infant's discharge and subsequent home care. Which of the following statements by the father would clue the nurse to explore the parents' need for more information?

a. "I have Lisa's complete home schedule here; she's going to hold her spoon soon!"

b. "I'm going to take one day at a time and enjoy her as she accomplishes more."

c. "I guess patience will become our most valuable asset."

d. "My wife and I know that sometimes we're going to need respite child care."

98. The day before surgery Mary asks the nurse if she could "try out the Stryker frame." This request would most likely indicate which of the following to the nurse?

a. Mary is still in concrete operational thought and bound by immediate physical reality.

b. Mary is fearful of losing control and needs to know how the bed feels and operates.

c. Mary is very immature and needs to play with the equipment.

d. Mary lacks abstract thinking since she cannot hypothesize how the Stryker frame will feel.

99. Follow-up care for Mary should continue until which of the following occurs?

a. her spine has completely matured

b. the lateral curve has been corrected

c. her iliac crests are parallel

d. the Trendelenburg sign is absent

100. Steven, aged 2 months, is admitted to the hospital with congenital hip dysplasia. Initial treatment would most likely involve

a. open reduction

b. flexion and bracing

c. tenotomy of the contracted muscles

d. osteotomy to reconstruct the acetabular roof

101. Steven is in a Pavlik harness for 6

months, after which his hip is still unstable and requires casting. He is placed in a plaster hip spica cast. The cast must be dry before he can be taken home. To facilitate drying of the cast, the nurse should implement all the following measures *except*

a. turning the child frequently
b. drying the cast with a fan or heat dryer
c. supporting the cast with pillows
d. keeping the cast uncovered

102. Becky Stevens, aged 7 years, is newly diagnosed as mildly retarded with an IQ of 65. Becky is the youngest of three children, unable to articulate well, and functions at a 3-year-old level. Becky's parents have recently separated. The best predictor of Mrs. Stevens' coping behavior in regard to Becky's problem would be

a. the state of the Stevens's marital relationship
b. Becky's birth order in the family
c. Becky's gender
d. Becky's developmental level

103. Mrs. Stevens is attempting to deal with Becky's diagnosis, minimize its impact on the family, and resolve her own marital problems. Progression of a stressful situation to a crisis situation commonly involves all the following variables *except*

a. available support systems
b. perception of the event
c. past coping behaviors
d. siblings' reaction to the diagnosis

104. Sarah Jenkins, aged 3 months, has a history of not being alert to sounds. For any child, all the following health history findings would indicate the need for hearing assessment between age 3 to 6 months *except*

a. congenital perinatal infection, such as cytomegalovirus or rubella
b. skeletal defects

c. birth weight less than 1500 g
d. severe asphyxia

105. Sarah is diagnosed as hard of hearing and will probably need the use of a hearing aid and assistance with her articulation when she begins to speak. Of the following plans for habilitation, which one requires attention *first*?

a. Encourage the child's independent development by emphasizing self-care.
b. Give the parents a list of approved programs for the hearing impaired.
c. Give the parents information on how to enhance communication with their child.
d. Assist the parents to accept the defect and actively engage in their child's care.

106. Which of the following comments by Sarah's mother would indicate the need for follow-up by the nurse?

a. "She is so quiet and sweet I have to be careful not to ignore her."
b. "When I hold her, I keep her face looking at mine so she can learn my facial expressions."
c. "She seems so independent—she pays no attention to me, her own mother."
d. "We're starting her early in an infant stimulation program."

107. When giving Mrs. Jenkins information on helping Luke develop security and independence, the nurse should explain which of the following?

a. She should room-in with Luke until he feels safe.
b. She should arrange home furnishings to provide maneuverability with key orientation objects strategically placed.
c. She should feed Luke to avoid spillage and embarrassment.
d. She should dress Luke so that he appears well groomed.

Answer Sheet for Comprehensive Exam

With a pencil, blacken the circle under the option you have chosen for your correct answer.

	A	B	C	D			A	B	C	D			A	B	C	D
1.	○	○	○	○	21.		○	○	○	○	41.		○	○	○	○
2.	○	○	○	○	22.		○	○	○	○	42.		○	○	○	○
3.	○	○	○	○	23.		○	○	○	○	43.		○	○	○	○
4.	○	○	○	○	24.		○	○	○	○	44.		○	○	○	○
5.	○	○	○	○	25.		○	○	○	○	45.		○	○	○	○
6.	○	○	○	○	26.		○	○	○	○	46.		○	○	○	○
7.	○	○	○	○	27.		○	○	○	○	47.		○	○	○	○
8.	○	○	○	○	28.		○	○	○	○	48.		○	○	○	○
9.	○	○	○	○	29.		○	○	○	○	49.		○	○	○	○
10.	○	○	○	○	30.		○	○	○	○	50.		○	○	○	○
11.	○	○	○	○	31.		○	○	○	○	51.		○	○	○	○
12.	○	○	○	○	32.		○	○	○	○	52.		○	○	○	○
13.	○	○	○	○	33.		○	○	○	○	53.		○	○	○	○
14.	○	○	○	○	34.		○	○	○	○	54.		○	○	○	○
15.	○	○	○	○	35.		○	○	○	○	55.		○	○	○	○
16.	○	○	○	○	36.		○	○	○	○	56.		○	○	○	○
17.	○	○	○	○	37.		○	○	○	○	57.		○	○	○	○
18.	○	○	○	○	38.		○	○	○	○	58.		○	○	○	○
19.	○	○	○	○	39.		○	○	○	○	59.		○	○	○	○
20.	○	○	○	○	40.		○	○	○	○	60.		○	○	○	○

	A	B	C	D		A	B	C	D		A	B	C	D
61.	○	○	○	○	77.	○	○	○	○	93.	○	○	○	○
62.	○	○	○	○	78.	○	○	○	○	94.	○	○	○	○
63.	○	○	○	○	79.	○	○	○	○	95.	○	○	○	○
64.	○	○	○	○	80.	○	○	○	○	96.	○	○	○	○
65.	○	○	○	○	81.	○	○	○	○	97.	○	○	○	○
66.	○	○	○	○	82.	○	○	○	○	98.	○	○	○	○
67.	○	○	○	○	83.	○	○	○	○	99.	○	○	○	○
68.	○	○	○	○	84.	○	○	○	○	100.	○	○	○	○
69.	○	○	○	○	85.	○	○	○	○	101.	○	○	○	○
70.	○	○	○	○	66.	○	○	○	○	102.	○	○	○	○
71.	○	○	○	○	87.	○	○	○	○	103.	○	○	○	○
72.	○	○	○	○	88.	○	○	○	○	104.	○	○	○	○
73.	○	○	○	○	89.	○	○	○	○	105.	○	○	○	○
74.	○	○	○	○	90.	○	○	○	○	106.	○	○	○	○
75.	○	○	○	○	91.	○	○	○	○	107.	○	○	○	○
76.	○	○	○	○	92.	○	○	○	○					

COMPREHENSIVE TEST—ANSWER KEY

1. **Correct response: d**
   The axillary method is safe, nonintrusive, accurate, and efficient.
   a. Use oral temperature measurement on children who can hold thermometer in mouth, usually 5 or 6 years.
   b. The rectal method is intrusive but can be used; there is increased danger of perforation if inserted too far.
   c. The skin method is not accurate in a 2 month old but can be used with premature infants who lie still.

   Knowledge/Physiologic/Implementation

2. **Correct response: b**
   There is no need to wean the baby yet; the supplemental formula and iron drops provide the necessary iron on a daily basis.
   a. Two supplemental feedings per day helps during the time that the mother is working.
   c. The iron drops can easily be added and are digested.
   d. Iron-fortified cereal also helps with the nutritional intake.

   Comprehension/Physiologic/Planning

3. **Correct response: c**
   36 oz of milk is still too much; need to limit to less than 1 liter (30 oz) so that the toddler is hungry for other foods.
   a. The diet includes iron-rich foods that can be cut up in "finger-food" size.
   b. Liquid iron must not come in contact with teeth to prevent staining; use straw or dropper.
   d. A written schedule is helpful for Ms. Jones to refer to at home for food ideas.

   Application/Health promotion/Planning

4. **Correct response: d**
   As the child grows and changes, it is helpful for the professional nurse to provide information of what to expect.
   a. The health care team is less successful with trying to change parenting styles than in working with them.
   b. There may not be a problem.
   c. This is individual counseling and guidance.

   Comprehension/Health promotion/Analysis (Dx)

5. **Correct response: a**
   The universality of this opening is that several parents have tried a similar approach or have experienced a similar problem.
   b. All parents do not approach a problem in the same way.
   c. This is a put-down, lead-off phrase.
   d. This might be acceptable but leaves the parent with fewer options.

   Applications/Health promotion/ Implementation

6. **Correct response: b**
   Socialization is an interactive process.
   a. Toys give fewer clues than interaction.
   c. Drawings are helpful from older children who draw, but the first step is the interaction.
   d. Some children are very social and do not like books.

   Knowledge/Psychosocial/Assessment

7. **Correct response: a**
   The pot-bellied appearance is due to less well-developed abdominal musculature, lordosis, and short legs.
   b. This is the characteristic stance of a preschool child.
   c. This is the characteristic sitting posture of an infant.
   d. Toddlers gain increased mobility

and learn to stand and then walk without assistance.

Knowledge/Physiologic/Assessment

8. **Correct response: d**
   This seems so obvious to avoid helping Aaron not feel "displaced" by the baby.
   a. Including Aaron in the discussion points out his achievements of growing.
   b. Including him in moving his security objects assures him that the "new" bed is his.
   c. Even though the bed changes, the ritual should not change to provide ongoing security.

Application/Safe care/Implementation

9. **Correct response: c**
   Limits provide the needed security for guidelines and protection from going beyond his or her own capabilities.
   a. Unlimited freedom leads to insecurity.
   b. Rigid rules allow for no creativity and adaptation to growth of child's capabilities.
   d. A child needs and craves guidance to learn from his or her significant others.

Application/Safe care/Planning

10. **Correct response: a**
    There is a curiosity to explore and little sense of inherent dangers; parents need to provide protection.
    b. Running and climbing are improving but still are done clumsily.
    c. Peer approval enters in later childhood.
    d. The drive is for activity to explore.

Analysis/Safe care/Analysis (Dx)

11. **Correct response: c**
    Assessment of the laboratory data; neurologic and behavioral changes support the diagnosis.
    a. This nursing diagnosis would be used with the assessment data from abuse or neglect.
    b. The assessment parameters would

include inflicted trauma as in an accident or abuse.
    d. There is an alteration in the family process; different assessment data would document this.

Analysis/Physiologic/Analysis (Dx)

12. **Correct response: d**
    The flaking paint chips are scraped and covered with nonlead paint or wallpaper.
    a. During the clean-up, Lakiesha and other family members may need to stay with relatives to avoid lead from the scraping and sanding process.
    b. Toddlers still like to taste things and need safe objects on which to chew.
    c. Understimulation is more the norm when there is lead ingestion with little else to do.

Analysis/Health promotion/Planning

13. **Correct response: b**
    She is most concerned about her parents. Their presence with her during the IV is best.
    a. The concept of time has no meaning for a toddler.
    c. The room is somewhat important but not of primary importance.
    d. The equipment can be shown to the toddler, but she will be more comforted by a brief explanation of what the "equipment" will do.

Comprehension/Safe care/Planning

14. **Correct response: a**
    This is necessary for identity with the parent of the same sex and to recognize their maleness or femaleness.
    b. Fear of darkness continues until the child's cognitive ability matures.
    c. Self-control is gained when the child is able to internalize and follow through with inner control during late childhood.
    d. This is Piaget's concrete stage at 7 to 11 years of age.

Comprehension/Psychosocial/Assessment

15. *Correct response: a*

Most preschool children are in this stage, which follows the reward and punishment mode (typical of toddlers).

b. This applies to middle childhood.

c. This applies to the toddler.

d. As internal controls and conscience develop, the middle to older child matures to a sense of right and wrong.

Analysis/Health promotion/Evaluation

16. *Correct response: c*

Cut implies pain to a preoperational child; better to describe it as taking pictures of your heart with a noisy camera, reassuring him or her that you will be there.

a. The outcome will make the child feel better; avoid the word *fix* because the child knows how difficult toys are to fix.

b. Any vital signs or laboratory tests should be described as being measured and not taken.

d. Radiographs are confusing, but most children like having a photograph taken by a special camera.

Application/Safe care/Implementation

17. *Correct response: b*

Varicella does not have a vaccine developed for widespread immunization (viral in nature).

a and d. Toddlers at 15 months receive a combined injection of mumps, measles, and rubella (MMR) (all viral).

c. HBPV is given at 24 months to toddlers to protect them from this bacterial infection (1985).

Knowledge/Safe care/Evaluation

18. *Correct response: d*

By 3 years most children say three- to four-word sentences.

a. Not able to alternate feet until 4 or 5 years.

b. Throwing requires large muscle development that develops later than age 3; can roll a ball.

c. By 3 years a child can be proficient with a spoon.

Analysis/Physiologic/Analysis (Dx)

19. *Correct response: a*

Two choices in how to drink the medicine allow some control for Jenny; positive approach.

b. Jenny is not taking the medicine to please the nurse, she takes it because it is needed.

c. It is difficult for preschool children to associate taking medicine and making them feel better, and it may not make them feel better for some time.

d. Competition works better for school-age children.

Application/Safe care/Implementation

20. *Correct response: d*

Information on driving can wait until drivers education class in high school.

a. Elementary children experience stress related to family, friends, and school activities.

b. Peer pressure plays an important role in getting a child this age to "try" these substances.

c. Sex education is important because of the need to have correct information for child's questions.

Application/Safe care/Planning

21. *Correct response: a*

Children need to understand that it is the individual's responsibility to exercise responsibility in healthy lifestyle choices.

b. Good nutrition is proved to help prevent certain illnesses.

c. Dressing appropriately is important to prevent hypothermia or hyperthermia with various temperatures.

d. Droplets from respiratory infections are highly contagious; handwashing is essential to prevent transfer of organisms through droplet spread.

Application/Physiologic/Planning

22. *Correct response: d*

a, b, and c. All these statements incorporate the child into the plan. When the child is a participant and understands his or her role, he or she is more likely to follow through with effective health care practices.

Application/Health promotion/ Implementation

23. *Correct response: b*

A cold pack decreases inflammation; a warm pack encourages spread.

a. Low Fowler's position localizes and prevents upward spread of infection.

c. Nothing per mouth is essential preoperative to keep stomach empty to prevent aspiration.

d. Palpation will determine degree of distention (if present) and indicate spread of peritonitis.

Application/Physiologic/Implementation

24. *Correct response: d*

At age 9, Susie can cope with separation from her family for periods of time; their presence, though, is important for her recovery during this situational crisis.

a. There will be discomfort from the incision; manage nonpharmacologically or with analgesics.

b. Dehydration occurs from not having any fluids by mouth, and fluid loss occurs during surgery.

c. Even without rupture, there is potential for infection developing with surgical incision.

Analysis/Physiologic/Analysis (Dx)

25. *Correct response: c*

The best "presents" is the nurse's "presence" and care of the child; not material presents, those are provided by family and friends.

a. The consistency of a familiar nurse is support and progression for the child.

b. Support from the family, (siblings, and agemates on a selected basis) provide "normalcy."

d. A sense of industry is enhanced by mastering this anxiety-producing situation.

Application/Psychosocial/Evaluation

26. *Correct response: b*

Teenage driving contributes substantially to vehicular fatalities; inexperience, peer pressure, and not using defensive principles.

a. Poisoning from alcohol and drug overdose are possibilities but infrequent occurrences.

c and d. Burns and firearm accidents occur but not at the rate of vehicular accidents.

Knowledge/Safe care/Assessment

27. *Correct response: a*

The infant triples his or her birth weight for a net gain of 12 to 18 lb that first year.

b. Toddler growth slows to 4 to 6 lb per year.

c. Preschool growth averages 5 lb per year.

d. School-age growth averages $5\frac{1}{2}$ lb per year.

Knowledge/Physiologic/Assessment

28. *Correct response: c*

The rate of sexual maturation is very individual; the sequence is predictable.

a. The rate differs; the age is between 9 and 16 years.

b. Girls finish maturation about 2 years before boys.

d. Girls mature faster than boys.

Comprehension/Physiologic/Evaluation

29. *Correct response: b*

Girls begin puberty between 8 and 14 years.

a, c, and d. Boys begin puberty between 9 and 16 years.

Knowledge/Physiologic/Evaluation

30. *Correct response: a*

Climate does not influence menarche.

b, c, and d. All three of these aspects play a part in the onset of menstruation.

Knowledge/Physiologic/Planning

31. Correct response: b
Crises intervention is based on the belief that the client has resources available to him or her that, when called on, will help them resolve the problem.
  a. This is a closeout response that is not helpful to the parents.
  c. The nurse can help but cannot solve for them.
  d. The community agency may be used after the parents' feelings of competency are established.

Analysis/Psychosocial/Implementation

32. Correct response: b
The prodromal signs and symptoms indicate that an adolescent is troubled and might attempt suicide; assessment data include preoccupation with death and giving away cherished possessions.
  a. Ignoring threats is not therapeutic for the adolescent who has a need to be helped.
  c. This is a nontherapeutic approach; talking out the problem is helpful to gather data to be manipulated.
  d. The crisis may not be temporary, and the act may be well planned; there may be a history of depression.

Analysis/Psychosocial/Implementation

33. Correct response: d
No assessment data given in the situation indicate that Tom has chronic depression; medications are not prescribed.
  a. Frequent counseling, initially, is important to reinforce Tom's self-esteem and provide support for his own resource development; counseling becomes less frequent as necessary.
  b. It is essential that he knows that he is valued.
  c. Fortunately, Tom has shown inter-

est in activities that he is good at and is willing to pursue.

Application/Safe care/Evaluation

34. Correct response: a
Symptoms of dehydration include concentrated urine with high specific gravity.
  b. Depressed fontanel is a symptom of dehydration.
  c. Decreased blood pressure is a sign.
  d. Decreased production of tears is a sign.

Analysis/Physiologic/Assessment

35. Correct response: a
Females have a 10 to 30 times greater risk of developing infection because of short urethral structure.
  b. Uncircumcised males have higher incidence of infection.
  c. Inadequate emptying of bladder predisposes to infection.
  d. Fluids are increased to prevent urinary tract infections.

Analysis/Physiologic/Analysis (Dx)

36. Correct response: b
Surgical intervention is indicated to prevent renal damage when there are recurring infections.
  a. Urine output is not affected by reflux.
  c. BUN is not elevated with reflux.
  d. Toilet training is not associated with the surgery.

Application/Health promotion/Planning

37. Correct response: d
There is a disturbance in the basement membrane of the glomeruli that leads to increased permeability to protein.
  a. There is decreased colloidal osmotic pressure that leads to a fluid shift causing fluids to accumulate in the interstitial spaces and body cavities.
  b. There is increased secretion of antidiuretic hormone.
  c. Fluid shifts lead to hypovolemia.

Comprehension/Physiologic/Analysis (Dx)

38. Correct response: d

Frequent position changes help prevent further skin breakdown related to edema.

a. Bedrest is maintained during phases of acute edema to control edema. Intervention is not directly related to skin care.

b. A tight diaper may cause further skin breakdown by rubbing against skin.

c. Child does not need to be flat in bed, and keeping him or her so would cause further skin breakdown.

Application/Safe care/Implementation

39. Correct response: c

Periorbital and generalized edema are a symptom of acute glomerulonephritis.

a. Hematuria is a symptom.

b. Mild to moderate elevations in blood pressure are common.

d. Seizures are a rare symptom.

Knowledge/Physiologic/Assessment

40. Correct response: c

Child may be stimulated by providing quiet play activities.

a. Child may be allowed to do simple self-care activities.

b. This intervention is not necessary although mother should be encouraged to participate in care as possible.

d. This is not necessary. The child may have a roommate as long as he or she is not exposed to infection.

Application/Psychosocial/Evaluation

41. Correct response: b

Amoxicillin or ampicillin are the drugs of choice for 10 to 14 days.

a. *Streptococcus pneumoniae* (pneumococcus) is the most common infecting organism.

c. Hearing loss may result from chronic infections.

d. Breast-fed infants have a lower incidence than bottle-fed infants. This is thought to be possibly related to the more horizontal feeding position of bottle-fed infants.

Comprehension/Physiologic/Analysis (Dx)

42. Correct response: d

The horizontal position promotes pooling of formula in the pharyngeal cavity. The child should be held upright for feedings.

a. Parents should be encouraged to complete the entire course of antibiotics even though symptoms may subside.

b. The physician might prescribe prophylactic antibiotic treatment for recurrent cases.

c. Gentle nose blowing only should be encouraged.

Application/Health promotion/Planning

43. Correct response: b

Clear liquids may be offered as tolerated. Fluid by the IV route is especially indicated during the acute phase and in the presence of tachypnea to lessen physical exertion and prevent aspiration.

a. Assess for airway obstruction by assessing respiratory status and monitoring vital signs closely.

c. Ease respiratory effort by keeping patient in a high-humidity atmosphere.

d. Administer oxygen therapy to alleviate hypoxia.

Application/Safe care/Implementation

44. Correct response: b

Undisturbed rest as well as long periods in the cool mist eases respiratory efforts and decreases oxygen demands.

a. The cool mist is not related to the hydration status of the child.

c. The child may be observed for respiratory distress without necessary frequent auscultation of breath sounds.

d. The child's respiratory status may be assessed without necessarily waking the child.

Application/Safe care/Planning

45. Correct response: b

The child demonstrates symptoms of epiglottitis. When symptoms of epiglottitis are present, physical examination of the throat should be done only by an otolaryngologist or anesthesiologist, and equipment should be available for performing an emergency intubation or tracheostomy.

    a. Stridor is not related to the throat examination.

    c. The child's irritability is not a factor in the decision to not examine the throat.

    d. Initiation of a respiratory tract infection is not an appropriate rationale for not examining the throat.

Application/Safe care/Evaluation

46. *Correct response: b*
Haemophilus influenza type b is a common organism causing epiglottitis. It may occasionally cause pneumonia in children.

    a. Staphylococcus is a common organism that causes childhood pneumonia.

    c. Streptococcus is a common organism that causes childhood pneumonia.

    d. Pneumococcus is a common organism that causes childhood pneumonia.

Knowledge/Physiologic/Analysis (Dx)

47. *Correct response: b*
Expiratory wheezing is common in acute asthma attacks and occurs as a result of narrowing of the airway due to edema.

    a. Periods of apnea are not a common manifestation of acute asthma attacks.

    c. Inspiratory stridor is more characteristic of a condition such as croup rather than acute asthma.

    d. Adventitious breath sounds such as wheezing are normally present rather than absence of breath sounds.

Analysis/Physiologic/Assessment

48. *Correct response: d*
The high sodium chloride content of the sweat in patients with cystic fibrosis can lead to problems with sodium

depletion, especially during hot weather.

    a. The child has sweat glands.

    b. The skin pigment of the child with cystic fibrosis is not affected.

    c. The temperature control center of the child with cystic fibrosis is not affected.

Analysis/Physiologic/Evaluation

49. *Correct response: c*
The patient is kept in an upright or side-lying position with head of bed elevated to prevent aspiration.

    a. The suture line is cleaned after each feeding to prevent infection.

    b. Elbow restraints are used to maintain integrity of the suture line.

    d. Feedings are slow with frequent burping to prevent regurgitation.

Application/Safe care/Implementation

50. *Correct response: a*
Infants with this surgery have the potential for respiratory difficulties. The nurse should monitor for any signs of respiratory distress. The infant should be placed on a side-lying position with head of bed elevated to prevent aspiration. The mouth or nasopharynx may be gently suctioned as needed.

    b. Although crying should be prevented because it places tension on the suture line, maintenance of a patent airway is of highest priority.

    c. This is not an appropriate intervention.

    d. IV fluids may be administered only until patient is tolerating oral fluids.

Analysis/Safe care/Planning

51. *Correct response: a*
Excessive vomiting results in a metabolic alkalosis with an increased pH and bicarbonate.

    b. A metabolic alkalosis is present.

    c. Hemoconcentration is reflected in increased hematocrit and hemoglobin levels.

    d. Hyponatremia is present.

Analysis/Physiologic/Analysis (Dx)

52. Correct response: c
Peripheral edema usually of lower extremities is present as a result of hypoproteinemia.
  a. Steatorrhea (fat in stools) is a clinical symptom.
  b. A general malnourished state is present because of malabsorption and vitamin deficiencies.
  d. Abdominal distention is present as a result of a weakened musculature, accumulation of intestinal secretions and gas, altered peristaltic activity, and fluid from altered osmotic pressure.
Comprehension/Physiologic/Assessment

53. Correct response: a
Parents and child should understand that diet restrictions are lifelong.
  b. Support parents and child by encouraging them to express their feelings and concerns.
  c. Emphasize positive changes as a result of adherence to diet.
  d. Focus on positive aspects (i.e., ways the diet can be normal) instead of on how the diet is restrictive.
Application/Psychosocial/Planning

54. Correct response: d
Intussusception is characterized by an invagination, or telescoping, of the intestine into the portion of the intestine immediately next to it.
  a. This describes pyloric stenosis.
  b. This describes gastroesophageal reflux.
  c. This describes Hirschsprung's disease.
Comprehension/Physiologic/Evaluation

55. Correct response: b
Elective surgery is scheduled for an inguinal hernia soon after it is diagnosed. Complications tend to be fewer when surgery can be done on an elective basis than when waiting until incarceration occurs.
  a. This refers to the management of umbilical hernias.

  c. This refers to the management of an incarcerated hernia.
  d. This refers to the management of a hydrocele.
Analysis/Health promotion/Evaluation

56. Correct response: b
Decreased resistance to infection is observed.
  a. Pallor is a symptom.
  c. Easy fatigue is a symptom.
  d. Growth retardation is a symptom.
Analysis/Physiologic/Assessment

57. Correct response: b
Dietary modifications are necessary in treatment of iron deficiency anemia. Compliance would most likely be achieved if client is a part of planning the diet.
  a. The client is not actively taking a part in planning the necessary diet modifications.
  c. The client is not actively taking a part in planning the necessary diet modifications.
  d. Because the client is an adolescent, the discussion of a plan of care should include him or her.
Application/Heath promotion/Planning

58. Correct response: a
Iron is best absorbed in an acidic environment.
  b. Milk is an alkaline, not an acidic, environment.
  c. Rest does not promote absorption.
  d. Medication should be given before meals in an acidic environment.
Knowledge/Safe care/Implementation

59. Correct response: a
Frequency of crises usually lessens as the child grows older.
  b. Parents can help and need to focus on the positive—the recognition and control of factors known to precipitate crisis.
  c. Parents need the opportunity to discuss their feelings regarding a potentially life-threatening disease.

d. The patient with sickle cell anemia experiences acute and chronic effects on organ systems as a result of sickling and crises.

Analysis/Psychosocial/Evaluation

60. *Correct response: c*
Hand–foot syndrome is a complication of sickle cell disease.

   a, b, and c. This syndrome is not seen in thalassemia major, in hemophilia, or in iron deficiency anemia.

Knowledge/Physiologic/Assessment

61. *Correct response: c*
Iron chelation therapy with deferoxamine is administered to eliminate excess iron and its side effects when deposited in tissues.

   a and b. Iron overload is the problem in thalassemia major.
   d. Splenomegaly is present and usually requires splenectomy, but it is not the reason for administering deferoxamine.

Comprehension/Physiologic/Analysis (Dx)

62. *Correct response: c*
Restraining the child from normal activities of growth and development is not encouraged. With close supervision during playtime, the environment for the toddler can be made as safe as possible to minimize injuries.

   a. Side rails may be padded to prevent injury.
   b. Clothes with padding over the elbows and knees may aid in prevention of joint injuries.
   d. Toys should be inspected to ensure safe play.

Application/Safe care/Implementation

63. *Correct response: d*
Tetralogy of Fallot is a cyanotic defect, and in cyanotic heart defects, desaturated blood enters the systemic arterial circulation. Cyanosis is caused by right to left shunting of blood.

   a, b, and c. Patent ductus arteriosus consists of left to right

shunting through an abnormal opening such as a patent ductus arteriosus, atrial septal defect, or a ventricular septal defect

Knowledge/Physiologic/Assessment

64. *Correct response: d*
The nurse should encourage the family to provide as normal a life as possible for the child and to stimulate the child with age-appropriate activities consistent with his or her activity tolerance.

   a. Inappropriate intervention with the child could cause detriment to the child's health although not change the defect itself. In working with parents, it is more appropriate for the nurse to emphasize the positive actions the parents can take to promote the child's development than to focus on the damage already done.
   b. The nurse should focus on educating parents rather than making statements about how much they do not know.
   c. The child needs activity within his tolerance to develop normally.

Analysis/Psychosocial/Evaluation

65. *Correct response: c*
The nurse is involved in assessing the child's hydration status and monitoring for signs of dehydration. The nurse should encourage intake once the child is awake.

   a. The nurse should observe and assess the puncture site for signs of hemorrhage.
   b. The nurse should auscultate the child's apical pulse to detect irregularities and arrhythmias.
   d. The nurse should observe for and teach the parents to observe for signs of inflammation or excessive tenderness that might indicate infection.

Application/Physiologic/Planning

66. *Correct response: c*

Surgical closure is accomplished with a dacron patch using cardiopulmonary bypass.

a. This is a correct description of VSD.

b. Most VSDs close spontaneously.

d. Surgery is possible to correct a VSD.

Knowledge/Physiologic/Analysis (Dx)

67. *Correct response: a*
The existence of the accompanying defect allows for the mixing of oxygenated and unoxygenated blood.

b. These measures are usually not necessary.

c. Infants with transposition of the great vessels usually do not undergo definitive repair until they are older. Initially, they usually rely on different palliative techniques to ensure adequate mixing of oxygenated and unoxygenated blood.

d. Administration of oxygen usually proves not beneficial.

Comprehension/Physiologic/Analysis (Dx)

68. *Correct response: a*
The nurse should stress measures to prevent and control infection, but this does not mean the child needs to avoid contact with people in general. The nurse should also stress avoidance of overprotection by parents.

b. The nurse should teach family regarding medications and potential side effects.

c. Initiation of a community health nurse referral should be made as appropriate.

d. The nurse should assure that the parents are knowledgeable about appointments for follow-up.

Application/Health promotion/Planning

69. *Correct response: b*
Digoxin increases cardiac performance by increasing the force of contraction.

a. Digoxin decreases the heart rate.

c. Digoxin directly affects the sodium–potassium pump in the muscle cell leading to hypokalemia.

d. Digoxin prolongs the PR interval.

Analysis/Safe care/Implementation

70. *Correct response: b*
The medication should be held if the heart rate is below normal, and the physician should be notified.

a. An unusually slow heart rate is a cardinal symptom of toxicity. It is therefore important for the nurse to check the apical pulse rate before administering.

c. The nurse should observe for signs of digoxin toxicity.

d. Because of the potent side effects of administering a wrong dose, it is appropriate for the nurse to check the dosage with another nurse before administering.

Analysis/Safe care/Implementation

71. *Correct response: d*
Kevin is neurogenic and susceptible to overwhelming infections.

a. Immunizations, particularly those of attenuated virus, should not be given until the child's immune system has recovered enough to respond appropriately to a vaccine.

b. Excessive bathing only dries out the skin and can lead to skin breakdown, a potential site of infection.

c. Platelet transfusions are used to control active bleeding

Application/Health promotion/ Implementation

72. *Correct response: c*
Lumbar puncture reveals types of cells, including leukemic cells in the cerebrospinal fluid.

a. Venipuncture is done to determine complete blood count and chemistry.

b. Bone marrow biopsy reveals maturity and type of white blood cells.

d. Peripheral blood smear gives estimation of the amount of hemoglobin and blood cell types, size, and shape.

Application/Safe care/Implementation

73. **Correct response: c**
Fear of body mutilation is a concern of preschoolers.
a and b. Toddler behaviors are ritualism and separation anxiety.
d. Finality of death is understood by school-age.
Comprehension/Psychosocial/Assessment

74. **Correct response: d**
Skin changes should not be referred to as *burns* because this word connotes too much radiation and causes undue emotional distress.
a. Exposure to sun should be avoided because the epidermis is sensitive and affords little body protection.
b. Daily baths are encouraged to keep the skin clean; however, soap is discouraged because it dries the skin too much.
c. Skin lubrication keeps skin pliable and avoids cracking.
Analysis/Psychosocial/Implementation

75. **Correct response: d**
Creatinine measures renal functions and does not give any information regarding intestinal obstruction.
a and b. Bowel sounds indicate movement through the intestines.
c. Distention is a result of localized edema as well as intestinal blockage.
Comprehension/Health promotion/Implementation

76. **Correct response: a**
Separation anxiety is a major concern for toddlers.
b. Magical thinking is characteristic of late toddlers and preschoolers.
c. Causality is characteristic of preschoolers.
d. Identity crisis is characteristic of preschoolers.
Comprehension/Psychosocial/Planning

77. **Correct response: b**

Idiopathic hypopituitarism is progressive linear growth retardation since birth or starting in the second year of life. This causes growth to be slow, and the child will wear out his or her clothes before outgrowing them. Usually children outgrow their clothes before they wear them out.
a. This growth pattern is characteristic of a pituitary tumor.
c. These symptoms of increased intracranial pressure indicate the possibility of a space-occupying lesion such as a craniopharyngioma.
d. This indicates a possible pituitary tumor with the sign of sudden growth retardation.
Analysis/Physiologic/Evaluation

78. **Correct response: a**
Children with hypopituitarism are prone to hypoglycemia, particularly when fasting before endocrine studies or having provocative tests stimulating growth hormone.
b. It is unlikely that a behavior disorder previously undetected would precipitate so rapidly.
c. Separation anxiety is most common with older infants and toddlers, protesting the loss of a significant other.
d. Hospitalism was a progressive depression disorder children experienced when parental hospital visits were severely restricted.
Analysis/Physiologic/Evaluation

79. **Correct response: b**
In addition to increasing linear growth, growth hormone in large doses increases vertical and transverse growth resulting in acromegaly.
a. An acute overdosage would lead to an initial hypoglycemia with a subsequent hyperglycemia.
c. There are few adverse reactions; however, among them is antibody formation to the growth hormone, which would be contradictory to the therapy.

d. High doses can cause side effects that are infrequent and mild, such as headache, localized muscle pain, weakness, mild hyperglycemia and glucosuria.

Application/Safe care/Implementation

80. *Correct response: c*

The adolescent period is a time stressing peer acceptance. Any condition that alters body image and stresses being different evokes considerable concern to the adolescent.

a. Fear of body mutilation is primarily a preschool phenomenon since preschoolers have little understanding of body boundaries.

b. Separation fears are primarily experienced during the toddler period when attachment to a significant other is of great importance.

d. Concern regarding school work and missing school is a primary concern during school-age period.

Comprehension/Psychosocial/Planning

81. *Correct response: d*

Significant physical and psychosocial problems can arise as a result of poor dietary control. Hypertension and water retention results from increased salt retention. Increased appetite and fat deposition cause truncal obesity, supraclavicular fat pads, and a "buffalo hump." Early dietary control may lessen effects of excess circulating free cortisol.

a. Adrenal insufficiency is a result of absence of adrenal corticosteroids; Cushing's syndrome is a result of excessive circulating free cortisol.

b. Although children with Cushing's syndrome are prone to infections, self-imposed isolation can cause unnecessary psychosocial problems. Children should practice constraint in being around large public gatherings or around people with known infections.

c. Children with Cushing's syndrome are prone to excessive bruis-

ing, petechial hemorrhage, and fractures, thus vigorous exercise is discouraged.

Analysis/Health promotion/Evaluation

82. *Correct response: d*

A child with ketoacidosis has severe glucosuria.

a. Blood pH 7.35 to 7.45 is normal; child in ketoacidosis have values above 7.45.

b. Normal blood glucose (euglycemic range) is 80 to 120 mg/dL; a child with ketoacidosis has values significantly above 120 mg/dL.

c. Normal bicarbonate level is 21 to 28 mEq/L; a child with ketoacidosis has values significantly below 21 mEq/L.

Comprehension/Physiologic/Assessment

83. *Correct response: b*

Regular insulin is given during ketoacidosis because it works quickly and can be given intravenously.

a. This is the *onset* of action for regular insulin rather than the time of *peak* action.

c. This is the *duration* of action for regular insulin rather than its *peak*.

d. This is the peak action for an intermediate-acting insulin such as NPH.

Comprehension/Physiologic/Assessment

84. *Correct response: c*

Julia is in the developmental stage of industry in which she enjoys accomplishing an assigned task.

a. Desire for peer acceptance increases as the child grows.

b. Formal operational thought is an adolescent, not school-age, cognitive development.

d. Development of a sense of identity is an adolescent task; Julia is in the stage of developing a sense of industry.

Comprehension/Psychosocial/Planning

85. *Correct response: d*

The defect location and amount of

nerve involvement will determine function. Nerve involvement results in stretching and pulling of the nerve through the defect, which results in dysfunction below the lesion.

a. Sensory and motor disturbances are parallel since the spinal nerves contain both major and sensory nerve fibers (dermatomes).

b. Denervation to bladder and bowel result in overflow urine incontinence and fecal incontinence detected in the diaper.

c. Joint contractures and hip dislocation are a result of partial denervation to the lower extremities. Partial denervation causes an uneven pull among extensors and flexors.

Comprehension/Physiologic/Assessment

86. *Correct response: b*

The defect does occur at about 4 weeks of gestation. The cause is unknown. The fact that it happens when a mother does not suspect that she is pregnant may help absolve the feeling of guilt.

a. It is only speculation that a virus might contribute to the development of myelomeningocele. The phrase "that the mother passes on to her unborn child" only heightens the feelings of guilt.

c. There is believed to be hereditary and environment factors that influence the development of the defect, but it is not a genetic defect; it is better described as a congenital defect.

d. This is incorrect because it could not have occurred at any time. There is a critical period when each organ and system is developing in which it is most susceptible to structural disturbances.

Analysis/Psychosocial/Implementation

87. *Correct response: b*

Hydrocephalus is a frequent development in a child with myelomeningocele, especially postoperatively since the absorptive surface for CSF is reduced.

a. Immediately postoperatively there is a sterile dressing covering the fresh wound to facilitate healing without trauma. Heat treatment is inappropriate at this time.

c. Diapers are contraindicated because the wound is not healed and there is a chance for fecal contamination.

d. The only positions allowed postoperatively are a prone or side-lying position (if physician allows). Sometimes a side-lying position, in children with myelomeningocele, aggravates a coexisting hip dysplasia.

Application/Physiologic/Implementation

88. *Correct response: c*

Dehydration would present with a depressed anterior fontanel.

a, b, and d. These all present with signs and symptoms of increased intracranial pressure as exhibited by a building anterior fontanel, irritability, and crying when moved or held.

Analysis/Physiologic/Evaluation

89. *Correct response: b*

Physical activity allows a child a means to express and deal with fear and fantasies and consequently reduce stress, especially at a time when the child is not very articulate.

a. Immobility thwarts one's expression of independence, especially during toddlerhood.

c. It has been found that children immobilized during the first 3 years of life have more difficulty with language development than do other children not experiencing restricted activities.

d. Sensory deprivation leads to behavior changes.

Application/Psychosocial/Implementation

90. *Correct response: c*

Although prenatal and postnatal history is important to ascertain any birth injury, trauma or infection, birth weight, height, and head circumference give little significant information.

a. Age of onset may help in identification of possible etiology.

b. Verbalized sensations indicate an aura prior to a seizure.

d. Precipitating factors help identify possible cause, epileptogenic focus, and eventual treatment.

Comprehension/Physiologic/Assessment

91. *Correct response: a*

Placing the child on the floor prevents additional injury.

b. Maneuvering a padded tongue blade into the mouth may cause injury to the teeth.

c. Restraining a child during seizure may cause additional injury.

d. Never leave a child alone unprotected during a seizure.

Knowledge/Safe care/Implementation

92. *Correct response: a*

Gum hyperplasia is a side effect of dilantin, which meticulous oral hygiene and gum massage may delay or prevent from occurring.

b. Thrombocytopenia occurs with depakene.

c. ACTH causes hypertension. No specific anticonvulsant drug causes hypotension.

d. Hirsutism is a side effect of dilantin, not alopecia.

Comprehension/Health promotion/Analysis (Dx)

93. *Correct response: d*

Coexisting learning disability does not hamper a child's need to engage in normal play activities.

a, b, and c. Criteria determining individual restrictions to normal healthy play activities depend on type of seizure, frequency of seizure, severity of seizure, response to therapy, and length of time in therapy.

Comprehension/Safe care/Planning

94. *Correct response: d*

School teachers should be instructed on the care of a child with seizures and what are and are not their limitations.

a. This indicates no behavior changes.

b and c. These indicate that Billy is in the home of a knowledgeable person if Billy should have a seizure.

Analysis/Safe care/Evaluation

95. *Correct response: a*

One third of children with cerebral palsy have normal intelligence; two thirds have mental retardation.

b. The goal of treatment is to improve motor functions, communication, and self-care.

c. Visual problems and hearing loss are frequently associated with cerebral palsy.

d. Seizures usually reach between 2 and 6 years and are most common with spastic cerebral palsy.

Analysis/Health promotion/Evaluation

96. *Correct response: c*

Walkers are discouraged because they pose a hazard; exaggerate abnormal motor patterns; delay normal balance and protective responses.

a, b, and d. Acceptable and useful mobilization devices.

Knowledge/Safe care/Assessment

97. *Correct response: a*

Parents should be encouraged not to place all of their focus on accomplishments of physical tasks; this can lead to frustration and a low self-esteem in the child.

b. Parents should be helped to avoid becoming overwhelmed and to find joy in their child's accomplishments.

c. Parents require patience because

their child will need considerable help to learn new tasks.

    d. Parents will need periodic respite care since there is minimal relief when caring for a child with cerebral palsy.

Analysis/Health promotion/Evaluation

98. *Correct response: b*
Adolescents can fear loss of control through enforced dependency, which the Stryker frame signifies.

    a. Anticipation of the next days events indicates Mary can transcend the here and now, a quality not found in "concrete" operational thought.

    c. Mary is not "playing" but rather requesting an opportunity to see how the bed works; maturity is the ability to wait for needed gratification.

    d. Hypothesizing about an event can help with problem solving, but it does not give tactile and perceptual sensations needed to reduce stress.

Analysis/Psychosocial/Evaluation

99. *Correct response: a*
When spine has matured, growth stops and curve no longer progresses.

    b. The curve may be corrected, but as a child continues to grow, the curve can progress.

    c. Parallelness of iliac crests is not a reliable indicator of scoliosis or its correction.

    d. Trendelenburg's sign is used to diagnose congenital hip dysplasia.

Knowledge/Physiologic/Assessment

100. *Correct response: b*
Initial therapy for congenital hip dysplasia is creating pressure on the acetabulum by bracing and flexion.

    a, c, and d. These are performed on older children whose deformity has resulted in limb shortening, hip contractures, and sec-

ondary adaptive changes.

Knowledge/Physiologic/Assessment

101. *Correct response: b*
This dries outside of cast while inside remains wet; heat can be conducted to underlying tissue, causing burns.

    a. Turning him frequently will prevent uneven pressure on the wet cast, which could result in indentations and pressure on underlying skin.

    c. Supporting on pillows exposes more surface to air; also reduces changes of creating pressure areas.

    d. Keeping cast uncovered allows for faster evaporation.

Application/Safe care/Implementation

102. *Correct response: a*
According to Frichrich, in 1979 the status of marital relationships is the best predictor of coping behavior. Single parents or poorly adjusted family units leave the family unit vulnerable to psychological and emotional trauma.

    b and c. Although Becky's birth order and gender affect how parents perceive a disability, they do not predict parental coping.

    d. Becky's developmental level, though different from her chronologic age, affect how the parents interaction with their child but does not predict their ability to cope in a stressful situation.

Comprehension/Psychosocial/Analysis (Dx)

103. *Correct response: d*
Siblings of chronically ill children can suffer negative or positive effects as part of the adjustment to the disability of a brother or sister; however, their behavior specifically would not precipitate a crisis.

    a, b, and c. All are variables that when absent or functioning on a limited basis can lead to a situation into becoming a crisis, creating disequilibrium.

Knowledge/Safe care/Assessment

104. Correct response: b

Skeletal defects usually do not have co-existing hearing loss except possibly those that affect the head and neck as with Treacher Collins syndrome.

a, c, and d. These are perinatal factors recommended by the American Academy of Pediatrics for hearing assessment by 6 months of age.

Application/Physiologic/Implementation

105. Correct response: d

Unless the disability is acknowledged and accepted, the family is unable to focus their energies on the care and treatment of the disorder.

a. Independent development is a later activity.

b and c. If the parents have not acknowledged that there is a problem, they will not use the tools the nurse gives them.

Analysis/Health promotion/Evaluation

106. Correct response: c

The hearing-impaired child is at risk of failing to develop the same degree of mutual deregulation or reciprocity between parent and child as the child without a hearing loss because of his or her unawareness of parental verbal cues; parent–infant attachment is vulnerable.

a. Parents need to take the initiative to make meaningful contact with the infant.

b. This supplements the child's stimulation needs with visual cues.

d. Early education programs prevent profound delays in normal developmental milestones as well as involve parents in the role as primary teachers.

Analysis/Health promotion/Evaluation

107. Correct response: b

This helps with orienting and mobility skills and development of feeling safe and secure; necessary feeling for development of autonomy.

a. This prolongs dependency.

c and d. This does not foster self-help skills necessary for independence.

Application/Safe care/Implementation

Index

Page numbers followed by *f* indicate figures; page numbers followed by *t* indicate tables.